Wake Tech. Libraries
9101 Fayetteville Road
Raleigh, North Carolina 27603-5696

WITHDRAWN

A DEATH RETOLD

STUDIES IN SOCIAL MEDICINE

ALLAN M. BRANDT & LARRY R. CHURCHILL,
editors

JESICA SANTILLAN,
THE BUNGLED TRANSPLANT,
AND PARADOXES OF MEDICAL
CITIZENSHIP
KEITH WAILOO, JULIE LIVINGSTON,
AND PETER GUARNACCIA,
EDITORS

A Death Retold

The
University of
North Carolina
Press
Chapel Hill

© 2006 The University of North Carolina Press
All rights reserved
Manufactured in the United States of America
Set in Scala types by Keystone Typesetting, Inc.
The paper in this book meets the guidelines for
permanence and durability of the Committee on
Production Guidelines for Book Longevity of
the Council on Library Resources.

Library of Congress Cataloging-in-Publication Data
A death retold : Jesica Santillan, the bungled transplant,
and paradoxes of medical citizenship / Keith Wailoo, Julie
Livingston, and Peter Guarnaccia, editors.
    p. cm.
Includes bibliographical references and index.
ISBN-13: 978-0-8078-3059-8 (cloth: alk. paper)
ISBN-10: 0-8078-3059-3 (cloth: alk. paper)
ISBN-13: 978-0-8078-5773-1 (pbk.: alk. paper)
ISBN-10: 0-8078-5773-4 (pbk.: alk. paper)
1. Heart—Transplantation—United States. 2. Lungs—
Transplantation—United States. 3. Blood—Transfusion—
Complications—United States. 4. Teenage immigrants—
Medical care—United States. 5. Santillan, Jesica.
I. Wailoo, Keith. II. Livingston, Julie. III. Guarnaccia,
Peter Joseph.
RD598.35.T7D43 2006
617.4'120592—dc22   2006013890

cloth   10 09 08 07 06   5 4 3 2 1
paper   10 09 08 07 06   5 4 3 2 1

CONTENTS

A DEATH RETOLD

INTRODUCTION

CHRONICLES OF AN ACCIDENTAL DEATH

KEITH WAILOO, JULIE LIVINGSTON, AND

PETER GUARNACCIA

In February 2003 Jesica Santillan, a seventeen-year-old Mexican immigrant living illegally in the United States, lay unconscious in a room at the Duke University Medical Center in Durham, North Carolina. She was dying because of a stunning medical oversight. As the hospital spokesman explained publicly, Jesica's surgical team had made a simple but tragic mistake in the hours leading up to her heart and lung transplant operation. Soon after replacing Jesica's failing heart and lungs with healthy ones, the team discovered that the transplanted heart and lungs had come from a patient of a different blood type. The donor organs were type A; Jesica was blood type O. As this frail young woman's immune system slowly rejected the organs and as doctors scrambled both to keep her alive and to find another set of compatible organs, her story attracted international media notoriety as the "bungled transplant."[1] For the next few weeks, the case became front-page news. But as more and more details of the Santillan story emerged, the meanings of the story compounded and reverberated in remarkable ways, gradually becoming a story about medical error, immigration, and alleged medical tourism. The organ transplant story also made for a toxic collision between a wider world of human commitments, cultural values, and political ideals.

Observers drawn from a wide spectrum of vantage points would come to characterize these events not only as an unfortunate personal tragedy for Jesica and her family but also as a prism through which profound problems in health care and American society came into focus. For some, the Santillan story was about illegal immigration and about foreigners taking resources that would otherwise have gone to American citizens. For other commentators, it highlighted an ongoing crisis of widespread error in medicine. The American media, cultural commentators, and politicians alike seized upon the Santillan story—for at the time (and still today) the story collapsed a range of pressing issues into one tragic narrative—questions about the promise and problems of high-technology (i.e., transplant) medicine, about the privileges of citizenship, about the principles that guide how we distribute scarce resources, about the right to sue for malpractice and about tort reform, and about the wider impact of such highly publicized high-profile media dramas on American society and beyond.

The collective media portrait that emerged in February and March 2003 figured the character at the center of the transplant story as a complex transplant herself: an immigrant moving from one place to the next, looking for a brighter future; a sick child in need of a new heart. Press accounts offered thinly developed sketches of Jesica as a person, plugging her tale into a pastiche of preformed American immigration narratives. As one observer later put it, she had journeyed "from the shacks of Guadalajara to the self-proclaimed City of Medicine, as Durham is known."[2] Another story recalled that she was born Yesica in the village of Arroyo Hondo, Mexico, that her schooling stopped in sixth grade, and that after graduating in 1997, "Jesica worked as a maid in a neighbor's house."[3] Work was scarce in this town of cane fields and a sugar mill. People were moving in the 1990s to larger cities like Guadalajara or looking for opportunities to cross into the United States. But the search for work was mentioned only rarely as an element in portraits of Jesica and her family. Most stories focused on the fact that her mother, Magdalena, had learned early in the girl's life that Jesica had a weak and failing heart, that little could be done for her in Mexico, and that the United States offered the promise of lifesaving medical care.

For some authors, the Santillan story was not only about a fateful medical error, it was about these broader demographic trends and the hopes of the immigrant community. In framing the story of the "bungled transplant," some accounts mentioned that three years before the operation, Santillan relatives had pooled money to pay a smuggler to bring the family across the border—with the goal of finding medical care. By 1999, the family had arrived in the small town of Louisburg, North Carolina, where Magdalena's sister and other relatives already lived and worked. They were part of a remarkable trend of "untraditional immigration" in the 1990s, as Mexican newcomers migrated to southern states like North Carolina, where jobs were plentiful in poultry processing, construction, and agriculture, and where many in the local population harbored strongly negative or mixed feelings about the unprecedented "influx of Hispanics."[4] News stories noted, for example, that "for much of America, the veil on this community was lifted last month with [Jesica's story] the saga of an undocumented teenager . . . at Duke University."[5] For those in North Carolina, this supposed veil was already long lifted. As Mexican and Latin American workers moved to North Carolina to find work, the foreign-born population climbed from 9,000 in 1990 to 172,000 in 2000; it was one of the largest rates of growth (1,865 percent) for any state in the nation.[6] As part of this trend, the Santillan family of five came to reside "in a relative's trailer parked near the 'cucumber shed'" where farmers sold their produce to a pickle company.[7] Like so many other immigrant workers, Magdalena found work as a cleaner; but unlike most cleaning jobs, the work at Louisburg College offered something that few other undocumented immigrants could obtain—health insurance for the family. This was a crucial fact that distinguished Jesica from so many other recent immigrants.

For most American commentators, the Santillan story was about America itself and about the attitudes and perspectives of its citizens. Evolving representations of Jesica in early 2003 produced a welter of conflicting attitudes about illegal immigration, regional labor trends, shadow economies, transplant medicine, and (perhaps most poignantly) the nature and limits of American generosity. Jesica enrolled in the local middle school; and, according to some accounts, it was the generosity and support of key people and institutions in the small town of only 3,500 that made Jesica's plight more widely known. The editor at the local *Franklin Times*, prompted by one of her teachers, published an "account of her life in a trailer without air conditioning" that then caught the attention of another recent newcomer to North Carolina from Dallas, Texas—a fifty-five-year-old businessman and builder of custom homes named Mack Mahoney.[8] As one national reporter later spun the story, "here in rural North Carolina, acts of generosity are not uncommon" and so it was that Mahoney not only paid for an air conditioner himself, but took up the cause of the "dimple-cheeked, suffering girl" and her struggling parents, and also "went on to found a charity to pay for her health care."[9] Other stories echoed these themes of local generosity and patronage— emphasizing how Jesica's case was referred by her school to the Franklin County Department of Health, which was the primary pathway to health care for many uninsured immigrants. But Jesica had her mother's insurance coverage and Mahoney's support and therefore stepped into a more comprehensive system of care. Jesica was referred to the Duke University Medical Center, where she was diagnosed with restrictive cardiomyopathy (a stiffening of the heart walls that resulted in poor blood flow and, ultimately, would mean heart failure). Even with the medical care provided at Duke, Jesica's heart continued to weaken, and in January 2002 she was placed on a heart transplant wait list—joining 275 children around the country.[10]

It is easy to see how such a story could take on broader cultural meanings in North Carolina and across America, for at the time of the transplant acci-

dent it highlighted powerful themes of immigration, adversity, the opportunity for a new life, and the magnetic appeal of America's high-technology
medicine. The family's illegal presence in the country only added to the
drama, generating an air of public ambivalence, paternalism, and, in many
cases, open hostility. For Americans, with their notoriously dysfunctional
health care system, the debate over issues of immigrant health care had taken
on a highly charged tenor at the national and the state levels. Critics of illegal
immigration blamed undocumented immigrants for bankrupting hospitals
and other public institutions; others bemoaned the declining public commitment and the increasing hostility toward these workers and their families.
Only a few years earlier, Californians had voted for Proposition 187—a measure restricting illegal immigrants' access to health care and schools. Intense
debate over the legality and morality of the measure lasted years. As the
national media followed the Santillan story, these themes of illegality, health
care access, and the morality of the citizen backlash would resurface.

In the days following the "bungled transplant," the story developed rapidly, taking new twists and turns. News accounts encouraged readers to identify with her, as a victim of a grave and seemingly unprecedented error. Jesica
Santillan sank into a coma. Then, days later, a new set of organs became
available. A desperate second transplant operation (which doctors publicly
gave a perhaps overly optimistic 50-50 chance of succeeding) failed to improve her condition. But by this point, the immigration theme had begun to
be featured more prominently in the coverage, and the themes of medical
error and patient victimization gradually were supplanted and eclipsed by the
question of her immigration status. Jesica's death soon afterward brought
waves of intense commentary about the deeper meanings of these events for
American health care. Sharp criticism and ideologically loaded invective radi-
ated through the Santillan case, and the story of the bungled transplant
played itself out in the American media in myriad ways and in locales too
numerous to mention.

For example, shortly after Jesica's death, in the halls of the U.S. Congress
where legislators were debating Republican president George W. Bush's proposals for medical malpractice reform (which, among other things, would
put a cap on "pain and suffering" jury awards), one Democratic senator
opposed to the physician-friendly legislation promised that the story of
Jesica's death at Duke "is going to be front and center in the evidence of why
we have to take medical malpractice reform very seriously."[11] As doctors
sought to draw attention to their perspectives on malpractice (the high cost of
insurance and proliferation, as they saw it, of "frivolous lawsuits"), Jesica

could be invoked effectively to reframe the debate. Many opponents of tort reform—from patients' advocates to plaintiffs' attorneys—seized on the story. One columnist in Pennsylvania remarked cynically "to the good doctors. . . . I know it has been a rough year for you, what with the spiraling cost of medical malpractice insurance forcing some of you to turn in your Jaguars and go slumming around town in leased Volvos. But let's take a momentary break from crying into your surgical masks to consider the case of Jesica Santillan."[12] Thus, long after the month-long drama had ended, commentators and politicians across the American cultural and political spectrum would continue to interpret the Santillan story as a story of privilege and slums—a modern parable not only about health care but also about America itself, and about whose perspective and pain mattered most.

Jesica herself became lost in much of the public commentary, and what emerged in full view was a menagerie of American attitudes. In the pages that follow, we revisit the accident, the subsequent events, the debates, and the cultural meanings generated by the "bungled transplant." Our purpose here in retracing Jesica's story is not to lay blame or to give voice to interested parties. To be sure, this book addresses many of the questions at the forefront of public and professional discussion then and now. Who was responsible for the error—the surgeon alone? The hospital? The United Network for Organ Sharing (UNOS)—the organization at the center of the American transplant system responsible for matching donor organs with recipients around the country? Or some other entity in the vast transplant system? What rules determined transplant eligibility for citizens, noncitizens, and people in the country illegally? Were these rules fair and just? What role did the hospital have in checking citizenship status? Was Jesica's second transplant obtained through normal channels or was she "jumped ahead" of other deserving people waiting for transplants (as some alleged)? Was the second transplant really medically and ethically defensible? The essays in this volume address such questions, but for us these questions are only starting points for exploration. Our aim is to go much further. By reflecting on this accidental death, and by examining the sharp lines of commentary and the web of critical issues that became refracted through the Santillan story, we explore profound questions of citizenship and justice that lie at the heart of contemporary medicine.

Many of the contentious and symbolically potent questions that emerged in the wake of the "bungled transplant" have no definitive answers. Indeed, the legal aftermath of the case and the legal settlement between Duke and the Santillan family would ensure that (in the absence of legal review) many of the "facts" of the case would never become public. Thus, from its outset and still today, the available evidence from the transplant mismatch case spawned unresolved questions and continuous debate about the values that shaped health care and society in America. What should our policies on illegal immigrants and transplantation be? Was it a sign of ungratefulness that Jesica's parents felt wronged by the hospital and considered suing, that they puzzled over when to declare her legally dead, or that they (allegedly) declined to donate her organs? The numerous allegations, rumors, and innuendo in the case are, in themselves, revealing. Jesica's story reveals a host of contradictory attitudes shaping American policies toward undocumented immigrants. While most analyses of immigrant health focus on access to basic health services like immunization and primary care, the Santillan case moved these familiar discussions into the realm of high-technology medicine with its own intense conflicts over questions of fairness and allocation in organ transplantation. It highlighted the seeming paradox of a high-technology medical system that is, at once, the envy of the world and characterized by an "epidemic" of life-threatening errors. One woman from Tennessee would capture the public anxiety quite nicely, noting with a glimmer of compassion and a healthy dose of ire, "I am a 37-year old single parent who is presently waiting on a heart. While I am glad that Jesica Santillan got a chance at a heart, I have to also say I am a little resentful. . . . It bothers me that these people who illegally crossed the border got what they needed, then sued the very people who tried to help them."[13] Other writers would link Jesica's travail to the dashed hopes of her natal community.[14] In looking beyond the bungled transplant, we look closely at this complex tangle of resentment, frustration, allegation, and representations about the young girl—untangling them and exploring their connections, we suggest, is a crucial step in understanding the Santillan story as a volatile microcosm of contemporary health care.

When the transplant mishap became widely known, the initial sense of public shock was palpable. Attention focused on the struggles of this young girl (as she was called), the plight of the family, and the fight to save Jesica's life. The rapid pace of the story and the intensity and immediacy of reactions prohibited careful reflection. Our first group of essays ("Medical Error and the American Transplant Theater") takes us back to the scene of the accident, to establish some of the major outlines, actors, and issues.

In "America's Angel or Thieving Immigrant?" communication scholars Susan Morgan, Tyler Harrison, Lisa Chewning, and Jacklyn Habib explore important changes over time in media representations of the main actors, tracking how themes of sympathy, horror, and hate characterized the public understanding. In this ambivalent public discourse, heated allegations of thievery, deception, betrayal, ungratefulness, and even murder often competed with careful discussions about the technical issues involved in the case. In "Hobson's Choices" (a reference to the take-it-or-leave-it choices faced in the transplant arena), transplant anesthesiologist Richard Cook offers an accident investigator's analysis of the internal discussions and dynamics within the transplant system, of the complex biological, administrative, and social issues involved in matching (and mismatching) donor organs and recipients, and of the embedded character of such errors.

The third essay, "The Transplant Surgeon's Perspective on the Bungled Transplant" by transplant surgeon Tom Diflo, provides insight into how surgeons have coped with such cases, how they (along with transplant centers and patients) maneuver for advantage within and around this complex system, and how the science and practice of transplant medicine has evolved over the past fifty years. Diflo's essay also draws our attention to a new and powerful phenomenon that turns the Jesica Santillan story on its head—the problem of Americans stepping outside the system, going abroad to purchase organs in the black and gray markets of other countries, a theme that is further developed in the next section in an essay by Scheper-Hughes.

In a fourth essay, "From Libby Zion to Jesica Santillan" (an account comparing the 1984 Libby Zion case of medical error with the Santillan story), physician-historian Barron Lerner describes the ways in which "easy truths" and competing narratives were generated in the public and private debate, and how the role of high-profile advocates like Mahoney or Libby Zion's father, Sidney, shaped the trajectory of these stories in key ways. It was Mahoney, a blunt-speaking, patriarchal presence throughout the Santillan story, for example, who became the public face for Jesica's Spanish-speaking mother, Magdalena, and who helped make the eventful decision to move Jesica's story into the glare of the public spotlight. He insisted that it was not the initial mistake itself but the failure of Duke to "fess up" early, to admit the error, and to publicize the need for donor organs that was now killing Jesica.[15]

One of the major historical developments that gave particular meaning to the Santillan story (in contrast to the Zion case years earlier) was the upsurge in the late 1990s in attention to error in medicine. Only a few years before the Santillan debacle, the Institute of Medicine had found that "medical errors kill more Americans than traffic accidents, breast cancer, or AIDS" and that "horrific cases that make the headlines are just the tip of the iceberg."[16] Jesica Santillan's story provided yet another human face for the hidden and anonymous crisis. The essay by medical sociologist Charles Bosk, "All Things Twice, First Tragedy Then Farce," looks closely at this problem of error, and at the main actors in the story (from Duke to Carolina Donor Services, from UNOS to the surgeon Jim Jaggers) in order to frame our understanding of medical mistakes as individual, institutional, and systemwide phenomena. Throughout these months, a disturbing question swirled around these major players (Duke, Jaggers, and UNOS)—did someone step outside of the system, were the rules violated, in order to get Jesica her first operation and her second transplant? How did the institution respond? asks Bosk. How did the elaborate dance between blaming individuals and reforming systems unfold in the searing heat of public controversy?

A second set of essays ("Justice and Second Chances Across the Border") delves into the deeper connections between the Santillan story and organ-matching policies, and the implicit and explicit rationales that govern how allocation and matching work in high-stakes life and death situations. The processes for deciding who receives which organs has changed dramatically over time, and they are being constantly revised in response to historical lessons, technical innovations, evolving tensions between small transplant centers and large ones, as well as a host of other regional, cultural, and political pressures. Throughout the controversial history of transplant medicine, then, questions of equity, justice, citizenship, and rights in the context of scarce resources have been highly politicized themes; and the process of shoring up public confidence in the system has always been a tricky one, especially as a troubling organ transplant trade has flourished abroad. In some ways, then, the Santillan story was an acute manifestation of this long-standing yet protean problem in transplant medicine and health care.

In the Santillan story, Jesica's second transplant became a crucial turning point, opening many new lines of reverberating criticism and commentary. The essay by historians Keith Wailoo and Julie Livingston, "The Politics of Second Chances," focuses on this controversial turning point, examining the public and professional discussions about whether Jesica received special treatment. The authors look closely at the "never say die" ethos pushing surgeons like Jaggers to fight for their transplant patients until the end and the problem of medical futility, and they examine the ways in which powerful American cultural myths about second chances suffused commentaries on the case. Within days of her second transplant, Jesica Santillan fell into a coma, and when she was declared brain dead her family began to grapple with the kinds of painful existential dilemmas confronted by people all over the nation, over the withdrawal of life support and the possibilities for organ donation. Like many other families in the wake of profound medical error, they also began a malpractice suit against Duke, a decision that inevitably colored future interpretations of the story. The essay also examines how border controversies had long been part of the puzzle of organ allocation. Only a few years before the Santillan story emerged, a heated controversy had flared from 1998 though 2000 about the appropriate rules for allocating organs across state lines, and between regions within America.[17]

In many respects, the Santillan story highlighted troubling inequalities and shifting lines between transplant "haves" and "have-nots," and exposed into public view how problems of justice and equity had long shadowed the transplant system. In "Tucker's Heart," medical historian Susan Lederer revisits an infamous and foundational case in the early years of transplant medicine. She documents the story of Bruce Tucker (an African American man whose heart was transplanted into a white recipient without his family's consent) and the lingering controversies over race and inequality that have shadowed transplant medicine in later decades. Although Tucker was a citizen of the United States, his case draws our attention to the fact that within national boundaries, the notion of citizenship can obscure the widely differing rights, opportunities, and claims implied by the term. In "Justice in Organ Allocation," philosopher and medical ethicist Rosamond Rhodes offers an analysis of how notions of justice should, and should not, influence organ matching. Her essay sheds light on UNOS policy in particular and on the ways in which issues of urgency, efficacy, equity, and the interests of small transplant centers are weighed in allocating organs; her essay calls attention to UNOS criteria as itself a fundamental problem in the Santillan case and in other cases. The following essay, "Playing with Matches without Getting Burned," by legal and historical scholar Jed Adam Gross, extends the discussion by Lederer and Rhodes into ideological terrain, examining the historical formation of UNOS and how the matching of available organs with worthy recipients has historically intersected with American debates over scarcity, abundance, fairness, equality, and public confidence. In his view, a range of technical and ideological factors have shaped the evolution of the matching process within UNOS and brought the system to this fateful collision with the life of Jesica Santillan. Such essays illuminate in a powerful way how questions of equity, fairness, and public confidence in organ matching have come to intersect with deep quandaries that are as much about ideology and cultural values as they are about biology and immunogenetics.

The section ends with an essay titled "Consuming Differences," in which anthropologist Nancy Scheper-Hughes offers a global analysis of the phenomenon often labeled "transplant tourism." She focuses not on Jesica Santillan per se, whose status as a poor immigrant made her transplant operation in America extraordinarily unlikely, but instead on many patients (Americans and citizens of other nations) with the financial means to increasingly circumvent the constraints of their national systems by traveling abroad to purchase organs. The essay discusses the collisions and contradictions produced by the current mix of national systems (like UNOS in the United States and the South African system), which, by law, define all donated organs as precious "national resources" and national property, and the relatively open (though still illicit) "organs markets" and closed and protectionist systems found elsewhere in the world. This international commodification of organs highlights how the economic inequities that propelled Jesica and her family to travel to the United States in search of health care also encouraged other poor people of the world to compromise their own health by selling organs to wealthy foreigners.

The global market in human organs and the medical migration of patients like Jesica remind us that citizens in diverse settings have widely different claims to medical care—and that their efforts to preserve health and bodily integrity can be read in different ways depending on the climate and political context.[18] A third group of essays ("Citizens and Foreigners / Eligibility and Exclusion") elaborates on these and other related themes. Historian of medicine Beatrix Hoffman, in "Sympathy and Exclusion," analyzes the ways in which the Santillan story fit and also did not fit into the larger politics of immigrant access to health care. Hoffman suggests that the apparently contradictory tensions in the case (between charity and generosity on one hand, and exclusion and hostility on the other) were not contradictions at all but characteristic of Americans' own contradictory attitudes toward immigration. In "Eligibility for Organ Transplantation to Foreign Nationals," medical ethicists Eric Meslin, Karen Salmon, and Jason Eberl discuss the extent to which "citizenship" should figure at all as a morally relevant policy criterion in America for determining access to this scarce treatment, and they identify this as a crucial moral and political question at the heart of the story. They also examine the place of humanitarianism, charity, and philanthropy in shaping allocation and access in the American system. The final essay in this section, by anthropologist Leo Chavez, "Imagining the Nation, Imagining Donor Recipients," explores the enduring impact of fundamental oppositions (such as citizen-noncitizen) in the American cultural imaginary, and the ways in which the vitriolic imagery, the major motifs, and the tragic details of the Santillan story tapped into preexisting narratives and representations about Mexican immigration and the immigrant threat. While many Americans saw innocence and error woven into the potent fabric of the case, others insisted that themes of illegitimacy and illegality were the central elements in the Santillan story line.

Lurking in the background of media discussions, Jesica's age was as unsettling as her immigrant status. As we see in a fourth group of essays ("Speaking for Jesica"), she was portrayed as a "child," referred to as a baby, and also labeled a minor and a teenager, descriptions that were also circumscribed by references to her femininity. These essays address many of the understated themes in the Santillan story—about the nature of transplant as experiment, about Jesica herself and her status as an adolescent, and about the silence of Jesica herself as she lay dying at the center of public controversy. In "Babes and Baboons," anthropologist Lesley Sharp examines the growing trend in high-risk, high-technology medicine toward using children and adolescents as subjects, and the problematic relationship between experimentation, transplantation, and children. The essay asks critical questions about how we should think about Jesica's role—was she agent, victim, heroine?—given the larger processes and imperatives driving transplant medicine, and it asks us to ponder the ethical challenges posed by bringing children into the transplantation arena.

One of the most obvious and troubling features of the story was the fact that the central actor herself remained silent and unconscious throughout most of the events. Even when she was alive and sentient, Jesica remained relatively invisible and apparently passive as a key actor. In "Jesica Speaks?" anthropologist Carolyn Rouse discusses the problem of adolescent agency and the profound cultural challenges involved in allowing young people like Jesica (not fully children, not quite adults) to create their own narratives and act for themselves. This is a particularly pressing problem as adolescent medicine has consolidated as its own subspecialty, and as parents, health care workers, and ethicists grapple with the in-between status of such patients.

A concluding essay by health lawyer and bioethics scholar Nancy King, titled "Fame and Fortune," turns to the question of how the case of the "bungled transplant" should be remembered. To be sure, the month-long public tragedy involved vivid, almost classically drawn, characters—there was the "Cinderella" figure of Jesica Santillan, the "fairy Godfather" Mack Mahoney, and allusions to the "cowboy" surgeons at the heart of the transplant process; the medical error had all the elements of a classical mystery and its own cast of bureaucrats and administrators sifting though the evidence in order to pass the buck or lay blame. King situates the Santillan story in the broad context of other high-profile "mediagenic" medical cases from the conjoined Bijani twins to Terri Schiavo, offering a comprehensive cultural commentary on the narratives generated in the media, in bioethics, and in public policy—narratives that are both terribly oversimplified and yet take on a powerful resonance.

Driving the story was a profound irony—an advanced technological system stretching from Boston to Durham and beyond, a complex operation where the patient's lungs and heart were removed even before the new organs had arrived (in order to reduce the transfer time to the bare minimum), and a basic mishap—characterized at one point as a "clerical error"—over blood typing. Equally ironic, because it was rarely mentioned, was the basic fact that a child had died in Boston and that this child's parents had donated the organs so that someone like Jesica might live. That other child never entered the public narrative, however, thus making for an unequal balance of anonymity and notoriety. It is a noteworthy silence in the Santillan story that while Jesica's individuality became a central focus of public discussion, the young child whose organs were donated after death only entered the story as a set of highly desirable parts—a heart and two lungs. Increasingly, the lines of anonymity that were drawn decades ago between donor and recipient have been breaking down. But we can only wonder about the ways in which the donor's parents grappled with the problem of death and donation, how they saw their role in the donation system, and how their own views about their child's life and Jesica's misfortune might have entered the public and professional conversation.

The Santillan story should be remembered as a portal into the complexities of American medicine and politics in our time, and it should rightly stand as an object lesson and a morality tale for those struggling to understand the cultural, political, and social values underpinning health care. The story of Jesica Santillan can stand alongside other cases in the annals of American medicine—next to the story of Barney Clark in which the first artificial heart transplant experiments gave rise to potent astronaut imagery, fearsome images of zombielike transplant patients, and vigorous ethical debates about the future of medicine; or part of a long lineage of silenced female patients, like Karen Ann Quinlan or Terri Schiavo, whose "right to die" stories opened new discourses about "vegetative states" and patients' rights, and continue to shape the American political and health landscape. Like other notable cases, the Santillan story unearthed problems that previously lay hidden within the system—revealing the processes and assumptions driving that system.

PARADOXES OF MEDICAL CITIZENSHIP

The Santillan story exposed a complex conversation about the problems and paradoxes of medical citizenship—a term that points to different dilemmas in the United States from those in other parts of the world. In many respects Jesica Santillan had a great deal in common with other North Americans maneuvering within and around their national health care system and making claims as citizens for access to drugs, information, procedures, and health care services while also looking across national and state borders to secure those services. In Jesica's time, some U.S. citizens would also routinely cross borders to secure services—heading into Canada and Mexico to refill their prescriptions, venturing into the so-called third-world or to China for organ transplants. And everywhere in the world, as many scholars are noting, bodily infirmity is becoming, more and more, a powerful vehicle for shaping relationships to the state and for establishing claims for equity, rights, and resources.[19] But the idea of medical citizenship, which might take on one set of meanings in the United States in 2005, carries widely different meanings, for example, in places with impoverished or hollow political structures, in places lacking resources or basic protections regarding the use of body parts, or in places where remarkable social inequities persist. Indeed, it is these regional and global disjunctions that account for many of the dilemmas encountered in these pages: the decision of Americans to travel abroad to obtain organs, the plight of Bruce Tucker, and the story of Jesica Santillan. In truth, then, there were large national forces and global processes moving people like Jessica into North Carolina to find work, moving Americans abroad to find lifesaving organ transplants, and moving the body parts of a deceased child in Boston to the Duke University Medical Center in Durham. Considered in this larger context, Jesica Santillan was not an indigent immigrant taking advantage of the American system; nor was she akin to wealthy world travelers and medical tourists who had become so problematic in the transplant community both in America and abroad.[20] Jesica was a kind of hybrid figure, a controversial, remarkably agile medical citizen.

We do not pretend that this book offers insight into the private realm of Jesica Santillan's experience or her family's painful plight. Nor does this book seek to recreate the perspectives of other major actors in the story of the "bungled transplant"—her surgeon Jim Jaggers, her patron Mack Mahoney, her friends, her teachers, or others intimately involved in the seventeen-year-old's life and death. Nor do we seek to judge patients, professions, or institutions currently navigating the therapeutic and moral terrain highlighted in this book. Rather, the book seeks to understand and analyze the story as it played itself out in key institutions and locales: in hospitals wary of committing such errors; in transplant organizations concerned with speeding organs from donors to recipients with as little waste of organs as possible; in the media with its concern for satisfying the public interest in questions of fairness, immigration policy, lifesaving medicine, scandal, and a host of other storylines; and on a global stage where transplantation had taken on a far more disturbing moral turn.

These vexing problems (medical error, medical citizenship, the ambiguities of high-tech medicine, immigration, and malpractice) do not exist in isolation but in dynamic relationship to one another. The Santillan story revealed this fact all too clearly, showing how debates and policy shifts in one realm inevitably altered policy in another. Therefore, one cannot pin a single meaning on this story of medical error. In the calm after the media storm, and in the wake of the 2004 legal settlement between Duke and the Santillan family, and with the benefit of analytical and historical hindsight, this book revisits the "bungled transplant," pausing from time to time to do what could not be done in February 2003. The book emerged from a series of intensive conversations held among all the authors and editors in June 2004 and again in May 2005. Our writings, coming from diverse vantage points, do not necessarily agree, but read as a whole the book must be understood as a unique, purposeful, and prolonged discussion of the significance of a crucial event by medical anthropologists, historians, medical ethicists, transplant surgeons, anesthesiologists, and others. And it bears repeating that our goal is not to lay blame or assign fault but to unearth and examine the underlying issues that made Jesica Santillan's story notorious, compelling, and memorable—truly a case for our time.

NOTES

1. As Jesica's health declined, press accounts began to refer to the transplant as "botched" and also as "bungled." One typical account in the *Washington Post* began: "A teenage girl who underwent a second heart-lung transplant after doctors bungled the first one by giving her mismatched organs died yesterday . . ." (Rob Stein, "Teenage Girl in Botched Organ Transplant Dies," *Washington Post*, February 23, 2003, A1). See also "Teen Near Death after Botched Organ Transplant," *Toronto Star*, February 19,

2003, A4; Jeffrey Gettleman and Lawrence K. Altman, "Girl in Donor Mix-Up Undergoes Second Transplant," *New York Times*, February 21, 2003, A1; "Transplant Victim, 17, Has Severe Brain Damage: Angry Benefactor Blames Hospital for Surgical Delays," *Ottowa Citizen*, February 22, 2003, A15; Emery P. Dalesio, "Public Anger Adds to Jesica Tragedy," *The Advertiser*, February 26, 2003, 32; and Martin Kasindorf, "Mexican Teenager Buried: Parents Considering Legal Action over Death," *USA Today*, March 5, 2003, 2A.

2. Jeffrey Gettleman and Lawrence Altman, "Girl in Donor Mix-Up Undergoes Second Transplant," *New York Times*, February 21, 2003, A1.

3. Will Weissert, "Mexican Village Was Ready, but Jesica's Funeral Not to Be," *Charlotte Observer*, March 6, 2003.

4. Rebeca Rodriguez, "Untraditional Immigration; Hispanics Flocking to Different States," *San Antonio Express-News*, March 2, 2003, 12A. The San Antonio newspaper's article focused on immigration trends in North Carolina.

5. Ibid.

6. Elizabeth Greco, "The Foreign Born from Mexico in the United States," Migration Policy Institute, October 1, 2003. Unofficial estimates would put the growth much higher. According to one 2003 United States Census study, the percentage of foreign-born people in North Carolina had climbed from 1.7 percent of the state's population in 1990 to 5.3 percent of the population in 2000. Most of that increase was fueled by immigration from Mexico and Latin America. Georgia also saw dramatic increases in its foreign-born population in the same period—from 2.7 percent to 7.1 percent of the state's population. In North Carolina, 56 percent of the 430,000 foreign-born population in 2000 were from Mexico and Latin America. See United States Census Bureau, "The Foreign Born Population: 2000 (Census 2000 Brief)," United States Department of Commerce, Economics and Statistics Administration, December 2003.

7. Jerry Adler, "A Tragic Error," *Newsweek*, March 3, 2003, 21.

8. Ibid.; Randal C. Archibold, "Benefactor Championed an Immigrant Girl's Cause," *New York Times*, February 26, 2003, A18.

9. Adler, "Tragic Error," 25; Archibold, "Benefactor Championed an Immigrant Girl's Cause."

10. Avery Comarow, "Jesica's Story," *U.S. News and World Report*, July 28, 2003, 51.

11. Editorial, "Legislative Battle Looms Over Medical Malpractice," *Tampa Tribune*, March 2, 2003, 2.

12. John Grogan, "Malpractice Caps? Think of Jesica," *Philadelphia Inquirer*, February 25, 2003.

13. Letter from Kim Lewis, Chattanooga, Tennessee, "Transplant Tragedy," *U.S. News and World Report*, September 1, 2003, 8.

14. See, for example, Alfredo Corchado, "Village Mourns Girl's Transplant Death," *Dallas Morning News*, February 24, 2003, A2. The author interviewed members of her

extended family, including her despondent great-uncle, Bernardo Torres, in Arroyo Hondo.

15. Mahoney stated in a press conference on February 20, "Had she not spent this much time on these machines it would not be a problem. Even if she did have to have another heart, if they had gone ahead and 'fessed up in time for us to find another one in time this would not be a problem." See "Girl has brain swelling after transplant" (statement by Mack Mahoney), *United Press International*, February 21, 2003.

16. J. Corridan, L. Cohn, M. Donaldson, *To Err is Human: Building a Safer Health System* (Washington, D.C.: National Academies Press, 2000). News coverage of this publication was extensive. See, for example, Bob Davis and Julie Appleby, "Medical Mistakes Eighth Top Killer," *USA Today*, November 30, 1999, 1A.

17. The existing rules required that donor organs would be shared first locally, then regionally, and only then offered nationally—in order to, it was said, to help those closest to home. The Clinton administration, supported by another Institute of Medicine report, pressed strenuously for a "sickest-first" policy where these borders would disappear, where the sickest person *in the country* would be first in line, and where (accordingly) existing disparities in waiting times across the nation would be reduced. In the end, the reforms failed, and doctors, transplant centers, and patients would learn to maneuver for best advantage within the borders and constraints of the system.

18. Asked in 1999, for example, about the care of ailing foreigners in U.S. hospitals, one emergency room director (at Bellevue Hospital in New York) could insist, "Should I wonder whether this guy is from Third Avenue who doesn't have any money or the guy from the third world who doesn't have any? That's not my job, I'm a doctor," while another spokesperson for a hospital in Miami would insist, "We have to draw the line somewhere, and we're doing it more and more. . . . The county has made it very clear that our first responsibility is to the people of Miami-Dade County." See Lewis Goldfrank, Emergency Services director, and Maria Rosa Gonzalez quoted in Randy Kennedy, "Ailing Foreigners Burden Emergency Rooms in U.S.," *New York Times*, July 1, 1999, A1.

19. See, for example, Adriana Petryna, *Life Exposed: Biological Citizens After Chernobyl* (Princeton: Princeton University Press, 2002).

20. These were two of the central images through which immigrants and foreign transplant patients were often understood in the American social imagination.

MEDICAL ERROR AND THE AMERICAN TRANSPLANT THEATER

AMERICA'S ANGEL OR THIEVING IMMIGRANT?

MEDIA COVERAGE, THE SANTILLAN STORY, AND PUBLICIZED AMBIVALENCE TOWARD DONATION AND TRANSPLANTATION

SUSAN E. MORGAN, TYLER R. HARRISON, LISA VOLK CHEWNING, AND JACKLYN G. HABIB

Organ donation has always faced a difficult battle in vying for positive media coverage. At the center of key tensions over how we tend to think about the goals of modern medicine and how we think about the human body, organ donation has often produced a profound ambivalence. Historically, print journalism and television coverage has often utilized almost Frankenstein-like images of "harvesting" organs to rebuild a defective human body while, at the same time, portraying organ transplants as miracles of modern science and the sole hope for life for the many thousands of people on the waiting list. Jesica Santillan's so-called botched transplant generated an intense media attention from February to March of 2003 that reflected this deep-seated ambivalence. News coverage first centered on a report of the clinical story: a terrible error and a failure to double-check medical tests lead to the near-death of a young Mexican girl at Duke University Medical Center in North Carolina. However, when a new set of organs became available almost immediately, the coverage began to question the fairness of the organ allocation system: how were doctors able to procure organs so quickly when thousands of other patients were waiting? These stories and commentary soon turned to ugly questions about why organs from an American citizen were used to save the life of an undocumented immigrant when so many American citizens were dying while waiting for transplants. In its slow transformation from a story of lifesaving transplant surgery into a vexing scandal laden with blame and accusation, the Jesica Santillan case added to the corpus of mixed messages in the media and throughout America about organ and tissue transplantation.

This essay examines shifts in media representations as the Santillan story unfolded in national and local media. We do not tackle critical questions about the motivations that shape these representations, nor are we interested in variations in how various newspapers and television stations across the United States covered the story. Rather, in the following pages we elucidate the overarching narrative of the Santillan transplant, how the story emerged into the public sphere, how it changed over time, and how authors and commentators articulated the meaning of this case. On such high-tech medical and scientific topics, Americans tend to rely heavily on representations in national media, especially because most readers have little personal experience with the issues; in these instances, then, such accounts play a disproportionately powerful role in shaping opinions.[1] Therefore, a national examination of the Santillan coverage provides a crucial starting point for understanding how key characters in the drama were presented to most Americans, and how these characters themselves came to embody different features of the publicized ambivalence toward organ donation and transplantation. Moreover, this national examination also allows us to follow the rapid shifts, instabilities, and ambivalences in the public discussion not only of the Santillan drama and organ donation and transplantation, but also of immigration—a theme that became a potent backdrop of the public commentary (see figure 1).

Remarkable events associated with a particular phenomenon create a spike in media coverage, and they also create potential turning points in representations of the phenomena.[2] The case of Jesica Santillan represented exactly such an extraordinary event that brought to the surface of public discussion deeper conflicts about donation and transplantation. While many other cases of organ donation have captured public attention for a few days at a time, in this instance media coverage lasted much longer than one or two days. The most intense reporting spanned approximately two weeks, from February 17 to March 5, 2003 (see figure 2); but articles referencing Jesica Santillan could still be found six months later. We used a television monitoring service called ShadowTV to gather data on this coverage, and we also performed routine online searches for national and regional newspapers stories. We focused principally on coverage of Jesica's story after the initial transplant on February 7. As a media event, the story was nevertheless short-lived, beginning with intense reporting on February 17 after the public disclosure of the error. By February 28, virtually all television coverage ended whereas heavy print coverage continued until March 27, 2003. Overall, our research uncovered 97 unique print stories and 65 unique television stories that featured or referenced the Jesica Santillan case, resulting in 162 stories for analysis.[3]

What were the major recurring patterns of coverage? And how did the themes (and the intensity of coverage) change over time? The telling of the

Santillan story produced a wide range of prototypical images of Jesica, her family (particularly her mother Magdalena), her patron Mack Mahoney, Duke University and its spokespeople, and other key actors such as the United Network for Organ Sharing (UNOS), and the coverage also produced linguistic themes that anchored the story. In the creation of social representation, processes of anchoring (that is, finding language to describe the new phenomenon) and objectification (in which key concrete images or prototypes are attached to the phenomenon) are crucial.[4] Over time, despite internal contradictions in the news reporting and commentary, despite wide variations in how the story was told in different parts of the country, and despite large differences between television and print media, a "consensual reality" of the case took shape.[5] A number of actors appeared repeatedly in news coverage, and as their influence on the circumstances changed, so did the media's portrayal of those individuals.

MEDIA REPRESENTATIONS OF JESICA SANTILLAN

The Santillan case played out like a drama in which media portrayals of concealment, deception, power, moments of joy, and tragedy captured the attention of the public. Yet, despite most of the action, the central actor, Jesica Santillan, was a silent symbol, characterized either as a victim/saint or, conversely, as an illegal immigrant. She would not be presented as a full person until after her death.

When television and print media first introduced their readers and listeners to Jesica in a comprehensive way, she had already undergone the first transplant with mismatched organs almost ten days earlier, and lay in critical condition. A second transplant offered her only chance for survival. While her family and her advocate Mack Mahoney petitioned the public for help saving Jesica's life, doctors contended that there was little that could be done. Jesica was small, frail, and barely clinging to life; and she was surrounded by a desperate family, apologetic doctors, and a chastened hospital. In one account after another, media accounts implicitly invited the public to pray along with Jesica's family. And when Jesica received the second transplants on February 20, her family and friends were portrayed as happy and grateful. At the same time, however, the coverage that had encouraged communal hope, began to question why a frail patient with such a slim chance of survival had received another transplant. Part of the explanation was the "sickest first" policy that determined eligibility; and Jesica clearly had become—because of her body's rejection of the first set of organs—extraordinarily ill. As ethicists and legal

Figure 1. Timeline of Jesica Santillan Events and Media Coverage Turning Points

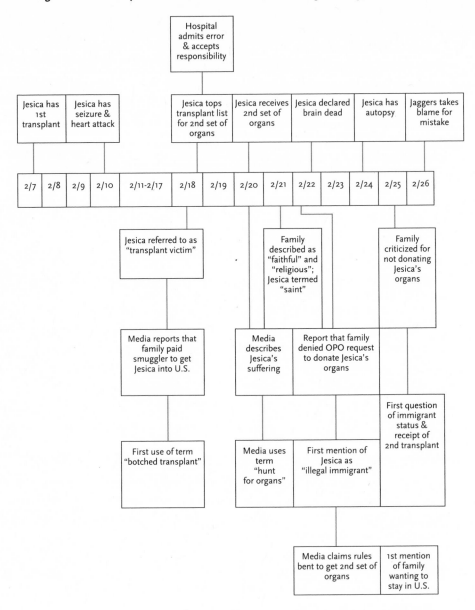

experts debated the wisdom of the "sickest first" allocation system and while others wondered why an illegal immigrant received a transplant in the first place, within days of the second transplant the story of Jesica Santillan was becoming more complex.

While, for some, Jesica became the face of an important issue—the short-

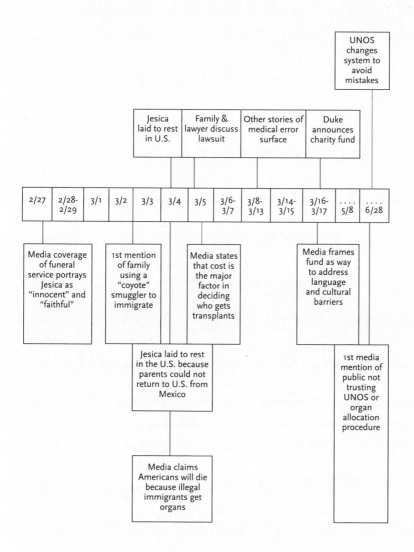

age of organs for children—she was also described as an unfortunate example of the toll of errors in cutting-edge medicine. But in the wake of the second transplant, her case would also become a potent immigration narrative. The media embraced Jesica through the well-trod narrative of immigrants chasing after the hope of a better life in America. A great deal of action—both real

Figure 2. Intensity of Media Coverage over Time (Number of Stories by Date)

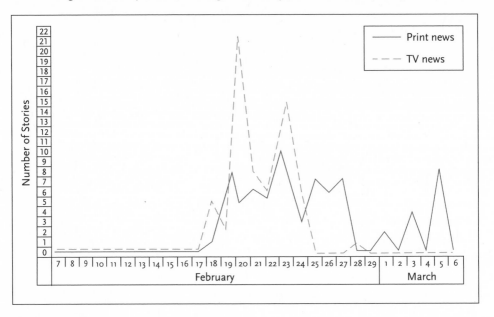

and symbolic—occurred around Jesica, and yet, because of the nature of her condition, she actually said and did the least in these news accounts. The lack of reportable action, then, left readers dependent on the various media attributions to link particular motives, sentiments, and feelings to Jesica. Where other characters might be allowed to speak for themselves, these actors in the drama (and the writers of the various news accounts) also spoke for Jesica in the unfolding media coverage.

Initially, accounts described Jesica in various and often conflicted ways. Some saw her as a seventeen-year-old, desperately ill patient with a grave prognosis. Others characterized her as a "botched transplant victim," and drew attention to her status as a poor, small-town girl. Elsewhere, Jesica was referred to as a "baby [that] needed some help," echoing her mother's characterizations, and some media stories further embellished her profile as the "world's sweetheart."[6] As Nancy King and Carolyn Rouse point out elsewhere in this volume, the media was drawn to her as a "mediagenic" individual— and these accounts quickly cast her as a young, pretty, "innocent," and sympathetic figure. The combination generally evoked positive public reactions.

At the same time, however, news stories rarely failed to mention her immigration status—albeit in various ways. Jesica was described as a "Mexican teenager," a characterization that eventually morphed into "Mexican immigrant," and later (by the end of the two-week period) into an "illegal immigrant from Mexico." The transformation in terminology reveals much about the shifting public meaning of the case. The "illegal immigrant" characterization invigorated controversy, for it shifted attention away from error and Jesica's victimization to her impropriety—put bluntly, to the question of whether an illegal immigrant should be allowed to receive transplants in the United States. As Beatrix Hoffman and Leo Chavez note elsewhere in this volume, long-standing concerns about immigrants' rights to health care shaped these public reactions to Jesica's case. And as we see in Jed Gross's essay, these anxieties could also emerge around cases of wealthy foreigners purchasing access to transplants in America. In such cases, immigration anxieties often commingled with barely submerged public mistrust about the allocation system.

Media claims of public outrage over Jesica's transplants peaked after her death, and a great deal of animus centered on claims of theft—or (as articulated by one college newspaper) that Jesica "[came] into our country and [took] the organs of not one, but two people, that could have gone to more deserving Americans."[7] By late February into early March, the tone of coverage had become inverted in crucial ways. When, early on after the first transplant, the outlook for Jesica had been most grim, stories cast her as an innocent victim; yet, just when events took a positive turn and Jesica received matched organs, questions of privilege and special consideration emerged. As her condition changed yet again and as her health declined, these conflicted characterizations would continue.

The often hyperbolic images of Jesica in the amalgam of news coverage traversed a spectrum between thieving immigrant and martyred saint. In the most vitriolic description, a caller to a radio show in the Southwest labeled her as a "wetback" immigrant who took organs from dying Americans.[8] On CNN, on the other hand, she was called "America's sweetheart" who had touched the hearts of many.[9] These images, of course, had little to do with Jesica herself, and much to do with popular American, even mythic, representations: the innocent victim, the underdog fighting the heartless system, on the one hand; and, on the other, the despised lawless outsider using precious resources intended for others, her greed resulting in the death of others.

PORTRAYING THE SANTILLAN FAMILY

In many respects, it was Jesica's family who bore the brunt of this characterization as conniving thieves (as we shall see later), but they themselves also played a role in shaping the public imagery of the case. The first days of media coverage saw the family's first appearance. The Santillan family spoke little English. Through a translator, they called the mistake "unforgivable," but Jesica's mother and father remained focused on obtaining a new transplant.[10] Their grief was evident but so too were the spontaneous bouts of anger toward the doctors and hospital. For example, when they called Duke Medical Center "piranhas," they evoked predatory and even vampiric images that had long circulated in social representations of organ donation and transplantation. The family's pronouncements in the media captured much about the public's sentiments about medicine and error. Magdalena Santillan, Jesica's mother, was reported stating bluntly that the "doctor should go to jail," and yet other stories showed her pleading for anyone concerned or anyone with a dying child whose organs might be available to help her find "the organs that my daughter needs to live."[11]

The Santillan family's direct appeal for public support and organs to save Jesica would have lasting implications. It foregrounded into public view another notion that had long been associated with transplantation: that public pressure, backroom deals, and the special status of patients were crucial factors in determining who received organ transplants. When Jesica received the second transplant days later, her mother's expression of gratitude to both the donor family and the media reinforced these sentiments. Magdalena suggested (and one CNN story translated her words) that "if it hadn't been for the support from . . . TV, from radios and newspapers . . . they would have let my baby die. I've seen a lot of cases where they don't pay much attention to Latinos."[12] But at the same time, Magdalena was also reported to have said that doctors had now done all they could.[13] And in the days after the second transplant, as Jesica's health began to deteriorate, the Santillan family receded from most news accounts.

But throughout the ordeal, the family's voices were often complemented by other actors who spoke for them. As the news commentary expanded, indeed more and more figures became involved in representing the family. There was, for example, the ever-present Mack Mahoney, and Renee McCormick (a spokesperson for Jesica's Hope Chest, which had been created to raise funds to pay for her transplant). Various reporters and television anchors also spoke for her family in a distant way, and even the Mexican consulate would represent the family's position at one point. Media coverage made continual references to the fact that the family relied heavily on translators and intermediaries to communicate with doctors, the hospital, and the public. The Santillans, in this view, were severely limited in their capacity to help

Jesica because of language; and, of course, the language difference (a frequently mentioned theme in news stories) reinforced the family's immigrant status. Early on, news stories reported, the family had granted power of attorney over Jesica's health care to Mack Mahoney. Mahoney himself, commenting on his role and their linguistic vulnerability, noted to a North Carolina journalist: "Nobody else can fight for her. Her family does not speak English. [The hospital] can bully them around and do all they want to, and I just refuse to let them bully me."[14] Such widely reported sentiments fostered an image of family dependency, need, and helplessness that would remain vital to the public story. Jesica's parents needed assistance in caring for their daughter. Media accounts portrayed them as adrift, confused, weak, easily influenced, and powerfully dependent on and beholden to patrons like Mahoney, and (by extension) to American goodwill writ large. That the family "only spoke Spanish" and relied on a translator constantly reminded readers and listeners that the Santillans were not Americans. Throughout the tragic story, as more and more of these intermediaries took center stage, it would become increasingly difficult for readers and listeners to discern whether the family had expressed particular ideas and sentiments, whether they originated with the friends or spokespeople, or whether they were merely free-floating, media-generated sketches presented as the family's attributes.

MACK MAHONEY AS RENEGADE COWBOY

It was not the family but Mack Mahoney who played the central protagonist in media accounts. Mahoney facilitated much of the action that was documented in news coverage. As the news later reported, it was Mahoney (after he first learned about Jesica's plight from a local North Carolina newspaper) who attempted to make an anonymous donation to the family in order to help her obtain her first transplant. When the family insisted on meeting him, an unusual relationship blossomed. In early accounts, then, Mahoney's closeness to the family came sharply into view; and stories characterized him as Jesica's "benefactor" and as the founder of Jesica's Hope Chest, a foundation to help critically ill children. Mahoney asserted himself with journalists as a credible family spokesperson, recounting the daily turmoil surrounding the transplant error and describing its impact on the Santillan family. Television coverage showed him criticizing the hospital for not admitting their mistake in public soon enough, and he was one of the prominent public faces in the family's appeal for a directed donation. Mahoney characterized himself as an irreverent cowboy of sorts, a Dallas native who seized the reins and took actions when the family could not and when the hospital *would* not. Some news accounts clearly found this image appealing and developed it fully in their profiles of Mahoney. One report in a Charlotte, North Carolina, newspaper noted, for example, that "Mahoney says if the hospital had gone public with the mistake immediately after the surgery, there might have been a better chance of finding a new donor."[15] In contrast to the hospital, which was criticized for allegedly delaying and dissembling, Mahoney was portrayed as blunt-spoken and ready to take action: "[W]e're gonna get everybody together and we're gonna find that baby some organs," he said on CNN on February 20.[16]

Such stories presented Mahoney as a man of action. Mahoney "took on the hospital," noted one account, drawing attention to the claim that he would not be bullied. Through the media, he issued stark challenges to the hospital's administrators, insisting at one point that "if she dies, Duke will have murdered her," and (later, as death neared) that "[the hospital] let my baby lay on that bed . . . and she's probably going to have brain damage, and, you know, guess whose fault that gets to be?".[17] Other stories reported that it was Mahoney who had pushed the family to go public with their appeal. And most accounts saw him as a positive if belligerent force in the story, "battling" with Duke as the hospital sought to avoid the bad publicity. As CNN put it, "Knowing that the time was running out for the girl [Mahoney] calls 'the world's sweetheart,' Mahoney sprang into action to get the word out to the media that Jesica needed a matching donor."[18] In some accounts, Mahoney's benevolent aggressiveness was even credited for getting Jesica the first transplant—and here, again, one sees the ways in which public ambivalence about organ allocation would be fostered. Other stories, however, such as the *New York Times*'s portrait of him as "a hand grenade in a china shop," offered less generous representations of Mahoney.[19] At times depicted as aggressive and benevolent, but also destructive, Mahoney was nevertheless portrayed as a necessary catalyst for action that could have saved Jesica's life.

After Jesica's death on February 23, Mahoney receded from the glare of the public spotlight with the simple statement: "I'm done. There's nothing more to say."[20] In the wake of his silence came a new type of coverage reassessing his role and sketching a less flattering profile of the man. Reflective essays and news analyses now described him as a "displaced Texan," as a "bearded 55-year-old with a white Panama hat and a raspy Texas accent," pointing more forcefully to his own uprooting and displacement.[21] Other accounts delved deeper into his own past, noting, for example (as one article did on the eve of Jesica's death), that he had lost his own son to medical error twenty years earlier.[22] The unearthing of this personal experience gave new significance to Mahoney's advocacy, his creation of a foundation in Jesica's honor, his role in applying for work visas for the Santillan family, and his fund-raising for Jesica's medical expenses. This notion of a hidden past evokes, of course, images of a lone ranger, championing the cause of the helpless, tired, and weary, taking on the powerful and pushing up to and sometimes beyond the limits of the law in service of a worthy cause. Such media stories, then, likened the Texan Mahoney to an iconic American character: the cowboy. His abrupt departure from the public eye after Jesica's death further reinforced this lone ranger image. His cowboy story, however, did not end happily. The image fostered ambivalence. And it is not altogether surprising that even while Mahoney could be characterized as a lone ranger, so too could Dr. Jaggers be figured as a renegade cowboy surgeon (as Nancy King and Carolyn Rouse note in their essays in this volume). Perhaps, in the media's perspective, it took one cowboy to effectively confront another.

IMAGERY AND INSTITUTIONS: DUKE UNIVERSITY HOSPITAL

Throughout the coverage of the Santillan case, competing representations of Duke Hospital vied with one another. Many accounts represented Duke as "one of the world's leading centers for organ transplantation" and as a medical institution involved in groundbreaking work.[23] The hospital was "well-known" and "renowned," making it all the more striking (in the media's perspective) that crucial safeguards had failed. From the outset, the focus rested on failing safeguards rather than on negligence per se. An "elite" medical institution, Duke appeared to be part of a large systemwide error, and thus the event was seen as a "grim reminder of what can go wrong even with top-rated surgeons at a first-rate hospital."[24]

But Mahoney and the Santillan family promoted a different characterization of Duke: an institution that was "very hard to deal with," one that failed Jesica once with the egregious error and a second time by not being forthcoming with the family and with the public.[25] Against this backdrop of elite medicine, error, and blame, Duke was presented on CBS News and in other outlets as "image conscious" and "insensitive," as "piranhas," or as bureaucrats who "dragged their feet" or who were most concerned with public relations and "wip[ing] the tarnish off their image." Expertise gone awry and arrogance was a major theme in some of these published stories. At one point, Mahoney bluntly asserted, "Duke is as arrogant as hell is hot."[26]

At the center of these widely varying and heated representations of the institution was the simple question of blame and fault. Who was directly responsible for the error, for the declining health and the death of the young Jesica? The question of culpability hung in the air around press conferences and in media stories, drawing attention to the inherent defensiveness of Duke's pronouncements. As media coverage of the case began, for example, administrators referred to the mistake as a "tragic error" even as they publicly accepted responsibility. Dr. Fulkerson, chief executive officer of the hospital, assured the family and the public that "[the hospital's] focus is really on her care here. And we have an extraordinary team of people that are working very hard to try and stabilize her."[27] In the context of heated accusations and the extraordinary error, Duke's apology could be read in different ways: was it admirable forthrightness under difficult circumstances? Or were their words read as superficial and unsatisfying attempts to shape future discussions about the institution's liability?

While the second transplant operation quieted the Santillan family's public condemnation of Duke, it opened another contentious line of public criticism, coming from new sources and focusing on whether or not the hospital should have attempted the second operation, on the motives of the hospital in working to secure a second set of organs, and on whether any extraordinary measures were taken to obtain these organs. By the time of the second transplant, the consensual reality of the case as represented in media stories held that Jesica's chances of survival were slim and declining. Duke's administrators remained optimistic in their public statements, asserting that her chances of surviving were 50-50. Other physicians and ethicists who were called into the public commentary disagreed, and another round of critical commentary on CNN, CBS, and other sources focused on the possibility that the hospital was wasting "scarce resources" and doing so only in a desperate effort to "fix their mistake."[28] (This topic—the second transplant and the debate over futility—is discussed at length in the essay by Wailoo and Livingston.) Without question, the second transplant served as a turning point in media coverage, for now much of the media commentary on Duke was centered on the fairness and wisdom of the second operation, and not exclusively on the original error.

Further controversy flared when Duke physicians declared Jesica (declining fast after the second operation) to be brain dead and pushed for removing her from life support despite her family's apparent resistance. Here was yet another conflicted image of the institution appearing toward the end of Jesica's life, and media attention swung to cover the acrimony and misunderstanding over the question of whether Jesica was dead. Bioethicists commented that Duke's actions (in this instance) were not only defensible but correct. Yet the new controversy only added one more facet to the conflicting representations of the high-tech institution, its motives, behaviors, and pronouncements, and the fate of patients within its doors. If the beginning of the public story cast Duke's high-technology facility in ambivalent terms (as both a mecca of modern medicine and as a site for unconscionable mistakes), then the concluding story about removing "life support" suggested another ambivalence about public concerns about premature declaration of death in service of organ donation. Duke hospital, throughout the Santillan drama, remained part of a complex array of stories touching on institutional and medical mistrust, on malpractice and institutional sensitivity, on error and its origins, and on the place of organ donation and transplantation in modern medicine and society.

JAMES JAGGERS: CONFLICTED PORTRAITS OF A DUKE SURGEON

When the error was discovered, Dr. James Jaggers—the surgeon who led the first transplant team and who had unwittingly transplanted the mismatched organs—was portrayed as forthright with the family. By all accounts, Jaggers took direct responsibility for the mistake, even as Duke's administrators suggested that a "clerical error" was responsible. Some stories delved deeper into the sequence of events, however, suggesting that Jaggers had failed to request information about the blood type of the donated organs and had failed to reconcile the organs' blood type with Jesica's. With one glaring exception, neither the family nor the media attacked or criticized Jaggers on a personal level. *Newsweek* later presented Jaggers as having the "courage to go out and tell the truth."[29] His remorse for the mistake earned much media attention. As the story broke, for example, the *New York Times* offered these quotes: Jaggers was "heartbroken about what happened to Jesica"; his "focus has been on providing her with the heart and lungs she needs so she could lead a normal life."[30] There was one stark exception to this trend, for initially the Santillan family had insisted that Jaggers be jailed for the error; but then they quickly acknowledged that he had done everything possible for Jesica, and they professed their complete faith in his ability as a surgeon. As news accounts later reported, they even insisted that Jaggers perform the second transplant surgery (although he was to be monitored). This tension over Dr. Jaggers—who he was, what his commitments were, what level of responsibility he would take, whether he was an exemplary surgeon or careless practitioner—dominated the media coverage throughout the public life of the case.

The news media and analysis quickly characterized Jaggers's failure to type the donated organs as a system error—thus shifting the focus away from the individual to the system and its multiple players and safeguards. Stories reported that the hospital and UNOS would conduct investigations to review the conversations and decisions leading to the error, but they insisted that such investigations would focus more on corrective action than individual punishment. Accordingly, most coverage cited Jaggers's decisions as contributing factors rather than the primary error. As one *Washington Post* article stated, "Most mistakes are not the result of incompetent or uncommitted doctors, nurses, or pharmacists . . . they are rather, the result of a failure in the system."[31] Yet, in such accounts, the line between individual fault and system error was not always clear. Another story on CBS concluded, "Dr. Jaggers never made any verbal confirmation that the organs were a match—a major oversight in the process."[32] In general, media accounts spread responsibility for the error to the large, complex, and diffuse administrative processes. These stories, therefore, relieved Jaggers of personal culpability, even as at the same time (ironically) he freely accepted responsibility. It is unclear to what extent his initial public display of remorse and his overt acceptance of accountability influenced the tenor of subsequent media coverage, allowing writers and commentators to grant him a kind of preemptory reprieve. (For more on this topic of individual and systems error, see the essay by Charles Bosk.)

Certainly, his status as a respected surgeon at an elite medical center, as well as the heated rhetoric surrounding Duke more generally, would have contributed to these media representations of the doctor. Stories were quick to point out that Jaggers was well-respected in the medical community. As one account on MSNBC noted, "From all accounts, Dr. James Jaggers is an exemplary surgeon . . . no one will say a negative word about him. He is apparently a very caring, compassionate person, and a family spokesperson says he wept after telling the family that he had made that tragic mistake."[33] This image of a exemplary practitioner, a compassionate man who was also capable of weeping at the bedside preemptively redeemed Jaggers in many media accounts. Another early report, for example, stressed that Jaggers "volunteered to go to Nicaragua to perform heart surgery on underprivileged children in that area. . . . [He was] known as the go-to guy here when dealing with babies with heart problems."[34] Such accounts of the surgeon's admirable character, found frequently in the coverage, insulated him from much of the public blame. Jaggers, however, did not escape blame everywhere. Some stories called for his resignation. Others noted that while he would be formally reprimanded, it was ironic that his work would continue: "Jaggers will still get up every morning and practice medicine and perform surgery . . . somewhere, there needs to be some sort of punishment. . . . A child died on his watch, and it was his fault because he did not double-check the blood type with that of the recipient."[35] In this telling, Jaggers was a reckless and powerful surgeon who would go unpunished for his extraordinary and deadly mistake. Yet such angry portraits were overwhelmed in numbers by positive and sympathetic images of Jaggers. One *Washington Post* editorial put the ambivalence toward Jaggers this way: "He's become a figure both noble and detestable, the captain of a sunk ship, a confirmation that Americans mythologize doctors while deeply suspecting them of the capacity for great arrogance and harm."[36]

Ambivalence pervaded media representations of the main characters in the Santillan story, but the media coverage of Jaggers was particularly fascinating, for it reinforced a particular mythology (that the doctors were compassionate and noble in their efforts to help patients) while also drawing attention to a competing set of notions—that they were not entirely trustworthy and often remained above normal systems of accountability.

BUREAUCRACY AND BARGAINING: PICTURING THE ORGAN ALLOCATION SYSTEM

If tension and ambivalence characterized coverage of Jaggers and Duke, then how did the organ allocation system fare in these media accounts? The case did provoke the media to explain key features of the complex U.S. organ allocation system, but media accounts also fostered many new concerns and anxieties about organ donation, allocation, and transplantation. At first, investigative news coverage sought to determine just how and where the mistake could have happened, and this involved detailed explorations of the blood-type matching and the role of organizations like UNOS in shaping the fateful error. After Jesica's second transplant, however, these examinations shifted to the broader-based ethical questions about how hospitals and UNOS determined eligibility of citizens and noncitizens, and about what criteria determined how patients rose to the top of the transplant queue. Reporters, commentators, medical ethicists, letter writers, and others raised questions of fairness in the wake of the second transplant—and media investigations of the transplant system took on a broader set of meanings. Was it fair, several stories asked, to give an individual like Jesica not one but two sets of new organs? The question provoked many to speculate that factors beyond clinical need influenced allocation, not just in this case, but more generally.

The coverage produced many accounts about the nature, location, and timing of the medical error, and about the character of the transplant system. All acknowledged that the process had broken down—but where and when? Some stories suggested broadly that "the system" was to blame; a few others highlighted UNOS's role (rather than Duke's) in attempts to discover where the miscommunication had occurred. Initially, such stories highlighted the slim likelihood that Jesica would be able to obtain a second set of organs; for example, one CNN story quoted a UNOS spokesperson's view that it would be an "uphill battle" because of the national shortage of donors.[37] Yet, because Jesica was now listed apparently as a "medical necessity," this designation ensured that her chances were quite good. Regardless of her designation, UNOS was compelled to explain that the rules of organ allocation prevented them from specifically searching for organs for Jesica. This was, they pointed out, simply not how the allocation system worked. (For more on this discussion, see the following essay by Richard Cook.) Clearly, however, Mack Mahoney and the Santillan family strongly believed that public pressure, media attention, and special pleading would be a factor in obtaining a second transplant. News accounts seldom questioned this notion; nor did they point out that the publicity could, indeed, have stimulated a potential parent from making a directed donation if their child was dying—thereby bypassing UNOS rules.[38] Directed donation was at the time, and still is today, a heatedly debated ethical issue in transplantation, yet this dimension of how organs are allocated remained invisible in public commentary. The silence around the difference between directed donation, standard UNOS allocation, and issues such as medical necessity was a missed opportunity in media coverage. Instead, the media's coverage spiralled off to investigate other hot-button ethical issues in organ donation.

Once Jesica received the second transplant (not through directed donation but through UNOS because she was listed as a "medical necessity"), commentary, speculation, and analysis dramatically shifted to the question of fairness. The organ allocation system was described as "complicated, often confusing, and certainly a highly controversial process."[39] To many, Jesica's receipt of two sets of organs and (despite this) her subsequent death "underscored a debate in medicine about the ethics of risky second-transplant operations at a time of grave shortages of human organs."[40] A range of new voices unconnected with the specifics of the case entered these stories. Reporters began turning to medical ethicists, who referred to the new situation as "an ethical dilemma with few precedents."[41] At the same time, the public commentary took many new forms as news writers also turned for commentary to people waiting on organ transplant lists and to "average citizens" for their views on the case. One MSNBC story, for example, speculated that people on organ transplant waiting lists might be perplexed, "sitting back and saying how come she got those organs so quickly."[42] *Newsweek* quoted a twenty-eight-year-old woman, a diminutive woman waiting for a heart-lung transplant, who suggested that "that could have been me [who could have received the transplant]."[43] The second transplant, then, led to a dramatic and qualitatively important expansion in the actors featured in the media coverage, many of whom led the charge in speculating about the motives of the main actors and many of whom positioned Jesica at the center of their own questions about the fairness of the allocation process and their own life-and-death chances. (Again, see the essay by Wailoo and Livingston for more discussion of this theme.) The ethics debate could turn heated at times. While one ethicist argued in the North Carolina–based *Charlotte Observer* that Jesica truly deserved the second transplant because she "never really got the first transplant" (because of the incompatibility of the organs), another on MSNBC pointed to the other silent actors off stage, insisting that "there are kids in the United States waiting for these organs and I don't [think] giving them to the person with the longest odds makes sense."[44]

Such outside commentators were among those leading the discussion about whether Jesica had received special privileges, and whether doctors manipulated the system in order to "fix their mistake." A few early reports had raised the possibility that Duke doctors had "pushed all the connections they had—not because of their mistake . . . but because Ms. Santillan's condition was so dire."[45] However, a growing number of sources developed this theme. One ethicist described it as a "horrible moral tension" in which doctors now perceived a special obligation to act because they made a mistake.[46] The perception of special manipulation on Jesica's behalf was only accentuated when, later in the year, other transplant scandals drew attention to the "impromptu bargaining" that occurred occasionally when a patient is not on UNOS's match-run list.[47] (Richard Cook's essay provides a detailed description of this issue of "bargaining," a term that carries a meaning in the context of allocation that differs somewhat from the public understanding of bargaining.) In the media, "bargaining" for organs could take on the appearance of a suspect and nefarious practice. Bargaining, as Cook makes clear, is a common part of the process of determining the clinical and biological fit between organ and potential recipient, even though it is discouraged by UNOS, which created the match-run list system precisely in order to prevent doctors from "gaming organs."[48] Other accounts went further, suggesting that doctors "admitted that they violated their own procedures and tried to correct their mistake with a new set of organs that matched her blood type."[49] Such depictions of the character of organ allocation unquestionably fostered mistrust not only of doctors and the hospital but also of the other actors in the process, and inextricably linked the Santillan story and Duke's doctors to ethical dilemmas that underlie the allocation process.

While ethicists, doctors, and would-be recipients questioned whether Jesica should have received a second set of organs, others used the opening to question whether she should have received even the first set. Late in the media coverage, as Jesica's condition declined, another debate ensued over whether immigrants should receive expensive organ transplants. UNOS publicly defended their standard practice, noting that immigrants like Jesica were indeed eligible for transplantation, and that a specific percentage of organs (5 percent) were allocated to immigrants. Moreover, UNOS insisted that immigrants in America actually donated *more* organs than they received. Investigative reports, however, pointed out that there were many conflicts within UNOS on the question of transplants for immigrants, nonresidents, and undocumented immigrants. As MSNBC reported, according to UNOS's definition, an eligible nonresident was an immigrant who is in the country legally. Jesica Santillan, of course, could not be considered to be eligible. However, media coverage made it clear that UNOS and hospitals rarely, if ever, adhered to this definition for practical reasons. As a UNOS representative noted, "We do not differentiate between whether a transplant patient has legal or illegal immigration status."[50] And a Duke hospital representative framed this decision in broader terms when he stated that "the duty of the hospital is to provide healthcare to all people, regardless of immigration status."[51] Such statements drew further attention to the role of such key players as UNOS—if not in the error itself, then in the decision to transplant. Reports on organ allocation policy highlighted how the shifting public discussion was coming to rest on questions of fairness and justice in transplantation. Organ allocation was truly a complicated process that the public and the media grasped imperfectly. It proved far easier to focus on cowboy surgeons, outspoken benefactors, troubled institutions, and illegal immigration (which became, by the end of the story, the dominant theme in the media commentary).

THE PUBLICIZED IMAGE OF IMMIGRANTS IN AMERICA

The topic of immigration served as a critical backdrop for most of the coverage regarding the Santillan case. Not only did the focus on immigration status shape judgments about Jesica and the Santillan family, but it also fueled the ethical argument regarding the allocation system.

Immigration aside, the narrative of the Santillan family resonated strongly in the American consciousness: a desperate family leaving everything behind, going to great lengths to get their daughter the medical care she needs to live. However, in the media coverage of the Santillan family a remarkable shift occurred as the story unfolded—a shift from portraying the family as heroes to portraying them as thieves. Initially, the Santillans' immigration status was a sympathetic framework for the media coverage of Jesica's dire condition and her need for advanced medical care. Monica Quiroc, an immigrant from Peru, was quoted in the *New York Times*, "They came for the reason why all of us come, because things are better here, or at least, they're supposed to be."[52] The *Washington Post* echoed this theme: "Jesica needed the transplant because a heart deformity kept her lungs from getting her blood. Her parents paid an immigrant smuggler to get the family into the United States from Mexico three years ago, in part for the better odds of landing a transplant for Jesica."[53] The Santillan family's experience was, in this telling, an epic journey of hope for a better life. The *New York Times* coverage, for example, described the Santillans as having "been on an odyssey to save their daughter's life that has taken them from the shacks of Guadalajara to the self-proclaimed City of Medicine."[54]

After her death, however, the description of their "odyssey" began to change to include other features of their immigration story—for example, that they "raised $5000 for a 'coyote' to smuggle them in."[55] Such details reinforced the view that the Santillans' immigration experience was a heroic journey that also involved sly and dishonest smuggling. The Santillan family's desperate journey of hope was also an act of criminal trespass. One account, notably from the Southwest, even portrayed the family as having "dared" to come into this country to take a heart-lung set away from others who may have died while waiting for transplants.[56] These accounts exploited stereotypical images of immigration—catering specifically to American fears of immigrants.

Retrospective accounts of the case continued to play upon the more negative or ambivalent immigrant stereotypes, offering images of a family who "stood on street corners with tin cans to collect money for their sick child."[57] Such images of solicitation and poverty were enriched by other descriptions of the Santillan family as "poor laborers" and portrayals highlighting that "the family of five was living in a relative's trailer parked near the cucumber shed where farmers brought their produce to sell to a pickle company."[58] Not only was the family living in a trailer near a shed, but they were living in a large Spanish-speaking community of "Mexican immigrants." Their reliance on others to accommodate their English language deficiency could further the belief that the Santillans were not interested in assimilation, even as (as some suggested) they simultaneously exploited the best that America had to offer. Images of the Santillans' "abuse" of the system, their opportunism, and their alleged exploitation of America itself continued even after Jesica's death, as coverage focused on the Santillan family's desire to bury Jesica in Mexico and their unwillingness to leave the country if it meant being barred from returning to America.

The constant discussion of the Santillans' immigrant status and the methods by which they smuggled Jesica into the United States conjured up images of the racialized foreigner sapping American resources. Ultimately, Jesica was portrayed as an illegal immigrant who robbed more deserving Americans of a new chance at life. To make matters worse, many stories suggested, not only were two sets of organs made available to Jesica, but, with her death, she herself did not become an organ donor. Whether the family was told that Jesica's organs were not viable for transplantation or whether the family *chose* to refuse to donate her organs was not entirely clear from the media coverage.[59] Nevertheless, it was said that, in the end, she deprived others of the chance she had been given. As Mahoney commented to one journalist on February 23, "We have received several scathing e-mails from people who are concerned that the family refused to donate Jesica's organs." He noted, however, that her body was "so saturated by medications and anti-rejection drugs" that most of her organs were not reusable.[60] Despite such assurances, however, by the end of the saga, the powerful allegations of their refusal to donate were left hanging, unproven and mostly unchallenged, in public accounts. Ultimately, the image that the American media dwelled upon was of the Santillans utilizing America's "precious resources" and not giving anything in return.

Through these shifting portrayals in the media, the Santillan family became both respected and detested, the subject of contentious media image-making reflecting two sides of the coin that is "the American dream." On one hand, they represented the belief that individuals could "make something of themselves" if only they worked hard enough. On the other hand, in trying to fulfill the American dream, they allegedly stood in the way of *Americans* who also wished to fulfill similar dreams; they robbed other American transplant patients, it was said, of the "dream of a chance at life." These themes of legitimacy, belonging, and community are further explored in compelling essays in this book by Leo Chavez, Beatrix Hoffman, and Eric Meslin et al.

American media enjoys a remarkably ambivalent relationship with organ donation and transplantation. While coverage in the news often presents a mixed picture of organ donation, very much like the one that appeared in the Santillan story, depictions of organ donation in the entertainment media tend to be even more problematic and negatively focused on scandal. Story lines in major motion pictures like the film *Blood Work* (2002), starring Clint Eastwood, or daytime dramas such as *One Life to Live* (May 2004) perpetuate many of the myths and fears about organ donation. In *Blood Work*, for example, a murderer targets people with specific blood and tissue types in an effort to obtain organs for a particular person on the waiting list. Other popular films in recent years revolve around similarly macabre story lines, like the one in which organ recipients take on the characteristics of their donors or another about the black market trade of organs in the United States.

As damaging as many fictional portrayals are, and as ambivalent as "normal" news coverage is, neither has as much potential for shaping attitudes and beliefs about organ donation as the real stories that stem from medical events or that contain as much hope, tragedy, and horror as the Jesica Santillan case did. The story would have been compelling and damning enough if it were covered as the story of a young American girl who suffered such a tragedy as the result of a medical mistake. That story line alone would have captured many of the current fears about organ donation and fed into broader issues of mistrust of the medical profession, fairness in allocation, and misunderstanding surrounding issues like brain death. But when this story line became intertwined with even more hotly controversial issues like illegal immigration, the potential for negative impact on ideas about organ donation was even greater.

The Jesica Santillan story contained all of the elements necessary to foster public ambivalence and trigger the development of conflicted social representations about organ donation in the American media. There was the controversial Mack Mahoney, the remorseful Jim Jaggers, the elite but "difficult to deal with" Duke University Hospital administrators, and the beleaguered Santillan family. And there was, of course, Jesica. As a beautiful but gravely ill young woman, Jesica Santillan elicited sympathy when she was portrayed as the victim of a series of medical errors. However, as the fairness of organ allocation became a public issue, she was represented as a beneficiary of ill-gotten benefits; and public fears emerged in the wake of her case—fears of corruption in the organ allocation system and of a "brown menace" of undocumented immigrants taking advantage of America's advanced medicine, leaving taxpaying Americans stuck with the bill, and resulting in worthy recipients dying on the transplant waiting lists. It was a story that captured many of the fundamental contradictions and ambivalences that society cultivated on a regular basis with regard to not only organ donation but also immigration and the American dream. Americans are often drawn to news about medical miracles and new technological approaches that can save lives. However, they are also often horrified by the image of arrogant doctors "playing God" and building human bodies from other people's body parts. And while the media trumpets a widespread public belief that everyone has the right to the American dream, there is also attention to the public's reluctance to share that dream with the "less deserving."

The Jesica Santillan case and its diverse elements created an overarching narrative that captured public attention and focused it, in an unusual and sustained way, on important issues in organ donation. It is unfortunate that this narrative also exposed a sometimes ugly attitude in various part of the nation about both organ donation and immigrants. Tragic as the story was, though, it did offer opportunities for constructive dialogue and forward-looking coverage about organ donation, medical ethics, and the allocation system. UNOS did successfully use the tragedy to change and improve the system of checks and balances. However, many other opportunities were missed. Whether this is the fault of the news media for focusing on the tragic and dramatic side of the story, or the fault of Duke hospital administrators (constrained as they might have been by issues of confidentiality and liability) for not being more proactive and forthcoming in their position, or the fault of others in the field of organ donation for not engaging more aggressively to dispel many of the myths or false assumptions that were presented, the fact remains that the most compelling media images portrayed were of incompetence and unfairness in the allocation process.

What, in the end, can we learn from the way in which the Santillan drama played out in these media accounts? According to Serge Moscovici, the writer Frank Kermode once stated, "A great narrative . . . is the fusion of the scandalous with the miraculous."[61] If that is the case, the story of Jesica Santillan is a perfect example of "a great narrative," and this fact may explain the intense media coverage. Few events could be portrayed as more miraculous than a heart transplant saving the life of the little girl, yet few events could have been more tragic or scandalous than her death and the charges that incompetence and corruption—in the very institutions that held her life in their hands—were responsible for her death. The real challenge that lies ahead is sorting through these media images to unpack and analyze them more thoroughly, and to dispel the intensely negative social representations of organ donation that are generated from frequently sensationalized media coverage.

NOTES

This study was supported by grant No. 1 H39 OT 000120–02 from the Health Resources and Services Administration's Division of Transplantation (HRSA/DoT), U.S. Department of Health and Human Services. The contents of this publication are solely the responsibility of the authors and do not necessarily represent the views of HRSA/DoT.

1. U. Flick, "Social Representations in Knowledge and Language as Approaches to the Psychology of the Social," in *The Psychology of the Social*, ed. U. Flick (Cambridge: Cambridge University Press, 1998); G. Gaskell, "Attitudes, Social Representations, and Beyond," in *Representations of the Social*, ed. K. Deaux and G. Philogene (Malden, Mass.: Blackwell Publishers, Inc., 2001); S. Moscovici and M. Hewstone, "Social Representations and Explanations," in *Attribution Theory: Social and Functional Extensions*, ed. M. Hewstone (Malden, Mass.: Basil Blackwell Publishers, 1983).

2. S. Moscovici, "The History and Actuality of Social Representations," in Flick ed., *Psychology of the Social.*

3. Data for this study comes from print and television coverage of the Jesica Santillan case. Data were obtained through subscription to ShadowTV and through daily monitoring of national coverage, as well as local print media for six different regions of the country. ShadowTV monitored ABC, NBC, CBS, FoxNews, CNN, MSNBC, CNBC, Bloomberg, C-Span, WCBS, and WNYW. Monitoring of print coverage included the *New York Times*, the *Washington Post*, Reuters, *USA Today*, *Newsweek*, the *Charlotte Observer* (North Carolina), the *Tuscaloosa News* (Alabama), the *Centre Daily Times* (Pennsylvania), the *Arizona Citizen* (Arizona), the *Battalion* (Texas), the *Star Ledger* (New Jersey), the *Daily Collegian* (Pennsylvania), the *Crimson White* (Alabama), the *Daily Targum* (New Jersey), the *Arizona Daily Wildcat* (Arizona), the *University Times* (North Carolina), the *Eagle* (Texas), as well as MSNBC.com, CNN.com, and CBSnews.com. These data, while not a complete list of all media coverage of Jesica Santillan, should provide a representative sample of the type of coverage presented. The selection of local media represents a counterbalanced sampling process that includes rural and urban local areas in the northeastern, southern, western, and southwestern geographic regions, in anticipation that media coverage in these areas may vary as a result of conservatism, religiosity, and diversity of each area's population.

Systematic thematic analyses of all actors in this case revealed themes for each actor that were consistent with coded categories, but as key events occurred, coverage shifted over time, revealing new frames that may trigger deep social representations. For instance, doctors may be framed as heroes and/or villains, common themes in organ donation stories. These shifts in framing were analyzed and linked to the timeline for the case and then cross-analyzed against broader categories such as immigration or ethical issues for organ donation as covered in all stories. This method provided not only systematic stories and representations of key actors but also wholistic pictures of key issues surrounding organ donation in relation to this specific case.

4. W. Wagner, V. Jose, and F. Elejabarrieta, "Relevance, Discourse and the Stable Core of Social Representations: A Structural Analysis of Word Associations," *Journal of Social Psychology* 35 (1996): 331–51; M. B. Brewer, "Social Identities and Social Representations: A Question of Priority?" in Deaux and Philogene, eds., *Representations of the Social*; W. Wagner and N. Kronberger, "Killer Tomatoes: Collective Symbolic Coping with Biotechnology," in Deaux and Philogene, eds., *Representations of the Social*; Flick, "Social Representations in Knowledge"; Gaskell, "Attitudes, Social Representations, and Beyond"; Moscovici and Hewstone, "Social Representations and Explanations"; M. Hewstone and M. Augoustinos, "Social Attributions and Social Representations," in Flick, ed., *Psychology of the Social*; D. Lupton, *Moral Threats and Dangerous Desires: AIDS in the News Media* (London: Taylor & Francis, 1994); T. A. van Dijk, "New(s) Racism: A Discourse Analytic Approach," in *Ethnic Minorities in the Media*, ed. S. Cottle (Philadelphia, Pa.: Open University Press, 2000); A. E. Eschabe and J. L. G. Castro, "Social Memory: Macropsychological Aspects," in Flick, ed., *Psychology of the Social*; C. M. Sommer, "Social Representations and Media Communications," in Flick, ed., *Psychology of the Social*; R. Matesanz, "Organ Donation, Transplantation, and Mass Media," *Transplantation Proceedings* 35 (2002): 987–89; S. Moscovici, "The History and Actuality of Social Representations," in Flick ed., *Psychology of the Social*; G. Maloney and I. Walker, "Talking about Transplants: Social Representations and the Dialectical, Dilemmatic Nature of Organ Donation and Transplantation," *British Journal of Social Psychology* 41 (2002): 299–320; D. A. Snow and C. Morrill, "Linking Ethnography and Theoretical Development: Systematizing the Analytic Process," Paper presented at the Midwestern Sociological Meetings, Chicago, 1993.

5. J. Potter and M. Wetherell, "Social Representations, Discourse Analysis, and Racism," in Flick, ed., *Psychology of the Social*. To be sure, there are many variations in media coverage. For example, so-called low-quality media (tabloid journalism) is associated with more negative attitudes toward the phenomenon. See Hewstone and Augoustinos, "Social Attributions and Social Representations," and Wagner and Kronberger, "Killer Tomatoes." Television images also can differ markedly from print media—and they also trace a rich variety that changes over time. See G. Maloney and I. Walker, "Messiahs, Pariahs, and Donors: The Development of Social Representations of Organ Transplants," *Journal for the Theory of Social Behavior* 30 (2000): 203–27; Maloney and Walker, "Talking about Transplants."

6. "Press Conference on Status of 17-Year-Old Jesica Santillan," CNN, February 20, 2003—08:13 ET, <http://edition.cnn.com/TRANSCRIPTS/0302/20/bn.06.html>; see also *American Morning*, Paula Zahn, CNN, February 20, 2003; "Teen's Family Grateful after 2nd Transplant," CNN, February 21, 2003, <http://www.cnn.com/2003/HEALTH/02/20/transplant.error/index.html> (accessed March 24, 2003); and Associated Press, "Adopted North Carolina Hometown Remembers Mexican Girl Who Died after Transplant Error," February 27, 2003, <http://www.msnbc.com/local/rtnc/adoptednojesi.asp> (accessed March 11, 2003).

7. Steve Campbell, "It's Time for Our Country to Change," *Arizona Daily Wildcat*, March 4, 2003, <http://wildcat.arizona.edu/papers/96/108/03—2.html> (accessed March 4, 2003.

8. Ibid.

9. "Teen's Family Grateful"; "Victim of Botched Transplant Declared Dead," CNN, February 22, 2003, <http://www.cnn.com/2003/HEALTH/02/22/transplant.error/index.html>. See also *Weekend House Call*, Heidi Collins, Elizabeth Cohen, and Lewis Teperman, CNN, February 22, 2003.

10. *CNN Live Today*, CNN, February 18, 2003.

11. "Teen's Family Grateful" ("doctor should go to jail"); Jessica Reaves, "Learning from a Tragic Transplant Mistake," *Time*, February 20, 2003 ("the organs that my daughter needs to live,"); "Hospital Seeks Clues to Transplant Error," AP News, February 19, 2003, <http://www.foxnews.com/story/0,2933,78851,00.html>. See also *MSNBC Live*, Donald Jones, MSNBC, February 19, 2003.

12. "Teen's Family Grateful."

13. Ibid.

14. Allen G. Breed, "Builder Battles Hospital for Jesica's Family," *Charlotte Observer*, February 22, 2003, 2A.

15. Scott Dodd, "Time Running Out for Sick Teen," *Charlotte Observer*, February 19, 2003, 1A.

16. *American Morning*, Paula Zahn, CNN, February 20 2003.

17. "Grim News for Jesica," CBS News Online, February 21, 2003, <http://www.cbsnews.com/stories/2003/02/22/health/main541588.shtml> ("if she dies, they [Duke] murdered her"; ". . . guess whose fault that gets to be?"). See also Jeffrey Gettleman and Lawrence Altman, "Girl in Transplant Mix-up Develops Brain Damage," *Tuscaloosa News*, February 21, 2003, 1A, 6A; CBS Broadcasting, "Anatomy of a Mistake," CBSnews.com, March 16, 2003, <http://www.cbsnews.com/stories/2003/03/16/60 minutes/printables544162.shtml> (accessed March 17, 2003).

18. "Teen's Family Grateful."

19. Randal Archibold, "Benefactor Championed an Immigrant Girl's Cause," *New York Times*, February 26, 2003, A3.

20. Karen Garloch and Peter St. Onge, "Jesica Loses Ill-Fated Fight," *Charlotte Observer*, February 23, 2003, 1A.

21. Jerry Adler, "A Tragic Error," *Newsweek*, March 3, 2003 ("displaced Texan"); Breed, "Builder Battles Hospital" ("a raspy Texas accent . . .").

22. Allen Breed, "Builder Battles Hospital for Jesica's Family," *Charlotte Observer*, February 22, 2003, 2A.

23. Editorial, "Best and the Worst for Jesica," *Rocky Mountain News* (Denver), February 25, 2003, 27A.

24. Lawrence Altman, "Even the Elite Hospitals Aren't Immune to Errors," *New York Times*, February 23, 2003, Section 1, 18.

25. "Teen's Family Grateful."

26. *CBS News*, Mark Strassman, CBS, WCBS, New York, February 24, 2003.

27. *Lester Holt Live*, Lester Holt, MSNBC, February 19, 2003.

28. "Autopsy Follows Transplant Mix-up," CNN.com, February 25, 2003, <http://www.cnn.com/2003/HEALTH/02/24/transplant.error/index.html> ("scarce resources"); *CBS Morning News*, CBS, WCBS, New York, February 21, 2003 ("fix their mistake").

29. Adler, "Tragic Error," 20.

30. Denise Grady, "Hope Only Glimmers for Transplant Victim," *New York Times*, February 20, 2003, A4.

31. Ellen Goodman, "The Banality of Screw-up," *Washington Post*, March 1, 2003, A19.

32. *CBS News*, Elizabeth Kaledin, WCBS, CBS, New York, February 20, 2003.

33. *MSNBC Live*, MSNBC, February 23, 2003.

34. Ibid.

35. Abbie Byrom, "Duke Doctor Should Resign His Position," *Technician*, February 24, 2003, <http://www.technicianonline.com/story.php?id=006934>.

36. "Editorial: Medical Checks and Balances," *Washington Post*, February 26, 2003, A22.

37. "Girl Tops Transplant List after Error," CNN.com, February 19, 2003, <http://www.cnn.com/2003/HEALTH/02/18/transplant.error/index.html>.

38. *MSNBC Live*, MSNBC, February 20, 2003.

39. Ashleigh Banfield, CNBC, February 20, 2003.

40. Randal Archibold, "Girl in Transplant Mix-up Dies after Two Weeks," *New York Times*, February 23, 2003, 18.

41. Sheryl Gay Stolberg and Lawrence K. Altman, "An Ethical Dilemma with Few Precedents," *New York Times*, February 21, 2003, A23.

42. *MSNBC Live*, MSNBC, February 20, 2003. See also Unmesh Kehr with Paul Cuadros, "A Miracle Denied: A Teenager's Death after Two Sets of Transplants Raises Questions of Procedures and Ethics," *Time*, March 3, 2003.

43. Adler, "Tragic Error," 20.

44. Jane Eisner, "More Donors Would Ease Organ Choices," *Charlotte Observer*, March 1, 2003, 19A ("never really got the first transplant"); *MSNBC Live*, MSNBC, February 23, 2003 ("longest odds makes sense").

45. Jeffrey Gettleman and Lawrence K. Altman, "Girl in Transplant Mix-up Undergoes Second Transplant," *New York Times*, February 20, 2003, A1.

46. Stolberg and Altman, "Ethical Dilemma," A23.

47. Associated Press, "Girl's Death Spurs New Transplant Rules," *New York Times*, June 29, 2003, <http://www.nytimes.com/aponline/national/AP-Transplant-Error.html?pagewanted=print&position=top> (accessed June 30, 2003).

48. Ibid.; M. O'Connor, "Transplant Scandal Hits Three Hospitals," *Chicago Tribune*, June 29, 2003, A1, A20; T. F. Murphy, "Gaming the Transplant System," *American Journal of Bioethics* 4 (1) (2004): W28; "Study Shows 'Gaming' in Heart Transplant System" *Science Daily Online*, March 9, 2004, <http://www.sciencedaily.com/releases/2004/03/040309072201.htm>.

49. Jeffrey Gettleman and Lawrence K. Altman, "Grave Diagnosis after Second Transplant," *New York Times*, February 22, 2003, A1.

50. "Report Claims Duke Violated Transplant Laws," WRAL-TV, Raleigh North Carolina, March 5, 2003, <http://www.wral.com/news/2018036/detail.html>.

51. Ibid.

52. Gettleman and Altman, "Grave Diagnosis," A1.

53. Emery Dalesio, "Hospital Seeks Clues to Transplant Error," *Washington Post*, 19 February 2003, <http://www.washingtonpost.com/wp-dyn/articles/A29838-2003Feb19.html> (accessed February 24, 2003); "New Hope after a Transplant Mix-up," MSNBC, February 19, 2003, <http://msnbc.msn.com/news/874197.asp?ocv=cb10>.

54. Gettleman and Altman, "Girl in Transplant Mix-up Undergoes Second Transplant," A1.

55. Adler, "Tragic Error."

56. Campbell, "It's Time for Our Country to Change."

57. Eisner, "More Donors," 19A.

58. Adler, "Tragic Error."

59. Associated Press, "Teen's Organs Too Damaged to Donate," February 25, 2003, <http://www.msnbc.com/news/874197.asp> (accessed February 26, 2003); "Autopsy Follows Transplant Mix-up"; "Services Set for Teen in Transplant Mix-up," CNN.com, February 25, 2003, <http://www.cnn.com/2003/HEALTH/02/25/transplant.error/index.html>.

60. Mahoney quoted and paraphrased in Emery P. Dalesio, "Public Anger Adds to Jesica Tragedy," *The Advertiser*, February 26, 2003, 32.

61. Moscovici, "History and Actuality of Social Representations," 247.

HOBSON'S CHOICES

MATCHING AND MISMATCHING IN

TRANSPLANTATION WORK PROCESSES

RICHARD I. COOK

The February 7, 2003, event at the Duke University Medical Center in North Carolina made clear the potential for donor-recipient mismatch during organ transplantation. This "celebrated case" changed the public perception of risk and hazard in health care. Like other celebrated cases, it played into a wide range of stakeholder concerns that includes U.S. immigration policies, tort reform, and the intrinsic fallibility of human performance. Like other celebrated cases, the "Duke event" was attributed to "human error" by a practitioner working at the "sharp end" of the system, in this case the pediatric cardiac surgeon. This attribution stands mainly because so little is known about the details of the event.[1] As with other celebrated events, in camera internal inquiries were undertaken but the data obtained are not available for review and what is known about the sequence and circumstances of this event comes mainly from the press coverage, much of it repetitive. As with other celebrated medical accidents, the absence of a detailed account based on an independent investigation is a critical limitation. We are left without a reliable assessment of the genesis and evolution of the event.

Rather than being simple occurrences arising from human error, medical accidents are complex systems failures. They result from the combination of multiple flaws, each individually insufficient to create an accident. All complex systems necessarily operate with such flaws in place. Each flaw is individually innocuous; only together are they able to produce the conditions needed for catastrophe. After accidents, the potential for these flaws to contribute to failure seems to be obvious, so much so that we conclude that practitioner error was "the cause" of the accident. The flaws seem obvious, however, because of the reviewers' hindsight bias.[2] The attribution of the accident to "human error" comes from the linking together of complex systems failure and hindsight bias during postaccident review.

A side effect of the impoverished account is that the accident functions as a kind of Rorschach test stimulus. The description of the event is provocatively ambiguous. The paucity of data makes interpretation a rich endeavor, one filled with possibility. Its gravity encourages stakeholders to search the event for specific meaning, but its ambiguity allows meaning to be layered upon it. Health care accidents are particularly suited to this imbrication of meaning. Because the stakeholders are sophisticates, their interpretations are fashioned quickly and elegantly, often within hours of announcement of the event. Because they are stakeholders attuned to particular interests, each interpretation is honed to bring out that interest. These are features that would attach to almost any similarly ambiguous event. The near-universal personal experience with health care, however, provides an opportunity for these interpretations to resonate with many people. This potential for resonance shapes the explanations and interpretations. Significantly, researchers and experts are no less susceptible to these influences; their biases and interests are as engaged as those of other stakeholder groups.

These "first stories" of celebrated cases make the events seem easily preventable, and, consequently, the human performances that preceded the event are judged as poor.[3] The dramatic quality of the event amplifies hindsight bias, which, in turn, makes it seem that the outcome could have been avoided and produces a series of "if only" inferences. If only the people involved had recognized the significance of some piece of data! If only they had been "more careful" in carrying out a potentially hazardous activity. The apparently flawed performances are treated as cases of "human error." This conclusion provokes efforts to rein in human capriciousness, most often through the application of rules, policies, or the interposition of mechanical obstacles.

The first stories we tell about accidents are deeply flawed and misleading. They are at odds with the results of scientific investigations of accidents occurring in complex systems. These investigations reveal complex but ultimately more useful "second stories" of complex systems failure. The second story of accidents involves multiple vulnerabilities, irreducible uncertainty, and practitioner adaptation and coping strategies. It addresses the ways that new technology, changing organizations, and procedures combine with economic pressure to create new paths to failure at the same time they create new paths to success.

We are engaged in a project to outline a second story for donor-recipient mismatches in solid organ transplantation.[4] This story is about the way that the variety of factors surrounding organ transplantation play out in the conduct of patient care. Although superficially routine, organ transplantation is exotic and fabulously complicated. It requires coordination and interaction across usually impervious organizational boundaries. It encompasses details from multiple disciplines and the coherent participation of many individuals who interact rarely and mostly under extreme time and consequence pressures. It inevitably engages vulnerable populations and inevitably does them calibrated harm in the hope of doing them calibrated good. The Duke event was not the first mismatch instance, and it will not, in all likelihood, be the last. Indeed, thoughtful examination of the vulnerabilities and capacities of the transplant system may lead us to conclude that the Duke event was not so much a spectacular failure as a nominal case in a working situation that is inherently and irreducibly fraught.

The rest of this essay provides a sketch of the solid organ transplantation process relevant to understanding the second story of the Duke event. The goal here is to ground our discussion of the Duke event in a socio-technical context or, at least, to characterize that context in a way that does not do violence to either the social or the technical. We need an expanded notion of technical because the technical context here is not so much a medical context as a technical work context.[5] Although much of the discussion of the Duke event involves details of immunology and heart disease, the technical substance of that event is not found in immunology or disease. Instead, the technical context for discussion of the Duke event and other such problems in transplant is the work process that bridges the space between medical science and a variegated set of goals, requirements, and forces that encompass the care of sick people, the use of scarce resources, and the critical need for equity in health care. The thesis of this essay is that Duke-like events arise from the predictable and unavoidable consequences of managing the tensions that accompany the shortage of organs for transplant.[6]

LIFESAVING ORGAN TRANSPLANTATION[7]

The transplantation of human organs represents a significant intellectual and organizational accomplishment. The complexity and hazards associated with each element of the process are substantial such that no individual would willingly take them on as either practitioner or patient. Yet the illnesses for which transplantation is undertaken are relentless and terrible. Indeed, transplantation is offered only to those patients whose current condition is precarious and whose future is known to be more terrible than the hazards of transplantation. Even when a transplant is initially successful in narrow medical terms, the long-term outcome for transplant recipients is not the same as for otherwise healthy people of the same age. Instead, the transplant recipient is committed to a lifetime of intrusive medical interventions and a future filled with new hazards. Post-implantation immunosuppression takes its toll on the patient, clearing the pathway for exotic infections and cancer, and these changes in the patient's lot are more of a burden than any healthy person would willingly undertake. And the transplanted organs themselves fail, sometimes within months of implantation. The eagerness of patients with end-stage kidney disease or heart failure to undergo transplant is as much testimony to the horrors of those illnesses as to the wonders of transplantation.

Transplantation experts distinguish between solid-organ transplants that are *life-enhancing* and those that are *lifesaving*. Life-enhancing transplants relieve the patient of some portion of the burden of their illness, slowing the deterioration of other organs and making the quality of life better. Patients with kidney and pancreas failure can have prolonged life span because there are effective therapies (dialysis and insulin) for the conditions. In contrast, there are few treatment options for end-stage heart, liver, or lung disease. Transplant of these organs is lifesaving because failure of these organs leads to death (table 1).

The Duke event patient's restrictive cardiomyopathy, for example, was a nonsurvivable condition, and the patient was already beyond the expected life span for that condition. The Duke patient had already developed elevated pulmonary vascular resistance, a condition found in the later stages of childhood onset restrictive cardiomyopathy.

The normal heart comprises two linked pumps, a right heart that pumps blood from the body to the lungs and a left heart that pumps blood from lungs to the body. In health, the right-sided circulation is a low-pressure/low-resistance circuit while the left-sided circulation is a high-pressure/high-resistance circuit. The right heart is normally less muscular and less powerful than the left, although both pump the same amount of blood per cardiac cycle. Slow increase in the pulmonary vascular resistance causes the right heart to become disproportionately muscular. Increasing pulmonary vascular resistance is an ominous sign, and early transplantation is advocated before the resistance becomes so high that a transplanted heart will fail. In patients who have already developed high, fixed pulmonary resistance, simultaneous heart and lung transplant—but not heart transplant alone—is lifesaving. In contrast with heart transplant, the outcome of lung and combined heart-lung transplantation is poor. The lung is more complex and delicate than the heart, and this plays out both on the donor and on the recipient sides of transplant.

Table 1. U.S. Transplants as a Percentage of Lifesaving Organs

	Lifesaving Organs	Liver	Heart	Lung	Heart-Lung
Total 2003	8,856	5,670	2,057	1,100	29
	100%	64%	23%	12%	1%

Source: OPTN National Data Reports, <www.optn.org> (accessed June 1, 2004).

The immediate and long-term success of organ transplantation varies across the organ types, disease types, regions, centers, and individual surgical teams. Two types of success measures are used: graft survival and patient survival. For lifesaving organs, patient survival and graft survival are similar. For nonlifesaving organs, graft survival is often considerably shorter. Long-term outcome statistics are difficult to use. The understanding of transplant immunology is changing so quickly that historical comparisons tend to measure the growth of knowledge and sophistication. More important, the transplantation process involves many people and processes so that reliable attribution to individual factors is difficult. Nevertheless, the immediate and five-year survival rate for adult heart transplant recipients (greater than 70 percent) is remarkable compared with that for heart-lung (less than 40 percent).

There is a more or less constant mismatch between the supply of lifesaving and life-enhancing organs and the number of potential recipients (table 2). Many people who would benefit from a transplant will not get one. Overall, only about a third of patients who meet the criteria for receiving solid-organ transplant will be transplanted each year. The majority of candidates awaiting transplant need kidneys (68 percent of the total waiting patients). Discussions of solid-organ transplantation tend to separate kidneys from other "extra renal" organs. Thoracic organs (heart and lungs) and abdominal organs (liver, pancreas, kidney, and intestine) are often distinguished from one another, in part because the associated physicians and surgeons come from different disciplines and training pathways.

In the United States there are eleven transplant regions and fifty-nine organ-procurement organizations that coordinate the donation and placement of organs from deceased donors using the United Network for Organ Sharing (UNOS; <www.unos.org>) as a central arbiter for matching. At present there are 258 certified transplant centers in the United States. Living-related organ donation is ex post facto reported to UNOS, but the process is managed at the transplant center level. Not all centers perform all types of transplant, as shown in table 3.

Table 2. U.S. Transplants Performed versus Recipient Candidates, by Organ, in 2003

	All Organs*	Kidney	Liver	Pancreas	Kidney-Pancreas	Heart	Lung	Heart-Lung	Intestine
Deceased donor	18,652	8,665	5,350	502	867	2,057	1,085	29	112
Living donor	6,807	6,464	320	0	4	0	15	0	4
Total 2003	25,459	15,129	5,670	502	871	2,057	1,100	29	116
Recipient candidates as of May 27, 2004	85,260	58,334	17,478	1,602	2,450	3,512	3,912	194	188
Expected to receive transplant in 2004	30%	26%	32%	31%	36%	59%	28%	15%	62%

Source: From combined OPTN National Data Reports, <www.optn.org> (accessed June 1, 2004).

*All organs not equal to sum of other columns because some patients received multiple transplants.

Table 3. U.S. Transplant Centers by Type of Organ

Organ type	Programs	Organs*
Heart-Lung	61	29
Heart	134	2,057
Lung	69	1,085
Liver	122	5,350
Intestine	46	112
Kidney	248	8,665
Pancreas	140	502
Total	820	

Source: UNOS Web site (<www.unos.org>).

*Organs from deceased donors transplanted in 2003; combined kidney-pancreas transplants not shown.

Matching donor to recipient is a social process that is constrained by technical factors, most notably the compatibility between the donor and recipient. Various technical factors determine compatibility. The size of the recipient versus the donor, for example, is particularly important for intrathoracic organs; an adult heart cannot be implanted into a newborn.

The most complex compatibility issues are those related to the immune system compatibility, technically known as histocompatibility.[8] The immune system is responsible for distinguishing foreign biological molecules from the self. It is this ability that allows the immunocompetent individual to fight off infection by bacteria and viruses. A primary goal in transplantation is to implant immunocompatible organs. Most transplanted organs are immunologically incompatible to some degree, and transplant recipients generally require immunosuppression with drugs (for example, steroids) to prevent rejection of the organ.

The prototypical immunocompatibility issue is ABO (blood) type. In general, donated organs need to be type compatible with the recipients. Blood cells created in the bone marrow may have two different antigens, one inherited from each parent. Three antigen expressions are possible: either A or B or none (O). A person whose blood cells express only A antigens is type A, one whose cells express only B antigens is type B, and one with both A and B antigens is type AB. A person without either antigen is type O.

The presence of a particular antigen on the blood cells generates tolerance in the individual for that antigen; the immune system in that person will not produce antibodies against that antigen. An AB person expresses A and B antigens on cell surfaces and, therefore, will be tolerant of foreign blood cells with either the A or B antigens or cells with both antigens. Such an AB blood type person is, with respect to the ABO system, a universal recipient and can accept blood or tissue from a donor of type O, type A, type B, or type AB. Similarly, a type A blood recipient may receive blood from a type A or type O donor while a type B recipient can accept blood from a type B or type O donor. A type O individual is, therefore, a universal donor. The distribution of antigens varies with race and region (tables 4 and 5).

The immune system is primed to recognize foreign antigens. Introducing a tissue (for example, blood) that expresses these antigens will provoke an immune response. The strength of this response can be quite startling, as anyone with an allergy to bee stings will attest. Transfusion of incompatible (that is, foreign antigen coated) blood is potentially life threatening. The

Table 4. ABO Compatibility

Donor "Type"	A	B	AB	O
U.S. white	40%	11%	4%	45%
U.S. blacks	27%	20%	4%	49%
Peruvian Indian	—	—	—	100%
Cells express antigens	A	B	A & B	None
Can donate to:				
A	Yes	No	No	Yes
B	No	Yes	No	Yes
AB	Yes	Yes	Yes	Yes
O	No	No	No	Yes
Has antibodies to:				
A	No	Yes	No	Yes
B	Yes	No	No	Yes

Note: Percentages are rough estimates of the frequency of these types; native Peruvian Indians shown for comparison.

resulting immune reaction can include a generalized allergic response, as well as a specific attack on the (detectably) foreign blood cells. Transplantation of an incompatible organ will provoke a similar immune system reaction that results in rejection of the organ and associated damage.

The ABO system is the best-known and most widely appreciated source of incompatibility between individuals. There are, however, numerous other types of antigens that may be expressed by blood cells. Some of these are so common that they have their own names (for example, "Christmas," "Kell"), and routine ABO typing is accompanied by a second test (the "screen" of "type and screen") to determine if common antibodies are present. The screening process does not guarantee compatibility but rather helps to narrow the search for a compatible unit of blood. The ultimate determination of compatibility in blood transfusion is the "crossmatch." In this test, donor blood is mixed with patient serum under specific conditions. If the potential recipient serum contains preformed antibodies to antigens on the blood cell surface, visible clumps of blood cells form, signaling incompatibility. Conversely, if the blood does not clump, the cells are compatible with the potential recipient's serum because either there are no antigens on the surface of the blood cells or the serum does not contain antibodies to the antigens present.

In some cases, the deterioration of incompatible organs is known to be

Table 5. Distribution of Blood Type O, A, B, and AB across Populations

People	O	A	B	AB
Aborigines	61	39	0	0
Abyssinians	43	27	25	5
Ainu (Japan)	17	32	32	18
Albanians	28	43	13	6
Grand Andamanese	9	60	23	9
Arabs	34	31	29	6
Armenians	31	50	13	6
Asian (in U.S.—general)	40	28	27	5
Austrians	36	44	13	6
Bantus	46	30	19	5
Basques	51	44	4	1
Belgians	47	42	8	3
Blackfoot (N. Am. Indian)	17	82	0	1
Bororo	100	0	0	0
Brazilians	47	41	9	3
Bulgarians	32	44	15	8
Burmese	36	24	33	7
Buryats	33	21	38	8
Bushmen	56	34	9	2
Chinese-Canton	46	23	25	6
Chinese-Peking	29	27	32	13
Chuvash	30	29	33	7
Czechs	30	44	18	9
Danes	41	44	11	4
Dutch	45	43	9	3
Egyptians	33	36	24	8
English	47	42	9	3
Eskimos (Alaska)	38	44	13	5
Eskimos (Greenland)	54	36	23	8
Estonians	34	36	23	8
Fijians	44	34	17	6
Finns	34	41	18	7
French	43	47	7	3
Georgians	46	37	12	4
Germans	41	43	11	5
Greeks	40	42	14	5
Gypsies (Hungary)	29	27	35	10
Hawaiians	37	61	2	1

Table 5. *Continued*

People	O	A	B	AB
Hindus (Bombay)	32	29	28	11
Hungarians	36	43	16	5
Icelanders	56	32	10	3
Indians (India—general)	37	22	33	7
Indians (U.S.—general)	79	16	4	1
Irish	52	35	10	3
Italians (Milan)	46	41	11	3
Japanese	30	38	22	10
Jews (Germany)	42	41	12	5
Jews (Poland)	33	41	18	8
Kalmuks	26	23	41	11
Kikuyu (Kenya)	60	19	20	1
Koreans	28	32	31	10
Lapps	29	63	4	4
Latvians	32	37	24	7
Lithuanians	40	34	20	6
Malasians	62	18	20	0
Maoris	46	54	1	0
Mayas	98	1	1	1
Moros	64	16	20	0
Navajo (N. Am. Indian)	73	27	0	0
Nicobarese (Nicobars)	74	9	15	1
Norwegians	39	50	8	4
Papuas (New Guinea)	41	27	23	9
Persians	38	33	22	7
Peru (Indians)	100	0	0	0
Philippinos	45	22	27	6
Poles	33	39	20	9
Portuguese	35	53	8	4
Rumanians	34	41	19	6
Russians	33	36	23	8
Sardinians	50	26	19	5
Scotts	51	34	12	3
Serbians	38	42	16	5
Shompen (Nicobars)	100	0	0	0
Slovaks	42	37	16	5
South Africans	45	40	11	4
Spanish	38	47	10	5

Table 5. *Continued*

People	O	A	B	AB
Sudanese	62	16	21	0
Swedes	38	47	10	5
Swiss	40	50	7	3
Tartars	28	30	29	13
Thais	37	22	33	8
Turks	43	34	18	6
Ukranians	37	40	18	6
United Kingdom (GB)	47	42	8	3
U.S. (blacks)	49	27	20	4

Source: L. Beckman, *A Contribution to the Physical Anthropology and Population Genetics of Sweden*, 1959, as revised by BloodBook.com 5/22/2004.

slow enough to permit deliberate implantation of an ABO incompatible organ under certain circumstances. ABO-incompatible liver transplantation has been done, for example, to forestall immediate death while awaiting a compatible organ. In one case of an unplanned ABO-incompatible heart transplant that occurred years before the Duke event, the patient was relisted for transplant and successfully retransplanted a few days later.

Determining compatibility between a potential donor and potential recipient requires ABO blood typing as well as tissue typing for some tissues, most notably for kidneys. Some of this work can be done well in advance; potential recipients are sampled and evaluated when they are entered onto the transplant list and at intervals as they wait for the organ-sharing process to address their need. But much of this work must take place under time pressure. Potential dead donors are seldom identified more than a day before the organs are removed, most often at a site remote from the recipient's. The flurry of activity needed to identify potential recipients and to assign the organ to a single patient takes place under an uncertain but inevitable deadline. The likelihood of technically successful organ procurement deteriorates inexorably with time.

The significance of compatibility is its technical complexity and the need to bring together and act on highly technical information under the conditions of time pressure, uncertainty, and high stakes.

The dominant feature of the organ transplantation system is the continuing mismatch between the number of potential recipients and the number of usable organs. Since the advent of practicable immunosuppression, there have been many more patients for whom the rigors of transplantation and the subsequent lifetime of medical interventions have been less daunting than the prospect of living with—or dying from—their disease. Human organs are the best means for dealing with the diseases for which transplant is undertaken and the most precious resource in the transplantation system. There is no practical substitute for human organs, and organs cannot be stored for later use but must be consumed by implantation within hours of procurement. Although many people die each year, medical progress has lengthened life span and promoted survival with concurrent illness so that only a few of those who die are potential organ donors. Motor vehicle accidents are an important source of donor organs, but mortality from motor accidents has been falling over the past two decades. The result is that, at every moment, the available supply of organs is smaller than the demand for them.

This disparity between supply and demand has shaped the entire transplantation system. From the number of transplant surgeons trained each year to the boundaries for regional organ sharing, every component is influenced by the number of organs available, and the great need of the potential recipients as a group translates into a great need to make sure that every usable donated organ is used. The need to cope with the technical and social consequences of this mismatch is constant and unremitting. The irreducible disparity between supply and demand fuels the strong social tensions around transplantation. The formal rules and administrative bodies that control the organ supply are responses to these tensions. The rules and procedures of the transplantation system are intended to distribute the imbalance between supply and demand fairly. These rules and procedures are the result of deliberate and thoughtful adaptations that have been made at intervals over the past four decades. The solution to this social problem is encoded, expressed, and discussed almost entirely in technical terms.

In contrast with the narrow technical notion of compatibility, matching donor organs with potential recipients is a socio-technical process. Compatibility is a necessary but not sufficient condition to matching organ donor and recipient. Matching also involves the pragmatics of procurement and implantation and a carefully constructed notion of what constitutes a socially

Figure 1. Utility vs. Justice in Organ Allocation

Utility	Justice
• Number of recipients	• Medical urgency
• Patient survival	• Time waiting
• Graft survival	• Medically disadvantaged
• Quality of life	• Geographic access
• Cost to benefit ratio	• Equitable access

Source: OPTN/UNOS NATCO Presentation, June 2003.

equitable process of organ allocation. Patient factors are prominent in determining equity, but it is clear that it includes the impact of allocation on donation decision makers, the consequent regional distribution of organs, the different organ procurement organizations, the transplantation centers within the system, and even individual surgeons.

The tensions that make equity a broadly contended issue are not usually visible to outsiders. There is competition—sometimes intense—across transplant centers and between surgeons. A center that implants more organs generates more income for its hospital. The higher volume adds luster to the surgeons' careers and makes them ever more sought after by other centers and creates opportunities to attract new research money. Organ procurement organizations, the corporate intermediaries between donors and recipients, benefit from increased volume of work. Thus, there are important economies of scale and political power within the transplant system.

Equity is also important to sustain the flow of donated organs into the system. Organ donation is voluntary, and donor families, who control access to the potential donor's organs, are financially uncompensated. At the time of donation, the donor family does not know which patients will receive the organs. Instead, the donation is made to the transplantation system. The appearance of equity in this system is an important incentive to donate one's own organs and also for one's family to confirm (as they must do) that donation when the moment comes.

The irreducible tension produced by the shortage of suitable organs shapes the process of matching like a magnetic field aligns iron filings. Deconstructing the matching rules and processes, in turn, provides a fine-grain map of that tension, for example in the allocation rules for thoracic organs (UNOS policy 3.7; figure 2). These rules address the disparities in frequency of different blood types by "spreading" blood group O organs

Figure 2. UNOS Policies Regarding Organ Allocation

3.7.8 *ABO Typing for Heart Allocation.* Within each heart status category, hearts will be allocated to patients according to the following ABO matching requirements:

(i) Blood type O donor hearts shall only be allocated to blood type O or blood type B patients;

(ii) Blood type A donor hearts shall only be allocated to blood type A or blood type AB patients;

(iii) Blood type B donor hearts shall only be allocated to blood type B or blood type AB patients;

(iv) Blood type AB donor hearts shall only be allocated to blood type AB patients.

(v) If there is no patient available who meets these matching requirements, donor hearts shall be allocated first to patients who have a blood type that is compatible with the donor's blood type.

Source: UNOS policies, <www.unos.org> (accessed June 9, 2004).

(universal donor) over type O recipients and blood group B recipients. There are few B organs available, so a strict one-to-one matching of organs by ABO group would tend to disadvantage blood group B recipients. For example, of the 2,121 hearts made available for donation in 2003, 213 (10 percent) were blood group B, but of the 2,057 recipients, 288 were group B. But note that the rules are not a statement of compatibility but of matching criteria. An O organ could be placed in any recipient, but this advantage of O organ donation is reserved for type O patients (who can receive only O organs) and blood type B recipients. By encoding this rule as a policy and incorporating the rule into the match-list-generation program, the process becomes, in an operational sense, equitable. But African Americans are more likely to be group B and it could be argued that this provides a differential advantage for African-American potential recipients (see table 4). Indeed, arguments based on statistical analyses are part of ongoing debates about race and equity in the United States.

Equity in the transplant system is embodied by rules and procedures to match the notions of equity that are present in the greater population on which the system depends. Inversely, the rules and processes encoded within the system in order to create equity map the understanding of what equity is in the various populations involved with transplant.[9]

The core feature of the matching process is the decoupling of the activities related to recipients from those related to the donor and donation. It is this decoupling that allows the management of the competition for the organs.

The structure of this process is intended to keep these intimately connected parts of the transplant process completely separate until a match is declared. To keep donation and recipient designation at arms length from each other, the management of that tension is turned over to a trustworthy intermediary that acts in a dispassionate, consistent fashion. The acts of the intermediary cannot be questioned because, although the rules that govern its behavior are public, the data on which it operates is private. Its behavior is oracular: it answers specific questions that are put to it, but the rationale for its decision is not provided.

Typically, the process for a deceased-donor heart donation happens this way:[10]

- Each transplant center has its own collection of registered potential recipients, enrolled through that center and committed to undergoing the implant operation in that center's facilities by that center's surgeons. Transplant centers "list" a potential recipient by entering that patient's data into a secure national computer database. To enter the list, patients must meet specific criteria and agree to receive organs in transplant. The computer database is structured so that a center can review only data on its own patients. Once listed, both patient and center wait for a contact from the organ procurement organization.

- When a donation becomes imminent, the hospital contacts the organ procurement organization (opo) and an opo transplant coordinator comes to the hospital and speaks with the donor family or guardians and obtains permission for the procurement of organs. Information about the donor is sent back to the opo, where data about the donor is entered into the national organ transplantation database and a match list is run. The criteria by which the match list is generated include compatibility, "objective" social features (for example, wait time), and medical factors (for example, the Model for End-Stage Liver Disease [MELD] score). The match list contains a rank-order list of potential recipients and associated transplant facilities for each organ. The list is sent to the opo coordinator at the donor hospital.

- *In rank order*, the opo coordinator contacts each local coordinator for the corresponding transplant facility and offers the organ. The facility coordinator has a limited time to respond to the offer.[11] If the offer is accepted, the organ is considered *placed* and the recovery and implantation process begins. In most cases, multiple organs are procured from the same donor and these organs may be placed at as many as six centers.[12]

- The transplant recovery surgery team travels to the donor's hospital, reviews the documentation, and begins the recovery. Typically, the recovery involves two surgical teams, one for the heart and lungs and another for the abdominal organs. Because the organ recovery requires an operating room, scrub and circulating nurses, and anesthesiologist, the timing of procurement may be delayed, sometimes until the evening after that hospital's regularly scheduled cases have been completed.
- The donor is brought to the operating room and the organs exposed and examined to make certain that they are suitable for implantation. After administration of appropriate drugs for organ preservation, the heart is stopped with an electrolyte solution and the organs are removed and preserved with cold solutions intended to put the cells into a hibernation state. The teams depart the hospital immediately and proceed to their own centers to begin implantation.
- While the recovery is going on, each transplant center arranges for its targeted recipients to come to the operating rooms for implantation. Typically, the recovery team communicates with the home operating room team to indicate that they have the organs and are returning. In the case of heart transplant, the short time that the heart remains viable while in preservation usually requires that the recipient be brought to the operating room, anesthetized, and put on cardiopulmonary bypass while the recovery team is in transit.[13]
- On arrival, the recovered heart is prepared and grafted into the recipient. As the heart begins beating again, cardiopulmonary bypass is terminated and the patient's chest closed and the patient returned to the intensive care unit. The entire process from entry of the donor into the database to chest closure of the recipient typically takes twelve to twenty-four hours.

The top-ranked potential recipient on the match list does not always end up being matched to the organ. Recipient conditions are constantly changing so that a recipient may not be a good candidate for the offered organ, but there are other factors, including some that are subtle and difficult to assess. Organs vary significantly in quality, and transplant surgeons may decline to use an offered organ for a potential recipient. A center's team, for example, may be already engaged in implanting an organ for a different recipient and not be able to perform two procedures simultaneously. Local factors such as weather in the donor or recipient hospital's region may make travel difficult or uncertain. If the first potential recipient is not matched to the offered organ, the OPO coordinator proceeds down the list, calling the different transplant center coordinators in the order in which the potential recipients appear on the match list. It is not uncommon for a single center to have more than one patient on the match list and the coordinator can identify lower ranked potential recipients at the time of the first call. Especially for less desirable organs (for example, those from older patients or from patients with coexisting diseases that may impair organ function), placing the organs may be difficult and the OPO coordinator may spend a large amount of time running through the match list without placing the organs.

The failure to produce a match has two consequences. First, it consumes valuable time during which the donor condition continues to deteriorate. Donor patients are seldom physiologically stable after death, and management of the donor tends to become more difficult and to involve interventions that may reduce the quality of the organs being donated. Second, it reduces the prospects for a "good" match because the first few potential recipients are the "best" candidates. Although every patient on the list meets the formal compatibility rules, the match-list order reflects equity and the quality of the match is reduced as one goes "down" the list.

It sometimes happens that early offers fail to produce a match even as the pressure to do so increases. This increasing pressure to produce a match may lead the OPO coordinator to shift from proceeding through the rank-order list to an "open offer."

In an "open offer" the organ is offered not to a specific *patient* but to a specific *transplant center* for use in any patient registered in that center. The open offer allows the transplant center coordinator and surgeons to select the recipient from the center's own list of patients. The particular advantage of an "open offer" is that the donated organs can be placed efficiently and the time to organ recovery can be shortened. The "open offer" is an escape mechanism from the tightly controlled transplant matching process.

The function of the match-list-generating program is to generate a rank-order list of potential recipients. By proceeding through the match list in rank order, the OPO coordinator is assured of equity in the placement of the organ. There is some risk, however, that proceeding through the match list in rank order will take so much time that the donor condition will have deteriorated to the point that the organs are unusable and the opportunity to transplant the donor's organs will be lost. Donated organs are something of a "use it or lose it" proposition. The result is that organ viability pragmatics trump equity. The entire process takes place under time pressure and uncertainty, both of which increase as time passes.

The "open offer" reverses the direction of information flow within the system. When the OPO coordinator calls transplant centers using the match list, the offer is made for a specific patient whose name appears on that list. During an "open offer," the transplant center proposes a patient to the OPO coordinator rather than vice versa. Rather than using the match list as source document to guide the sequence of offers, the match list becomes a secondary document that may or may not contain the patient proposed by the transplant center.

Because the match list is produced by an oracle, it cannot help the OPO and transplant center coordinators understand why a patient does *not* appear on the list. When the coordinators move to an "open offer" they step outside the list-driven process and find themselves without much support. The oracular nature of the list creation is critical to managing the social tensions that arise because of the shortage of organs. When the list works as intended it gives the OPO coordinator assurance that the resulting match will be equitable because the formal rules that encode equity are used to create the list. But the same features that make the list work also make it harder for operators to "see" into the workings of the system when it becomes necessary to step away from the oracle's guidance in order to work out problems directly.

THE DUKE EVENT RECONSIDERED

The foregoing sets up a reconsideration of the Duke event. In particular, we want to understand whether, as some have proposed, the event represents a "blunder." Reconstruction of the Duke event, based on information from a variety of sources, indicates that the failure was not the result of "human error" in the sense that the term is conventionally used. Instead, the failure appears to be entirely in keeping with the complex systems failure model of accidents.[14] The accident occurred because a number of individually innocuous conditions combined to create the opportunity for the process of matching to lead not to a compatible match but to an incompatible one.

The recipient was type O and the donated organs type A.[15] Only a type O heart-lung would have been compatible with the recipient. The recipient blood type was, at the time of running the match list, correct in the database, and the recipient's name and number were not in the match list delivered to the OPO coordinator.

Based on multiple sources, we believe the sequence of the Duke event is as follows:

1. At the Boston Children's Hospital, a seven-year-old child's heart and lungs became available for donation when that child was declared dead. The donor was listed with UNOS, and the match list was run by the local OPO, the New England Organ Bank (NEOB).

2. The heart-lung combination was not suitable for local recipients, and a coordinator at the New England Organ Bank began, in accordance with the organ sharing rules, to search for other potential recipients outside the local area. The organs were compatible with two potential recipients ("[Pt A]," a child, and "[Pt B]," an adult) at Duke. These were the only patients who seemed to be realistic potential recipients given the conditions and geography involved.

3. Via a Carolina Donor Services (CDS) coordinator, an intermediary OPO, the NEOB coordinator contacted an adult cardiac transplant surgeon at Duke to offer the organ for [Pt A].

4. The surgeon referred the CDS coordinator to the pediatric cardiac transplant surgeon at Duke. The CDS coordinator called the pediatric transplant surgeon at home and offered the organs for [Pt A]. The surgeon told the coordinator that [Pt A] was too sick to be a candidate for the transplant but asked if the organs could be used for the ultimate recipient ([JS]), saying, "Could another child have the heart and lungs?" Pertinent information about the potential recipients was kept in a binder for the surgeon's immediate use, but the surgeon was at home and the binder was in the office. The CDS coordinator said he would check.

5. The CDS coordinator contacted the NEOB coordinator to ask whether the organs could be used for [JS]. The CDS coordinator was told that the patient was not on the match list in hand at the NEOB and was advised to contact UNOS directly to find out why.

6. The CDS coordinator called UNOS to check on the status of [JS] but misspelled [JS]'s name and gave the blood type as A. The UNOS operator could not find [JS] on the match list for the NEOB's organ donor. The UNOS operator discovered [JS]'s name on a different transplant recipient waiting list and confirmed that [JS] was listed as Status 2, that is, that she was listed in the computer system as a candidate. A discussion ensued about the reason that [JS] did not appear on the match list that the NEOB and UNOS had available, but the possibility of ABO incompatibility was not considered.

7. The CDS coordinator called another adult cardiac surgeon at Duke and offered the organs to him for [Pt B]. That surgeon declined the offer.

8. The CDS called the Duke pediatric surgeon and offered the organs to him for use in [JS]. He accepted the offer. The CDS coordinator called the NEOB coordinator and obtained a "release" of the organs for [JS].

9. The pediatric surgeon began the process of recovery of organs by contacting the local pediatric cardiac transplant coordinator, a nurse practitioner who was relatively inexperienced in that position. The local coordinator called [JS]'s family and had them come to the hospital.

10. The cardiac surgery fellow who would normally travel to the donor site to procure the organs was not available. The pediatric cardiac surgeon contacted another cardiac surgery fellow and instructed him to arrange procurement with Boston Children's Hospital.

11. The cardiac surgery fellow and the coordinator from CDS flew on a chartered aircraft to Boston, where they examined the donor and reviewed laboratory data relevant to the quality of the organs to be recovered. Telephone conversations took place between the fellow in Boston and the pediatric cardiac surgeon at Duke regarding the implications of these data for the use of these organs. The pediatric cardiac surgeon decided to accept the organs for transplant into [JS].

12. In Boston, the organs were procured by the fellow and placed in a cooler. The cooler was taken, along with a packet of information regarding the donor, by the fellow and coordinator to the airport for the chartered flight back to North Carolina. De-icing of the aircraft consumed forty-five minutes. The flight left for North Carolina.

13. [JS] was taken to the operating room, put on cardiopulmonary bypass, and her diseased heart and lungs were removed.

14. The donor organs arrived and were grafted into [JS]. The technical aspects of the procedure went smoothly despite the relatively long ischemic time. The heart began to beat and cardiopulmonary bypass was terminated. The chest was closed.

15. A laboratory technician elsewhere in the hospital was running routine tests on donor blood and noticed that there was a discrepancy between the donor and recipient blood types. The laboratory technician called the coordinator.

16. The surgeon, who was still in the operating room, was notified by the coordinator of the incompatibility.

The pediatric cardiac surgeon later acknowledged that the event was his responsibility. This announcement was greeted with approval from the media and clearly served the public relations needs of Duke at the moment. It does not, however, correspond well with our current understanding of the way that the event unfolded.

Instead, it is clear that the Duke event was a likely consequence of the necessary conjoining of the socio-technical features of the transplant system within an automated system structured to produce and defend equity in the allocation of organs. The system's design provides highly reliable *forward* transfers of information in ways that usually produce a compatible match between donor and recipient. In the Duke event, the system failed because it did not support, indeed was intended not to support, the type of exchanges that took place between the CDS, NEOB, and UNOS.

The transplant match process prevents recipient advocates from determining why their patients are not on the transplant match list. Access to the transplant match list is restricted to prevent one transplant center from learning about another center's patients. The opacity of the system is intended to decouple the process steps in ways that make the equity of the system easy to assess and to defend both in public and in private.

The need to short-circuit this carefully and elaborately constructed system comes not from a desire to undermine equity but from the need to make certain that organs do not go unused. The Duke event was not an "open offer" in the usual sense but something of a hybrid. The event was a series of quite reasonable queries and responses that were intended to make use of an irreplaceable resource, a dead child's organs. The practitioners were reaching into the system in order to create the conditions that might allow these organs to be used. There was no hesitancy here, and equity was not at issue. What mattered is that these organs should be placed and placed quickly.

The precise language used between CDS and UNOS is preserved on the tapes made of all the phone conversations with UNOS operators. We do not have access to the tapes, but the presentation of their contents on which our chronology is based is certainly consistent with what we have discovered in studying the transplant process and what information has been made available from different sources. The UNOS operator and the CDS coordinator's conversation led the CDS coordinator to believe that the UNOS operator had confirmed that the Boston organs were compatible with the Duke patient.

The situation is akin to that of the Pink Panther movie scene in which Inspector Clouseau (Peter Sellers) enters a hotel in the Alps and comes upon an elderly man, smoking a pipe behind the desk and a small dog lying on the carpet in front. After arranging to rent a "rheum," Clouseau says to the pipe smoker, "Does your dog bite?" The man replies succinctly, "No!" Clouseau leans over to pet the dog and is immediately bitten. "I thought you said that your dog does not bite!" exclaims Clouseau. "That," says the elderly man, "is not my dog."

CONTINGENCY, CAUSE, AND "ERROR" IN MEDICAL FAILURE

The sequence details demonstrate the highly contingent nature of this event. The account calls attention not only to the multiple opportunities to prevent the ultimate outcome that were missed but also to the multiple conditions needed to produce failure. The Duke event, like other celebrated medical failures, is not a case of human error but a case of systemic failure. The "first story" of error is a sufficient one to satisfy most reviewers and, indeed, becomes the grist for a host of scholarly and popular media mills. The first story is a Rorschach test, and the result is that stakeholders—including researchers—are able to understand the event as meaningful to them in their own terms.

The Duke failure shows how delicate the balance is between reliability and equity. The rules that insure an equitable distribution of donated organs took decades of work. These rules are embodied in a computational artifact that regulates and guides the process. But the pragmatic features of placing organs can lead to situations that require departing from the prescribed sequence. The apparatus of the system is not constructed to support them in this departure. It was developed to preserve the equity that is such an integral part of its function.

The Duke event, then, is not so much of a blunder as the nominal functioning of a system carefully created to preserve a balance between competing requirements. The current "solution" to the presentation of a Duke-like problem is to force rerunning of the match-list-generation process until the intended recipient appears on that list. But this is not so much a solution as a reinforcement of the existing system. There are no tools present in the system to support reversing the process leading from donor to recipient, because this is precisely the activity that could undermine the mechanical application of equity-producing rules and raise doubts about equity!

The difficulty facing those who would devise defenses against yet another Duke-like event is this: the event itself arose not from human error by practitioners but from *deliberately* embedded features of the system itself. It may be possible to create effective defenses against Duke-like failures, but doing so is likely to require disassembling the portions of the system that are presently combined to make the process opaque and immune to tampering, or accepting an increased potential for organ loss.

The desperate condition of potential recipients coupled with the limited supply of donated organs make protecting equity an essential function of the system of transplantation. The system produces equity by carefully structuring the process of matching donor to recipient. That structure controls the flow of information within the system, insuring that the workings of this expensive, valuable process remain equitable. However, the same structure that insures equity creates a tiny vulnerability to wrong blood type accidents. It was this vulnerability that became evident in the Duke event, an accident that was not the result of human error or some foible of human nature. It came instead from the deeply rooted features of this socio-technical system.

NOTES

1. Richard Cook and David Woods, "Operating at the Sharp End: The Complexity of Human Error," in *Human Error in Medicine*, ed. M. Bogner (Hillsdale, N.J.: Lawrence Erlbaum, 1994), 255–310.

2. D. D. Woods and R. I. Cook, "Perspectives on Human Error: Hindsight Bias and Local Rationality," in *Handbook of Applied Cognition*, ed. R. S. Durso et al. (New York: Wiley Press, 1999), 141–71.

3. R. I. Cook, D. D. Woods, and C. Miller, *A Tale of Two Stories: Contrasting Views on Patient Safety* (Chicago, Ill.: National Patient Safety Foundation, April 1998), <www.npsf.org/exec/report.html>.

4. PRACTIS (Probabilistic Risk Assessment Chicago Transplant Inquiry Study); this project is funded jointly by the University of Chicago and the Agency for Healthcare Research and Quality (AHRQ).

5. S. R. Barley and J. E. Orr, *Between Craft and Science: Technical Work in U.S. Settings* (London: ILR Press, 1997).

6. A note on the vocabulary of transplant: Organ donors are not, in the conventional sense, patients, and the term "patient" is usually reserved for a living person, whereas the donor is simply called "donor." In the past, the term "harvest" was used to describe the process of removing organs from the donor. Transplant donor family members have objected to the use of the term "harvest," and the word "procurement" is now preferred. In the past one would speak of "harvesting the heart from a donor," whereas one would now describe the activity as "procuring the heart from a deceased person." The deliberate caretaking of vocabulary marks the emotional and social character of the activities being described.

7. Transplantation also includes tissues and structures other than the solid visceral organs. "Non-solid" organ transplant, for example bone marrow transplant and blood and blood products transfusions, are considered transplants, as are use of preserved bone, cornea, skin, tendon, etc.

8. From the Greek *histos*—meaning tissue or web. The description of transplant immunology that follows is substantially simplified.

9. It may be that notions of equity within professional populations, including surgeons, transplant coordinators, and their organizations, weigh more heavily than notions of equity within the population at large. Few people undergo transplant, and for most the experience is a one-time event. In contrast, the professionals are in constant contact with the system, and dependent on it for access to organs, and the prestige, authority, money, and recognition associated with transplantation. Because of this, professionals tend to be notably sensitive to equity and versed in its subtlety.

10. The details vary slightly with the organ and are described in detail here for the lifesaving organs; live-donor organ donation is not discussed nor are complex processes such as multi-organ transplants or splits.

11. In some heart transplant centers, the transplant surgeon acts as facility coordinator. This allows the surgeon to communicate directly with the OPO coordinator in order to determine the donor characteristics and avoid time delays. This offers the surgeon a measure of direct control over portions of the process and is tractable because the number of potential heart recipients is, in contrast with the number of potential kidney recipients, limited.

12. Heart, lungs, liver, pancreas, and two kidneys constitute the primary collection of organs potentially transplantable. Other transplantable tissues may also be recovered, although the recipients for these are not typically identified before recovery.

13. The time pressure for implantation of other organs is less than that for hearts. In the case of kidneys, the viable time is long enough that the implantation operation can be worked into the next day's regular operating room schedule.

14. Charles Perrow, *Normal Accidents* (New York: Basic Books, 1984); Cook and Woods. "Operating at the Sharp End"

15. Significantly, type A and type O are the most frequently occurring types (see table 3). Indeed, by chance alone a type A organ would work in slightly over half of the recipient population; an O organ would work universally.

On the evening of February 6, 2003, Dr. James Jaggers received a telephone call from Carolina Donor Services, the local organ procurement organization (OPO) that services Duke University Medical Center and the surrounding area.[1] Dr. Jaggers was the head of pediatric heart and heart-lung transplantation at Duke, and a donor had been identified in New England for one of the patients on the Duke heart-lung transplant list. Heart-lung transplants are rare—only 39 were done in the United States in 2004, as compared to 6,200 liver transplants and 16,000 kidney transplants.[2] This is partly due to the relative paucity of conditions that require a combined heart-lung, and partly due to the stringent requirements for matching the donor and recipient. Not only is it a requirement that the blood types be compatible, but there also must be a rough correlation between the body sizes of the donor and recipient. A heart-lung bloc from a large donor may not even fit into the chest cavity of a small recipient, and a small donor's organs may not be large enough to function adequately for a bigger recipient. In addition, not infrequently the first people on the list for any organ prove untransplantable for any of a variety of reasons—they may be too sick, or even too well; they may have a cold or other infection, or they may refuse.

For whatever reason, the number one patient on Duke's list was not transplantable on that night. Dr. Jaggers thought that the organs would be appropriate for another of his patients, Jesica Santillan. When Dr. Jaggers heard back several hours later that the organs were Jesica's if he wanted them, two tragic assumptions had been made. The first was on Jaggers's part when he assumed that the organs would only be offered to Jesica if the blood type were compatible. The second was on the OPO's part when it assumed that Jaggers had a good reason for using the organs from a blood-type incompatible donor. There certainly is precedent for the use of such donors, but usually in a dire life or death situation or in a living-donor transplant in which the recipient has undergone an exhaustive and rigorous preconditioning regimen. This case clearly did not fall under either of these conditions.

THE SURGEON'S ROLE

We have all made mistakes, some trivial, some tragic. Many, if not all, surgeons have at one time made a mistake that proves to be significant and irreversible. It may be a fraction of a second slip of the knife, or an agonizing hours-long ill-fated operation. Once realization sets in, the reaction is almost instantaneous, and quite visceral. In polite terms, I would characterize this as the "Oh, No!" moment. One immediately becomes light-headed, short of breath, sweaty, and nauseated. Being surgeons, who are used to handling disasters and tragedies quickly, our "fix-it" mode kicks in. Sometimes, however, there is no "fix."

If there is indeed no "fix," the next line of thought is "damage control," mostly for the patient, but also, eventually, for the surgeon. Over the past decade or so, a key concept in the operative management of severely injured patients has moved away from the "let's fix everything" approach and toward the "let's just fix the life-threatening problems" approach. This "damage control" technique allows the patient to be taken to the intensive care unit, warmed up, transfused, and otherwise optimized and made a better candidate for further operative therapy. There was no "damage control" possible for Jesica.

I write this essay as a busy clinical transplant surgeon, having performed almost 1,000 kidney, liver, and pancreas transplants. My clinical experience and involvement with various transplant organizations makes me acutely aware of the astonishing complexities of transplantation in the United States. In addition, a major interest of mine is the international trade in organs, and donors. Therefore, my perspective is that of both a practitioner and an analyst, similar to several of my co-authors in this volume.

THE ORGANIZATION OF TRANSPLANTATION

Much has been made of the "experimental" nature of transplantation— common perceptions exist that the field is in its infancy and that we are still finding our way, technically, scientifically, and ethically. In some sense, since every patient is unique, and since we never know beforehand how an individual transplant procedure will turn out, every transplant could be considered an "experiment," although no more so than any other surgical or medical procedure. However, while the ethical issues continue to proliferate, the scientific and practical aspects of the field have become well established in the fifty years of modern transplantation history. Transplantation in the United States, particularly deceased-donor transplantation, has become an exquisitely choreographed dance between the listed patients, their transplant physicians and surgeons, the OPOS, the hospitals where the donors have been treated, and the donor families. The logistics are staggering, and I am frequently amazed that the system works at all. In fact, it not only works, it works quite well. It is worthwhile to look into the evolution of organ transplantation in the United States (see also Jed Adam Gross's essay in this volume) to give us some perspective on "the system."[3]

The first successful kidney transplant in the world was performed in Boston on December 23, 1954, between two identical twins, the Herrick brothers, by a team at the Peter Bent Brigham Hospital led by Dr. Joseph Murray, eventual Nobel laureate. In these early days the numbers of transplants were few, since there were relatively few identical twin pairs with one-half in need of a kidney. In 1961, azathioprine was introduced as one of the first antirejection medications, and in 1962 the first deceased-donor (cadaveric) kidney transplant was performed. The first successful liver and heart transplants followed in 1967 and 1968, respectively. Also in 1968 the South-Eastern Organ Procurement Foundation (SEOPF) was formed to help standardize transplantation procedures, exchange scientific information, and organize the way in which deceased-donor organs were allocated.

By 1977 the advances in computer technology allowed SEOPF to introduce the first computer-based matching system, which was called the United Network for Organ Sharing. By 1982 SEOPF established the Kidney Center, which operated twenty-four hours a day, seven days a week, to provide assistance in placing donated organs. The year 1984 was a landmark in transplantation in that the National Organ Transplant Act (NOTA, or "The Gore Law," after its sponsor, Senator Al Gore) codified into law the various aspects of transplantation. One of its provisions involved the separation of the United Network for Organ Sharing (UNOS) from SEOPF into a nonprofit entity with responsibility for overseeing transplantation in the United States. Two years later, UNOS was given the federal contract to operate the Organ Procurement and Transplantation Network (OPTN). By 1992, UNOS had begun to gather data on transplant rates, survival rates, and other such information, which it reported and made available to the transplant centers and the general public. As time has gone by, UNOS has become the most recognizable authority in transplantation in the United States. It sets and modifies policy after exhaustive internal and external review, certifies transplant centers and transplant surgeons and physicians, and, in a very real sense, "runs" transplantation in this country. It is a crucial and exceedingly complex role, a role required to maintain credibility of and trust in the system (see the Gross essay in this volume).

Transplantation worldwide has become very big business, for hospitals, practitioners, OPOs, and governments, not to mention the thousands of patients who benefit annually. The business trades not only with common currency but also with the currency of prestige and innovation. Transplant programs can bring their sponsoring hospitals a great deal of money, as well as the type of recognition that can set them apart from other similar institutions that do not have such programs. This quite naturally leads to competition between centers for patients and practitioners. There is also significant competition among them for the scarce and precious resource of donor organs. Larger centers can overwhelm smaller centers, but, perhaps not surprisingly, they frequently have better survival and graft function statistics. Programs open and close based on their success rates, and UNOS plays a crucial role in collecting these results and policing programs. Not surprisingly, UNOS has had a great deal to say about the Santillan case.

WHERE DID THE SYSTEM FAIL?

During Jesica's transplant procedure, after the organs had been implanted but before the incisions were closed, the blood bank at Duke informed the operating room and Dr. Jaggers that there was a blood type incompatibility— the donor was blood type A, and the recipient was blood type O.[4] This clearly would have been Jaggers's "Oh, No!" moment. In certain rare circumstances this seeming incompatibility might be inconsequential (a small percentage of blood type A patients have a so-called subtype A2 blood type that, immunologically, acts like blood type O). Unfortunately, this was not the case with Jesica. When organs of an incompatible blood type are transplanted, the recipient experiences a rare type of rejection called "hyperacute." This is distinguished from the more common "acute" rejection, which has a time course on the order of five to seven days and is mediated or controlled by cells of the immune system. Hyperacute rejection occurs within minutes to hours after the transplant and results when antibodies that already exist in the recipient bind to the cells of the transplanted organ, initiating a cascade that can destroy the organ rapidly. In this case, the antibodies were the "anti-A" antibodies that all people with blood type O have.

When facing a situation involving hyperacute rejection, the usual approach in attempting to save the organs and the patient involves reducing the antibody levels. This is generally done, as in Jesica's case, by using plasmapheresis—a technique akin to dialysis that removes plasma from the patient (in which antibodies reside) and replaces the plasma either with donated plasma from the blood bank or with human albumin. If the organ cannot be salvaged, it needs to be removed (in the case of a non-life-sustaining organ like a kidney), or the patient must be retransplanted, to save his or her life. After Jesica's first transplant, her team made the wildly optimistic assessment that, when the second set of organs became available, she had a 50-50 chance of recovery with the new organs. Unfortunately, by the time Jesica was retransplanted, she was already too far gone, and shortly thereafter she expired. In some circles, much has been made of the fact that Jesica's mother refused to allow her daughter to be an organ donor when she died after her second transplant.[5] First, it is not clear that the mother understood what was being requested. From a more pragmatic point of view, however, the organs of a person who had just undergone two transplants and who had been critically ill in the intensive care unit are frequently unusable in any case. Castigating her mother for this seems harsh, particularly since she has subsequently become a spokesperson for organ donation in speeches and advertisements.

From all accounts, the surgical procedures performed on Jesica were perfect, her care in the intensive care unit top-notch, and the rapid institution of plasmapheresis completely appropriate. In fact, Duke has objected to the use of the term "bungled transplant" because they maintain that the operation itself was flawless.[6] This notion plays into the popular misconception that transplantation is "just" an operation. Certainly a perfect operative procedure is helpful for a good outcome, but the other crucial aspects of transplantation, such as immunosuppression, peri-operative care, the prevention of infections, and the like are as important, or even more so, than the technical aspects of the operation. In Jesica's case, the cause of her demise was not poor care in the hospital, it was the error made at 3 A.M. on February 7.[7] This was an egregious error in and of itself, akin to failing to ascertain a donor's age, cause of death, comorbidities, or HIV status.

However, most medical errors are not the result of one person's mistake or incompetence. They are a result of a failure of the systems, as eloquently described by Charles Bosk in his essay in this volume, as well as his other works on the topic. Now when medical errors are detected, they are not dealt with by finger-pointing or assigning blame—they are subjected to "root cause analyses," which attempt to ferret out where and how the systems broke down and, more important, how to prevent the same errors in the future (see also Cook this volume). The root cause analyses at both Duke and UNOS revealed how the systems, both locally and nationally, broke down.

The Jesica Santillan story raised other, more common issues in organ transplant—"transplant tourism," the purchasing of organs and "beating the list." Some commentators speculated that there was some impropriety in Jesica's first transplant, and particularly in her second.[8] Unfortunately, transplantation is not infrequently the subject of such speculation, especially in the situation of famous patients receiving transplants "ahead of others." The well-publicized cases of Mickey Mantle and Larry Hagman come to mind, even though both of those transplants were performed in a completely appropriate and legitimate way. There are, however, many people who have found ways to circumvent the organ allocation system and, in some way, "beat the list."

HOW TO BUY AN ORGAN, AND OTHER NEFARIOUS DOINGS

As of May 2005, there were 88,068 candidates for transplantation enrolled with UNOS, and in 2004 there were a total of 27,033 transplants performed in the United States, according to the UNOS Web site.[9] Given the wide, and widening, discrepancy between the number of people on our transplant waiting lists and the number of transplants done, many patients have lost faith in the system and have taken matters into their own hands. Those who have are generally the wealthy and the well connected. The transplant community works hard at maintaining equity, but the system, as it exists, is inherently inequitable. The country is divided into eleven geographical regions by UNOS, and organs are generally allocated within regions. The rapidity with which a patient is transplanted after being listed can vary markedly from region to region and is based on two variables: the number of patients enrolled on the list within the region, and the number and rate of donations in the region. Because these figures vary widely from region to region, so do the transplant rates and waiting times. It is not unusual for some renal failure patients to wait eight or nine years for a kidney transplant in some urban centers in the Northeast, whereas the same patient might wait half that time only thirty miles away in a nearby state, or one-quarter of that time at some southern centers.

Anyone who has access to the Internet can easily find these figures, and many patients use the information to their own advantage. While I mentioned above that there are 88,068 *patients* enrolled with UNOS, there are a total of 95,508 *registrations* with UNOS.[10] A patient who is listed at more than one center is counted only once, but each registration is counted separately. This means that as many as 7,440 patients are enrolled at more than one center. In all likelihood, the number is smaller, in that many patients who enroll at more than one center enroll at more than one additional center.

Who are these patients on multiple lists? Put simply, most are the ones with money. In order to be listed at a center other than the local one, patients have to have either insurance to cover the procedure or the ready cash to pay for the evaluation and transplant. They also have to have the ability to travel to other centers and pay for lodging and other expenses. Any patients with Medicaid as their primary insurance are out of luck—Medicaid will only cover patients within the state in which they are enrolled. Many of the diseases for which we transplant, particularly liver failure and renal failure, have significantly higher incidences in the poorer population. Effectively this prevents the vast majority of patients from pursuing the multiple listing option.

That being said, why do we allow it? The simple answer is that, over time, it just happened, and it became a part of the system without anyone really taking notice, or taking action. Periodically UNOS has floated the concept of eliminating the possibility of multiple listing, only to be roundly rebuffed by many transplant centers and patient advocacy groups. Basically, momentum is carrying the multiple listing concept along.

Far more sinister is the participation of some patients in the buying and selling of organs from living donors, as described by Scheper-Hughes in her essay in this book, where she chronicles her remarkable studies of the worldwide organ trade. There are many variations of the theme, but the underlying engine driving the trade is the flow of organs from those economically less fortunate toward those more fortunate. There are numerous reports of Americans traveling worldwide for organs—to the slums of Central and South America, the Philippines, India, the Middle East—and even to China, to benefit from the particularly egregious practice of using the organs of executed Chinese prisoners for transplantation.[11]

In China in the mid-1980s it became clear to the government and some hospitals that a possible resource was being wasted by burying potentially useful organs in the bodies of prisoners who had been executed. In 1984, the government issued a directive giving instructions for the disposition of the organs from these prisoners ("The 1984 Provisional Rules on the Use of Dead Bodies or Organs from Condemned Criminals"),[12] which allows the removal of the organs under three conditions: the prisoner's body is not claimed, the prisoner has given prior consent, or the prisoner's family has given prior consent. Investigating all of the details of this practice is best left to another forum, but most commentators consider this a gross violation of human rights. Nonetheless, it has proven to be very popular both in China and throughout the world. Numerous patients have traveled from the United States (most are Chinese American immigrants) in order to purchase a prisoner's organ from the state or the hospital. In many ways, there are parallels between those patients who have traveled to China and Jesica and her family. Both were immigrants who traveled to America in the hopes of improving their lots in life. Both had acquired enough money (or had enough insurance) to allow transplantation to occur. Jesica, however, stayed within the system.

Unfortunately, American medicine cannot declare itself free of these practices. Some American physicians actively encourage their patients to pursue such options. In addition, there are well-documented reports of Americans receiving kidneys at American transplant centers from "relatives" who have been brought to this country by brokers solely for the purpose of selling their organs.[13] The great irony in the Santillan case is obvious. Usually the story would be that of a young Latino woman who had sold her kidney to a wealthy American for enough money to buy some clothes, some food, and maybe a television set; or, even more commonly, the story would be that of a young illegal immigrant who had suffered some terrible accident and had become a deceased multi-organ donor.

ADDRESSING THE PROBLEM

Clearly the Santillan tragedy could have been avoided by the simple question, "What's the blood type?" Anyone could have asked: Dr. Jaggers, the procuring surgeon, the team from the New England opo, the team from the North Carolina opo, the transplant coordinator at Duke, the circulating or nurse, the anesthesiologist, the transplant fellow. . . . No one did.

Duke performed a root cause analysis for both their own quality assurance and to fulfil unos's requirements.[14] Simply put, the facts were as follows: the transplant surgeon did not recall either receiving or requesting blood type information from the procurement coordinator, the procuring surgeon went to New England and procured the organs, also without specifically noting the blood type, and back at Duke, no confirmation of donor and recipient blood type was made until the transplant was almost complete.[15]

Duke's response to these findings was rapid, substantive, and very comprehensive. unos, in addition to placing specific requirements on Duke, instituted numerous changes in procedures nationwide, most of which incorporated redundancy into the systems. In summary, Duke implemented the following changes:[16]

In the transplant division:
- The divisions of pediatric cardiac transplantation and pediatric lung transplantation were reorganized and integrated into the respective adult divisions.
- The requirements for certification as a procuring surgeon were made more stringent.
- Two attending transplant surgeons are required to perform all pediatric thoracic organ transplants.
- The transplant surgeon will accept an organ based on recipient characteristics (including blood type) available in an online database. The transplant coordinator will independently confirm these characteristics.
- The procuring surgeon will confirm donor and recipient compatibility with source documents at the donor hospital.
- Dedicated parking spaces are defined for the procuring team, to solidify the chain of custody of the procured organs.
- On arrival at the OR suite, the donor organs will be logged in at the operating room desk.
- Prior to induction of anesthesia in the recipient, the attending anesthesiologist and transplant coordinator will have a "time-out" during which ABO compatibility will be confirmed. The confirmation will be recorded by the circulating OR nurse.
- On arrival of the organs at the OR, a second "time-out" will occur, to reconfirm the donor UNOS number, the integrity of the organs, and the blood type of the donor and recipient.
- Donor blood will be delivered to the Duke blood bank for a final reconfirmation of the donor's blood type.
- In the circumstance when a transplant will be done with an incompatible organ, a second transplant surgeon will confirm that this is the case in the medical record.

In the Medical Center, the administration:
- Established a Patient Safety Action Task Force.
- Initiated a safety review of patient procedures.
- Established a pediatric safety program.
- Hired a full-time expert in patient safety.
- Hired an associate chief information officer for patient safety.
- Hired a senior executive patient safety officer.

- Expanded the Board of Directors Patient Safety and Quality Assurance Committee.
- Established a partnership with the quality improvement organization for the local region designated by the Centers for Medicare and Medicaid Services.
- Developed a computerized drug order entry system.
- Developed a computerized monitoring system for adverse drug events.
- Launched an Internet site for anonymous reporting of medical errors.

In addition to the wide-ranging changes instituted at Duke, UNOS changed numerous policies and instituted several new policies, which have been implemented at all transplant centers nationwide, for all organs transplanted.[17] In sum:

- Potential transplant recipients will have their blood types checked at least two separate times during their evaluations.
- When recipients are registered in UNET (UNOS's Web-based registration tool), the blood type will need to be entered twice, by two separate individuals.
- At the time of organ procurement, the blood types of donor and recipient will be verified by at least two different staff members at both the host OPO and the transplant hospital.
- Transplant programs will check the donor blood type on arrival of the organ and compare it to that of the recipient.
- The attending transplant surgeon will re-check the blood types of the donor and recipient, and document the results in the recipient's medical chart.
- Transplant centers and OPOS must keep records of these verification procedures, which will be examined during UNOS audits.

Clearly Duke and UNOS took seriously their responsibility to address the systems errors; the changes are comprehensive and thorough, perhaps even overwhelming. Most of the recommendations and new rules are appropriate, but some seem to have spilled over into the outlandish, and certainly the unenforceable. It is difficult to imagine that providing a dedicated parking space to the procuring team will enhance patient safety more than it will make the transplant fellow's life a little easier. Some of the recommendations won't even work—the second "time-out" when the organs arrive will occur well after the recipient's surgery has begun. In addition, although it might prevent the placement of inappropriate organs into a patient, it will not prevent the operation from happening at all, which is obviously what should happen.

Jesica Santillan is not the only patient who has undergone an errant transplant with incompatible organs, but she is certainly the most famous. The remedies put into place after her heartrending death, both locally at Duke and nationwide through UNOS, highlight the complex issues of protecting patient safety and improving outcomes in the transplant community. In his essay, Bosk makes the trenchant observation that, as is frequently the case, these changes have been made to address the last disaster, not the next one. Unfortunately, few of us are sufficiently visionary to anticipate the unimaginable.

NOTES

1. DukeMedNews, "Background Information on Jesica Santillan Blood Type Mismatch," 2004, <http://www.dukemednews.org/mediakits/detail.php?id=6498>.

2. UNOS, transplants by organ type, 2005, <http://www.optn.org/latestData/step2 .asp>.

3. United Network for Organ Sharing, "Timeline of Key Events in U.S. Transplantation and UNOS History," 2005, <http://www.unos.org/whoWeAre/history.asp>.

4. DukeMedNews, "Background Information on Jesica Santillan."

5. Stormfront White Nationalist Community, "How Little Yesica Got Bumped Ahead of White Kids & on TV for 2 Heart/Lung Transplants, 2003, <http://www .stormfront.org/forum/showthread.php?t=57159>.

6. K. Wailoo, personal communication, 2005. In an email communication with Wailoo, a Duke University news office director wrote that the term "bungled transplant" was incorrect. He noted: "To correct the record on the title of your conference, this was an organ blood-type mismatch case. The transplants were not bungled or botched, because the surgeries were performed up to appropriate surgical standards" (Correspondence from Jeffrey Molter to Keith Wailoo, January 12, 2004).

7. DukeMedNews, "Background Information on Jesica Santillan."

8. M. Malkin, "Tough Questions about Jesica's Transplants," 2003, <http://www .jewishworldreview.com/michelle/malkin022103.asp>.

9. UNOS, 2005, <http://www.optn.org/latestData/step2.asp>.

10. Ibid.

11. E. Baard and R. Cooney, "China's Execution, Inc.," *Village Voice* 46 (2001): 36–40; J. D. Briggs, "The Use of Organs from Executed Prisoners in China," *Nephrol Dial Transplant* 11 (2) (1996): 238–40; C. Chelala, "China's Human-Organ Trade Highlighted by U.S. Arrest of "Salesman," *Lancet* 351 (9104) (1998): 735; T. Diflo, "The Use of Executed Prisoners' Organs for Transplantation in China," In *Ethical, Legal, and Social Issues in Organ Transplantation*, edited by T. Gutmann, ASD, R. A. Sells, and W. Land, 500–506 (Lengerich, Germany: Pabst Science Publishers, 2004). T. Diflo, "Use of Organs from Executed Chinese Prisoners," *Lancet* 364 (2004): 30–31.

12. Diflo, "Use of Executed Prisoners' Organs"; Laogai Research Foundation, "Communist Charity: A Comprehensive Report on the Harvesting of Organs from the Executed Prisoners of the People's Republic of China," 2001, p. 16.

13. N. Scheper-Hughes, personal communication, 2004.

14. DukeMedNews, "Background Information on Jesica Santillan."

15. UNOS News Bureau, "OPTN/UNOS Statement Regarding Jesica Santillan's Transplant," 2003, <http://www.unos.org/news/newsDetail.asp?id=249>.

16. DukeMedNews, "Background Information on Jesica Santillan."

17. UNOS News Bureau, "OPTN/UNOS Review of Transplant Error Continues," 2003, <http://www.unos.org/news/newsDetail.asp?id=251>; UNOS News Bureau, "OPTN/UNOS Recommends Additional Safeguards for Patient Safety in Organ Transplants," 2003, <http://www.unos.org/news/newsDetail.asp?id=273>; UNOS News Bureau, "OPTN/UNOS Continues to Improve Accuracy in Donor/Recipient Matching," 2004, <http://www.unos.org/news/newsDetail.asp?id=308>.

FROM LIBBY ZION TO

JESICA SANTILLAN

MANY TRUTHS

BARRON H. LERNER

At first glance, the Jesica Santillan case is a textbook example of how experts believe that medical errors occur. There was a human error, when no one at Duke University Medical Center checked that the donor heart and lungs matched Jesica's blood type. But, in fact, this error actually masked a larger systems flaw, which was an inadequate strategy for preventing organ mismatches. What needs correcting, according to this paradigm, is the system. "The most important problem identified through this whole sad story [of Jesica Santillan]," stated Thomas Murray, president of the Hastings Center, "is the failure to build a system that would prevent such a disastrous thing from occurring in the first place."[1]

Yet while this is a reasonable conclusion regarding the events in the Santillan case, it is not necessarily the "truth."[2] This essay, by revisiting the case of Libby Zion, who unexpectedly died at New York Hospital in 1984, demonstrates how difficult it is to draw simple lessons from individual cases of medical error. Four reasons are given for this phenomenon: 1) different participants and commentators construct different narratives of events beginning immediately after the mistake occurs; 2) explanations of catastrophic medical errors, like any past events, are historically contingent and therefore reflect the era in which they were constructed; 3) as witnessed by the legacy of malpractice litigation, issues of blame and responsibility—not systems flaws —tend to be the enduring legacy of medical error cases; and 4) the randomness of disease complicates efforts to prove that errors occurred and that they produced bad outcomes. Although the Santillan case was, in some ways, more straightforward than that of Libby Zion, these factors also interfered with efforts to draw definitive conclusions about what had occurred at Duke.

The first three of these factors draw primarily on my knowledge as a historian of medicine. To explicate them, I reviewed standard historical sources, ranging from scholarship on the history of malpractice and medical errors to contemporaneous newspaper clippings and correspondence about the Zion case. The fourth factor stems more from my knowledge as a physician experienced in caring for patients and reading medical charts. Although these approaches differ epistemologically, I believe that they are complementary.

Before studying the ways in which the Libby Zion case has been told and retold, here are the skeletal "facts" of what happened.[3] Zion was an eighteen-year-old student at Bennington College when she became ill in early March 1984 shortly after a tooth extraction. Her symptoms included a low-grade fever and an earache, for which a private doctor had prescribed erythromycin. At home, Zion got worse instead of better and began acting strangely, with periods of agitation and jerking motions of her body. This led her parents, Elsa and Sidney Zion, to bring her to the emergency room of New York Hospital on the night of March 4, 1984. Sidney Zion was a well-known investigative journalist originally trained as a lawyer.

The emergency room physician could not determine a clear source for Zion's temperature, which was 103 degrees, but found an elevated white blood cell count of 18,000, possibly indicative of bacterial infection. He also learned that Zion was taking an antidepressant known as Nardil. Aside from marijuana, she denied any use of cocaine or other illicit drugs. The emergency room physician notified Dr. Raymond Sherman, who Sidney Zion had called before the family left for the hospital. Sherman was an attending physician who had treated both Libby Zion and other family members in the past. The decision was made to admit Zion to the hospital given her fever and strange body movements.

On the floor, a nurse noted that Zion was lucid at times but had periods of delirium. Two resident physicians, Luise Weinstein, an intern, and Gregg Stone, a junior resident, evaluated her. Neither knew exactly what was going on, but they were not extremely alarmed. Stone's admission note raised several possible diagnoses, but highest on his list was "a viral syndrome with hysterical symptoms." Stone touched base with Sherman. The main plan was to hydrate Zion and to give her Tylenol for her fever, while awaiting the results of other tests.

Sidney and Elsa Zion went home around 3 A.M., having been reassured that their daughter was all right. Although what happened subsequently remains contested, some facts seem clear. Zion was given a shot of Demerol, an opiate medication, to help control her shaking movements. But she grew more agitated, swearing and trying to climb out of the hospital bed. The nurses, Myrna Balde and Jerylyn Grismer, called Weinstein and recommended some type of restraint. Weinstein ordered a Posey restraint that covered Zion's torso. When this did not work, the nurses also tied down her ankles and wrists. Balde called Weinstein again and asked her to come and evaluate Zion, but Weinstein declined, indicating that she was with another sick patient and had seen Zion recently. Weinstein prescribed an injection of Haldol, a tranquilizer, which the nurses administered around 4:30 A.M.

Finally, Zion fell asleep. At 6 A.M., Balde later said, she awakened her patient and got her to take two Tylenol tablets, although this was not registered in the chart. One-half hour later, during the routine morning temperature checks, a nurses' aide found Zion's temperature to be extremely high, somewhere between 106 and 108 degrees. The nurses immediately swung into action, calling Weinstein, who ordered cold compresses and a cooling blanket. But ten minutes later, Zion was in cardiac arrest, presumably due to her extremely high temperature. Despite a fifty-five-minute attempt at resuscitation, Zion died.

Although the Zion family and their lawyers would try for more than a decade to determine what had happened to their daughter that night, no definitive answers were forthcoming. As has already been suggested, poor documentation and contradictory memories made a clear-cut account of the events impossible to produce. In contrast to Jesica Santillan, whose survival for two weeks after the first transplant led to some urgent fact checking, Libby Zion's rapid deterioration prevented any dispassionate assessment of what had occurred by the medical staff. That is, attempts to document the truth were immediately influenced by the people who had participated in the encounter and who sought to explain away the events in question. There was never a definitive story that got spun in various ways; the first accounts were themselves spun, both consciously and unconsciously.[4]

What narratives thus emerged about Libby Zion's death? It is worth noting that amid Sidney and Elsa Zion's terrible shock and grief, one of the first persons they contacted was a malpractice lawyer, Theodore H. Friedman. Therefore, from the start, Sidney Zion was thinking in terms of a medical error. How else could one explain the death of his daughter from what doctors had told him was a viral infection? After Libby Zion's funeral, her psychiatrist later recalled, Sidney framed her death not as an act of God but due to a series of mistakes.[5]

Although it is not clear exactly when Sidney and Elsa Zion decided to sue, the combination of presumed medical errors, a call to a lawyer, and Sidney's legal background suggest that the notion of malpractice reared its head almost immediately. After all, lawsuits were (and are) the most common way to try to avenge or set right a bad outcome stemming from medical care perceived as substandard. This was, then, the first narrative of the Libby Zion case: a stunned and outraged family seeking legal and financial recompense for presumed malpractice.

And the situation might have stayed this way except for what Sidney Zion subsequently learned about his daughter's care. What truly stunned him was that Raymond Sherman, his daughter's doctor and the senior physician on the case, had not been consulted when Libby worsened and never saw her before she died. Rather, it was Luise Weinstein, an intern nine months out of medical school, who was in charge of her care and had single-handedly made the decisions that had either caused or not prevented the death. Gregg Stone, although still on call, had not been roused from his bed to assist Weinstein. Finally, Zion learned, it might have been the combination of Nardil and Demerol, known to be toxic, that led to Libby's death.

At this point, the Zion family's story of what happened to their daughter began to evolve. The manner in which New York Hospital cared for its patients, at least at night, appeared gravely flawed. And the more the Zions learned, this impression was reinforced. It was routine, apparently, for senior physicians not to come to the hospital at night to see newly admitted patients. House officers not only covered the hospital at night, but they often did so in thirty-six-hour shifts and with little or no sleep.

From the vantage point of 2006, with over twenty years of discussion of these topics in the medical and lay press, such revelations are hardly startling.[6] But in 1984, to most people outside of the medical profession, they were. No doubt other aggrieved families had learned this information when researching their loved ones' deaths. It was Sidney Zion, however, who chose to make the issue of overworked, unsupervised residents central to his lawsuit. As a journalist, Zion knew a good story when he encountered one, even amid his grief. And he was especially well-equipped, because of his connections, to transform a malpractice claim, a claim of what might be termed a "private error," into a claim of "public error," or a crusade against the medical profession. In the months after Libby's death, Sidney Zion called everyone he could think of, ranging from powerful journalists like the *New York Times*'s Tom Wicker to New York City Council president Andrew Stein.

The new story that the Zions were crafting thus had a different focus—not so much on bad individual doctors but on a bad system, an analytic progression that is commonplace in cases of error, as Richard Cook notes in his essay in this book. For Sidney Zion, this new perspective dramatically elevated the hospital's culpability. He relentlessly charged that New York Hospital had "murdered" his daughter and sought criminal charges against her physicians.[7] What had happened, Zion stated, was not a "human mistake," which was forgivable, but an "inhuman mistake."[8] What had occurred was both misdiagnosis and misconduct.

Meanwhile, within hours of Libby Zion's death, the staff of New York Hospital had begun to construct its own narrative of her death. The doctors and nurses who initially spoke to the family were apologetic but did not indicate that anything had gone wrong. Luise Weinstein told Elsa Zion, "I want you to know we did everything we could for Libby."[9] It is likely that the doctors did not initially view what had happened as a "mistake" or "error"; circa 1984, this type of language was rarely used on the wards and almost never with family members. Two decades later, and in the glare of media spotlight, Duke could not avoid such words when the story went public. But New York Hospital was able to use a more neutral phrase to describe Libby Zion's death. It would be characterized as a bad (and unfortunate) outcome.

The hospital's assessment of the case began on the morning of March 5, 1984. Having heard what had happened, the medical chief resident reviewed the chart and found nothing unusual except for the fact that Zion was on Nardil, a medication known to have many potentially dangerous interactions with other drugs. When he checked a book known as the *Physicians' Desk Reference*, he learned that Demerol was contraindicated in someone taking Nardil because the combination of the drugs could lead to hyperthermia, an extremely high fever. But there was no report of this ever having happened with the small dose of Demerol—25 milligrams—that Zion had received. Thus, concluded both the chief resident and the physician-in-chief of the hospital, R. Gordon Douglas, Zion had not died from a drug reaction. In this manner, one potential medical error was explained away.[10]

Other aspects of the hospital's story began to come together. Although the nurses would later state that they had told Weinstein that Zion had become more agitated after the Demerol, Weinstein denied having clearly been told this. And Weinstein defended the use of restraints as appropriate. There was even a growing consensus among hospital staff that Zion had been improving up until the time that her temperature dramatically increased. This consensus may have explained why the hospital did not hold a formal morbidity and mortality conference on the Zion case. Even though the mysterious death of an eighteen-year-old would have made for an instructive presentation, it might have opened questions that were no longer being asked.[11]

At one point in time, New York Hospital appeared to take responsibility for what had occurred. In March 1987, three years after her death, the New York State Department of Health fined the hospital $13,000 for its "woeful" care of Libby Zion.[12] In addition, the state required the hospital to file monthly

reports on unexpected deaths and submit to periodic inspections of its nurs-
ing and medical staffs. By agreeing to this arrangement, the hospital was, in a
sense, admitting its guilt; but it had also insisted on a clause indicating that
this agreement could not be used in any civil or criminal hearings related to
the case. And Raymond Sherman announced that he still did not believe that
the hospital had done anything wrong. The hospital's initial narrative of the
Libby Zion case, therefore, was crafted to avoid guilt and, as best as possible,
to put the matter to rest.

But even as this story was being told, another one was being constructed:
Libby Zion had died by using cocaine, probably shortly before her admission
to the hospital, and then concealing this fact from the doctors despite repeated questioning. The cocaine, according to this theory, proved toxic when
combined with Nardil and other drugs that Zion did not admit she was
taking, such as the opiate Percodan. It is not quite clear when this theory was
first advanced. As part of its routine, the New York City medical examiner's
office, which performed Zion's autopsy, tested for cocaine and other drugs in
her bodily fluids. The blood test revealed a trace of cocaine, which evidently
led doctors at New York Hospital to factor it in as contributing to Zion's death.

It is reasonable to conclude that the inevitable lawsuit that was going to
result from the case encouraged the hospital—and its lawyers—to make the
issue of cocaine a major part of its defense. According to Natalie Robins, the
author of *The Girl Who Died Twice*, a book on the Zion case, there was already
a buzz at New York Hospital as of July 1984 that Libby Zion would be blamed
for her death.[13]

By January 1987 there was no doubt that this would be the strategy. The
previous month, a grand jury convened by New York District Attorney Robert
Morgenthau had declined to indict Libby Zion's doctors on murder charges
but had issued a scathing report criticizing what had happened at New York
Hospital and the general state of graduate medical education. (This report
would lead to the formation of the Bell Commission, which would outline a
strategy for revamping the training of house officers in New York State).[14] In
response, New York Hospital issued a press release on January 14, 1987,
objecting to the grand jury's findings and instead warning of the ramifica-
tions of illicit cocaine use. The claim that Libby Zion died as a result of
cocaine use would become a centerpiece of the 1994–95 malpractice trial,
and a major factor in the jury's split decision, even though the additional tests
of both Libby Zion's blood and urine came up negative for the drug. The issue
of cocaine will be discussed in further detail below.

There were, therefore, at least four competing narratives of what had happened in the Libby Zion case: 1) she had died due to a medical mistake, probably a fatal drug interaction, or a series of errors; 2) she had died because of the improper patient care system at New York Hospital, which left Zion in the hands of inexperienced and overtired physicians; 3) she had died of a mysterious illness despite excellent care; and 4) she had died in part or completely because of her use of cocaine.

Although different individuals and groups would attempt to prove that one or another of these stories was the "truth," none of them was; that is, all of them involved some degree of spin from the start. This is not to say that efforts to learn the actual events were of no value. For example, an enormous amount of information was presented at the trial, *Zion v. New York Hospital*, which surely shed light on what had occurred. Such disclosure would never occur in the Santillan case against Duke, as it was settled out of court in June 2004. To some degree, the goal of Robins's book on Libby Zion's death was to use the voluminous material amassed for the trial to try to come to some approximation of the "truth."[15]

However, various narratives may appear to be more truthful than others based on the historical times in which they are introduced. That is, certain versions may obtain more credibility and durability due to concurrent historical trends. This was certainly true in the Libby Zion case. Zion was only one of thousands of patients who had died under questionable circumstances in a teaching hospital. But the case would engender a unique legacy because of when it occurred.

As of 1984, the issue of medical error had been discussed for decades in the medical literature. Although occasional physicians argued that mistakes were an inevitable part of medical practice and should be openly discussed, the vast majority of commentators called for discretion. Errors, they believed, should be discussed quietly by the doctors involved and internal solutions devised.[16]

While other patients and family members who had filed high-profile malpractice suits had surely brought the issue of medical error to the public, few had done so as overtly as Sidney Zion. Thanks to his column at the *New York Daily News* and the help of other journalists and prominent friends, Zion continually pushed the possible Nardil-Demerol interaction, which had been overlooked by Zion's doctors. But the issue of medical error did not become the legacy of the Zion case. For whatever reasons, it was not until the 1994 Betsy Lehman case and the 1999 Institute of Medicine report, *To Err Is Human*, that medical mistakes became perceived as a major hazard of hospitalization and a threat to the public's health.[17]

The issue that did "stick," however, was that of overworked house officers. This, too, had been quietly discussed within the medical literature for years. But when Sidney Zion, Tom Wicker, and other journalists revealed that doctors-in-training routinely worked over 100 hours weekly and had questionable supervision, the revelation came at a historically propitious moment.[18] By this time, other industries charged with keeping customers safe had begun to adopt procedures to ensure that their employees were well-rested and properly supervised. In addition, with the rise of civil rights, feminism, and the antiwar movement in the 1960s and 1970s, organizations that potentially abused their labor forces were increasingly suspect. And the entrance of more women into medicine, along with a growing inclination of men to become more active in raising their children, had rendered the venerable notion of "residing in the hospital" highly problematic. The degree to which the issue of overworked residents was ripe for attention was demonstrated by the unprecedented decision of the Manhattan grand jury to issue a report recommending whole-scale revisions of medical education. As the abolitionist Wendell Phillips stated in 1852, "Revolutions are not made, they come."[19]

One of the ironies of the Libby Zion case was that the story that won the day—that overtired, unsupervised residents were killing patients in teaching hospitals—may have not even been particularly relevant. Although Weinstein and Stone had both been working for roughly sixteen hours when they first saw Zion, they were nowhere near the thirty-six-hour mark that Sidney Zion and the grand jury report publicized in the media. There is no direct evidence that fatigue impaired the doctors' decision-making regarding Libby Zion (although the large number of patients that Weinstein was covering may have).[20] Nevertheless, once the issue of overwork was outed, this story became the "truthful" explanation of why Libby Zion had died.

Another irony of the Zion case was that the role played by cocaine in her death—while debated as if it held the key to the truth—actually served as a blinder to more important issues.[21] The central issue in the Zion trial was the standard of care received by an eighteen-year-old girl with a history of depression and new-onset fevers, thrashing movements, and periods of confusion. The main interventions Zion received were hydration and Tylenol and, when she became more agitated, physical and chemical restraints. Despite these efforts, Libby Zion died. Should the doctors have suspected cocaine or other drugs as an explanation for her strange combination of symptoms? Should they have suspected such drugs even if their patient denied having used them? And, regardless of the cocaine, shouldn't the doctors have detected the potentially deadly interaction of Nardil and Demerol, evaluated Libby Zion more carefully when her unexplained agitation persisted, and sent her to the intensive care unit for closer monitoring? The answer to all of these questions, I believe, is yes. In contrast, the answer to the question of whether cocaine contributed to Zion's death is unknowable. Thus, the only really relevant question about cocaine that the jury should have considered was whether it was a mistake to take at face value Zion's word about not using the drug.

Why, then, did the case get sidetracked trying to answer the question about the possibility that cocaine killed Libby Zion? As we have seen, New York Hospital viewed the discussion of this topic as a good strategy for swaying the jurors. But Sidney Zion also fostered this line of questioning by flatly denying the possibility that his daughter was a cocaine user. Had the plaintiff's lawyers spoken more frankly about the possibility of cocaine use, they might have made an even stronger case that New York Hospital missed the boat when assessing the patient.

The resulting emphasis on Libby Zion's guilt or innocence—was she or was she not a cocaine user—should remind us what factors propel these types of court cases. For hundreds of years, examples of medical mistakes have come to light most often as malpractice cases in which doctors and hospitals are pitted against patients and families. This adversarial framework is the one in which we have traditionally understood the concept of medical error: the patient says errors or mistakes were made, the doctor says he or she met the standard of care. Or, in other words, the patient says that the doctor was culpable and the doctor disagrees.

Within a conceptual framework that searches for and assigns blame, it is hard to impose a new and different one that explicitly discourages finger-pointing at specific individuals: that of systems error. The importance of applying the systems concept pervades both the Institute of Medicine report and the vast majority of the current scholarship regarding medical errors (see also the Cook essay).[22] Indeed, by calling attention to the issues of house staff hours and inadequate supervision, the Zion case identified a systems issue. But there are always one or more human errors that cause medical mistakes, regardless of how good a system of error prevention is in place. And it is these human gaffes that we continue to pursue on an emotional level. Blame and absolution are powerful notions that, rightly or wrongly, enable us to process medical tragedies.[23] This was surely true in the Libby Zion case. And the ability to raise the issue that the patient herself was to blame—for using cocaine and then denying it—was too powerful a moralistic tale for the defense or the plaintiffs to pass up. The pursuit of this supposed truth, however, obscured the fact that both sides were in fact constructing competing stories designed to win the jurors' hearts.

The fourth and final factor that impeded the search for truth in the Zion case is the randomness of disease and its symptoms. When Libby Zion came to the emergency room, she was treated just like any other young person with an obscure fever and complicating features, receiving a physical examination, blood and urine tests, and a chest x-ray. When these did not reveal anything specific, the decision was made to admit her to the hospital for observation and to await additional test results. The admission diagnoses reflected this mind-set. Luise Weinstein suspected some type of infection but was not sure what kind. As noted above, Gregg Stone wrote, "viral syndrome with hysterical symptoms."

At the trial, Stone was criticized for having implied with this diagnosis that Libby Zion was only mildly ill and, given her psychiatric history, overreacting, or, as chief plaintiff witness Harold Osborn put it, that she was dismissed by the hospital as a "ditsy redhead with a lot of complaints" who should not have been in the hospital and would simply get better by herself.[24] The implication made by the plaintiff's lawyers was that Stone and Weinstein did not take Zion's deterioration seriously and thus medicated her and tied her to the bed instead of reevaluating her. These actions, in turn, led to her death.

While the Libby Zion story is a compelling one, it ignores the wider population of patients who receive similar diagnoses and care. If one could obtain the charts of 100 of the previous young patients admitted to New York Hospital with similar symptoms, it is likely that all of them would indicate that the patients had survived. That is, Stone's initial diagnosis, even with its implication that Libby was malingering, may have been reasonable. It is also reasonable to argue that Weinstein was not obligated to make a personal appearance at Libby Zion's bedside every time something changed in her condition. A hospital could not function if this were the expectation for busy interns.

The larger point is that all medical cases are based on probabilities and hunches, backed up, when possible, by the medical literature. That is, as Nancy King argues in the concluding chapter of this volume, the stories of Libby Zion, Jessica Santillan, and the conjoined Bijani twins, who died during corrective surgery, all reflect "the complexity of uncertainty" in medicine. The initial assessment of Zion's condition was based on similar cases that the doctors had seen or read about. But the main question, which the jury was never really asked to consider, was when did Zion's case become *atypical* enough to warrant more aggressive intervention. In defending her decision not to go see her patient despite the nurses' requests that she do so, Weinstein noted that she had just seen Zion. That is, she already knew the situation. She was still thinking within the initial construct that she, Stone, and Sherman had devised.

In retrospect, of course, the Zion case was anything but typical. The question thus becomes: at what point, if any, should Weinstein have realized this, called Stone and/or Sherman and sent Zion to the intensive care unit? What I am arguing is that the errors in the Zion case were errors of judgment and thus the hardest to evaluate and the least identifiable with the "truth." And it is this type of error that permeates medicine. While it is relatively easy to acknowledge flagrant mistakes, such as the accidental administration of the wrong drug or ten times too high a dosage of medication, errors of judgment will always inspire multiple and competing stories.[25]

How does this discussion of errors and truth in the Libby Zion case inform the Jesica Santillan case? First, it is worth noting several differences. The Santillan case occurred at a historical time in which medical error had become a familiar public topic, thanks in large degree to the publicity surrounding the 1999 Institute of Medicine report. In contrast to 1984, there was a template for what was "supposed" to happen in such cases: media coverage was expected, as was some type of official institutional acknowledgment of what had taken place. Thus, when the press originally learned that a patient had received the wrong set of organs, Duke Chief Executive Officer William Fulkerson gave numerous interviews describing what had occurred.

Moreover, Duke officials readily admitted that something had gone very wrong. Whereas New York Hospital argued that Libby Zion's death had been unavoidable, Fulkerson readily admitted that an error had occurred.[26] Meanwhile, Jesica's surgeon, James Jaggers, who had informed the family of the mistake right after the first operation, issued a public statement indicating his personal culpability for not having checked the organs for compatibility. "As Jesica's surgeon," he stated, "I am ultimately responsible for the team and for this error."[27]

Yet closer scrutiny of the Santillan case reveals many more similarities with the Zion case. As this book demonstrates, a seemingly clear-cut example of a medical error can generate several different, and at times competing, stories. If Libby Zion's death could cause a public outcry over the quality of graduate medical education, Santillan's case could become a cautionary tale about the limited ability of technology to "fix" disease, particularly among disenfranchised groups such as immigrants. In addition, just as the uncertainties of medicine, in retrospect, led Zion's doctors to make several bad clinical decisions, so, too, did they contribute to questionable decisions regarding Santillan's first and second transplants. Was it wrong for Jaggers to have pushed for the first set of organs when Jesica was not gravely ill? Is there any chance the second heart and lungs could have worked given the first rejection and what Jesica's body had already endured? These are hard, perhaps unanswerable, medical questions that complicate discussions of errors.

But the major parallel between the two cases focuses on the issues of blame and publicity. Although it initially appeared that Duke had been highly forthcoming, it actually misled the press at first, according to an article in Newsweek.[28] For example, a hospital spokesman made no mention of the mismatched organs four days after Jesica's first surgery, implying that she was undergoing immune rejection characteristic of all transplant cases. In addition, like those made by New York Hospital, Duke's admissions of guilt were carefully worded, designed from the start to limit the institution's culpability. "This was a tragic error," Fulkerson said after the first operation, "and we accept responsibility for our part."[29] This caveat was Duke's way of immediately deflecting some of the blame from the medical center. The implication was that Jaggers himself was primarily accountable for the mistake. Such a decision is ironic, as Charles Bosk points out elsewhere in this book, since a systems approach, which Duke implemented in the wake of the Santillan scandal, supposedly avoids blaming specific individuals, who themselves should be seen as victims of bad systems.

And just as Sidney Zion had unabashedly used his New York media connections to reveal the "truth" about his daughter's death, Mack Mahoney mobilized a similar response among local and national journalists covering the Santillan case. Mahoney was a North Carolina businessman who had been an early champion of Jesica, raising hundreds of thousands of dollars to pay for her medical care at Duke. Like Zion, Mahoney was an older male who became the spokesperson for a younger, silenced female, reasserting her innocence in the face of tragedy.

It was Mahoney who had angrily revealed to the press that the institution was not being forthcoming about the mismatched organs. "I'm mad. I'm enraged. I'm horrified," he announced.[30] He asserted that if Jesica died, the cause would be Duke's secrecy. That is, honesty would have led to prompt identification of a second set of organs that would have saved her life. Mahoney's words were full of condemnation and accusations. Echoing Sidney Zion, he threatened that "if she dies, they murdered her."[31] The Duke administration, he charged, was a group of "piranhas" that wanted to silence him.[32]

Was such hyperbole, with an eye toward creating a scandal, justifiable? Not if one believed that the way to remedy the problem of medical errors was to implement a systems approach. And Duke did, announcing after Jesica's death that, for both transplantation and all medical services, it had to develop "the kind of systems that we need to be able to catch errors—and prevent errors."[33] In other words, rather than focusing on the gaffes of specific individuals, Duke would install systems that would automatically "red flag" human errors.

But this approach, however theoretically sound, was just what Mack Mahoney had little tolerance for. For him, the worthy goal of eliminating future medical errors was much less important than achieving justice and recompense in Jesica's specific case. If Duke was spinning events in its behalf, limiting its accountability and shifting blame, the public deserved to know. Sidney Zion, the former prosecutor, would surely have agreed. As he loved to say, "No names, no accountability."[34] This sort of calculus also worked for the press. A story assigning blame for a little girl's death would always be preferable to one on the need to implement better error-prevention systems.

In arguing that the stories of Libby Zion and Jesica Santillan can be told in multiple ways, this essay does not suggest that there is no reality to the stories. Specific events took place both before and after their deaths. Similarly, while Charles Bosk is correct to argue that celebrated cases of error cause all stakeholders to craft opportunistic versions of what happened, some of these accounts are more or less opportunistic than others. It is the job of historians to investigate and describe the events in question, explore motivations, and, if appropriate, affix blame.[35] But history is even richer when it also explores the feelings that such events evoke, "the interpretations they invite [and] the meanings they embody."[36] Such history may be messier, but, to paraphrase the historian David Greenberg, it is the stuff of experience.

NOTES

1. Tim Friend, "Fatal Transplant Mix-up Not 1st Time Duke Has Had Errors," *USA Today*, February 24, 2003, 5A.

2. There is now a large literature on the issue of whether historians can truly pursue the "truth" about past events. See, for example, Peter Novick, *That Noble Dream: The "Objectivity Question" and the American Historical Profession* (Cambridge: Cambridge University Press, 1988); Joyce Appleby, Lynn Hunt, and Margaret Jacob, *Telling the Truth about History* (New York: W. W. Norton, 1994); Robert F. Berkhofer Jr., *Beyond the Great Story: History as Text and Discourse* (Cambridge, Mass.: Harvard University Press, 1995); and C. Behan McCullagh, *The Truth of History* (New York: Routledge, 1998).

3. This information comes primarily from "Report Concerning the Care and Treatment of a Patient and the Supervision of Interns and Junior Residents at a Hospital in New York County," Grand Jury Report, Supreme Court of the State of New York, December 31, 1986; and Natalie Robins, *The Girl Who Died Twice: The Libby Zion Case and the Hidden Hazards of Hospitals* (New York: Dell, 1995).

4. On the construction of stories, see Marita Sturken, *Tangled Memories: The Vietnam War, the AIDS Epidemic, and the Politics of Remembering* (Berkeley: University of California, 1997), 5; Mark Roseman, *A Past in Hiding: Memory and Survival in Nazi Germany* (New York: Picador, 2000), 368–73.

5. Robins, *The Girl Who Died Twice*, 80.

6. "No Shock Here: Interns' Long Hours Cause Medical Errors," *USA Today*, November 10, 2004, 11A.

7. Robins, *The Girl Who Died Twice*, 174; "Docs Killed My Daughter—N.Y. Writer," *New York Post*, August 26, 1985, 4.

8. Robins, *The Girl Who Died Twice*, 233.

9. Ibid., 35.

10. Ibid., 185–89.

11. Stephen Brill, "Curing Doctors," *American Lawyer*, September 1985, 1, 12–17.

12. Robins, *The Girl Who Died Twice*, 266.

13. Ibid., 229.

14. On the Bell Commission regulations, see Howard W. French, "In Overhaul of Hospital Rules, New York Slashes Interns' Hours," *New York Times*, July 3, 1989, 1, 24. The legacy of the Bell Commission cannot be discussed in detail in this essay but it served as the template for recent nationwide reforms in medical education implemented by the Accreditation Council on Graduate Medical Education.

15. Although I argue that several stories emerged from the Zion case, I am not suggesting that all of the stories are equally plausible. It is simply beyond the scope of this essay to evaluate the various accounts. However, as I note later in the essay, Libby Zion's caretakers completely missed the fact that she was undergoing a serious deterioration. And then they chose not to acknowledge this point after the fact. In doing so, I believe that they erred twice, thus justifying Sidney Zion's fury. Thanks to Ted Marmor for pushing me on this point.

16. Louis J. Regan, *Doctor and Patient and the Law* (St. Louis: C. V. Mosby Company, 1956).

17. Linda T. Kohn, Janet M. Corrigan, and Molla S. Donaldson, eds., *To Err Is Human: Building a Safer Health System* (Washington, D.C.: National Academies Press, 1999).

18. Tom Wicker, "Blaming the System," *New York Times*, February 4, 1987, A27; Sidney Zion, "Doctors Know Best?" *New York Times*, May 13, 1989, 25.

19. Quoted in Robins, *The Girl Who Died Twice*, 300.

20. "Deadly Dosage: Who's at Fault?" *Court TV*, May 1995; Dennis Murphy, "A Father's Story," *Dateline NBC*, May 25, 1997, NBC News Transcripts.

21. Robins, *The Girl Who Died Twice*, 331–34.

22. See, for example, Lucian L. Leape, "Error in Medicine," *Journal of the American Medical Association* 272 (December 21, 1994): 1851–57; and Troyen A. Brennan and Michelle M. Mello, "Patient Safety and Medical Malpractice: A Case Study," *Annals of Internal Medicine* 139 (August 19, 2003): 267–73.

23. See Charles L. Bosk, "All Things Twice, First Tragedy, Then Farce," in this volume.

24. Harold Osborn used this phrase at the Zion trial to criticize what he believed was New York Hospital's pejorative attitude toward Libby Zion. See Robins, *The Girl Who Died Twice*, 323.

25. Barron H. Lerner, "Final Diagnosis: The Death of Eleanor Roosevelt," *Washington Post*, February 8, 2000, Health Section, 1, 12–17.

26. "Duke University Hospital Implements Additional Transplantation Safeguards," *Duke Medical News*, February 17, 2003.

27. Quoted in "Statement from Dr. James Jaggers Concerning Jesica Santillan," *Duke Medical News*, February 22, 2003.

28. Jerry Adler, "A Tragic Error," *Newsweek*, March 3, 2003, 20–25.

29. Quoted in "Duke University Hospital Implements." See also David Resnick, "The Jesica Santillan Tragedy: Lessons Learned," *Hastings Center Report* 33 (July–August 2003): 15–20.

30. Quoted in "Botched Transplants Lead to Brain Damage," *Windsor Star*, February 22, 2003, A1.

31. Quoted in Jeffrey Gettleman and Lawrence Altman, "Grave Diagnosis After 2nd Transplant," *New York Times*, February 22, 2003, A11.

32. "Jesica Santillan's Mother Claims Doctors Would Have Let Her Daughter Die If It Weren't for Media Attention," quoted on CNN's *Crossfire*, February 20, 2003.

33. William Fulkerson quoted in "Anatomy of a Mistake," on CBS's *60 Minutes*, March 16, 2003.

34. Sidney Zion, "Stop the Killing in Hospitals," *New York Daily News*, December 2, 1999, 12.

35. In my forthcoming book, *When Illness Goes Public*, to be published by Johns Hopkins University Press, I specifically discuss who was "right" and who was "wrong" in the Zion case.

36. David Greenberg, *Nixon's Shadow: The History of an Image* (New York: W. W. Norton, 2003), xxv.

ALL THINGS TWICE,

FIRST TRAGEDY THEN FARCE

LESSONS FROM A TRANSPLANT

ERROR

CHARLES L. BOSK

In a recent book on capital punishment, Scott Turow reversed his long-standing support for the practice. While the reasons to oppose capital punishment are numerous, there was one in Turow's brief that I found particularly intriguing. Celebrated cases, those that attract the public's attention because the crimes in question stand out as particularly loathsome instances of a hanging offense, those cases that most cry out for a guilty verdict and punishment by the death penalty as part of a collective stampede for retributive justice, are precisely those cases where errors occur most frequently. Fueled by public outrage and extensive media coverage, a network of actors, connected only by their shared desire to make certain that justice is neither delayed nor denied, collude, albeit unwittingly, to reach a hasty, foregone conclusion.

Police investigators discount evidence that points to other suspects or that exculpates the defendant. Prosecutors suppress evidence that they are required to share with the defendant's attorneys, suborn perjury, or otherwise overlook procedural rules that would normally be followed as a matter of course. Judges ignore past precedents in overcoming objections to the introduction or suppression of evidence or in providing instructions to jurors. Members of the jury, having witnessed a constricted adversarial contest, have little difficulty determining guilt and then settling upon the death penalty. Turow argues that public attention creates pressures that encourage mistaken judgments in those circumstances where their consequences are the gravest, least reversible, and most likely to undermine public faith in legal institutions once they come to light.

Celebrated cases of error in medicine are much like celebrated capital cases in law. There is a premature rush to judgment about what happened and why. As a consequence, as many of the contributors to this volume point out, our ability to learn from such events is limited by a number of factors: (1) our major source of data is repetitive media coverage of dubious accuracy and of uncertain relevance; (2) critical data from official inquiries is often "confidential"; results, presented in summary form, form the basis for new policies and procedures. However, without the ability to inspect the data, we are unable either to challenge the wisdom of "official" conclusions, to fashion alternatives to conventional wisdom explaining the case, or to determine which new vulnerabilities the newly adopted measures create; (3) the rush to restore public confidence and to provide reassurance in the face of what looks to be at first glance breathtaking incompetence or negligence stifles any efforts to acknowledge obdurately irreducible vulnerabilities, uncertainties, and limitations that are embedded in the provision of technologically complex care to desperately sick, brittle patients with multiple-system problems in a resource-constrained environment; and (4) multiple stakeholders have an interest in celebrated cases of medical error; they are not shy about using these cases to promote those agendas, however tangential they may be to the central issues raised by the case.

The Duke transplant error—"the case of Jesica Santillan"—illustrates how creative stakeholders are at transforming celebrated cases into vehicles for delivering issues to a mass audience. For example, stakeholders have used the transplant error as a dramatic example of the seriousness of and the need to control medical error; of anxieties about immigration; of the increasing coarseness of a market-driven, global economy that views body parts as just one more commodity to be bought and sold; of the disparities and inequalities within our chaotic health care system, both nationally and internationally; of the need for tort reform; of the difficulty distinguishing experimental from therapeutic interventions; and of the barriers to achieving a genuine informed consent when the patient is an adolescent.

The coarse opportunism of a crowded field of stakeholders makes it a certainty that celebrated cases of error provoke discussion in public arenas; but whether that discussion is productive is another question, one that is considerably more difficult to evaluate. The question of how to measure the efficacy of policies formulated in the wake of celebrated, spectacular errors in medicine is a vexing problem, its difficulty indexed, in part, by the general inattention paid to it. If we grant three propositions, the difficulties of assessment are more easily apprehended and appreciated. First, one of the things that makes a case celebrated is that it is a rare event, and oftentimes this rareness is indexed by the adjectives used as epithets to mark the event, terms such as "unprecedented," "unthinkable," or "previously unimaginable." Not much is needed in the way of preventive policy to keep improbable events that are so rare that they are unthinkable from recurring. Second, if we think of sustained attention in social organizations as a scarce resource, we might ask what new possibilities for mishaps are created when we redirect time, energy, and attention from their normal pathways to guard against the recurrence of the previously unrecognized, but now overappreciated, danger. Third, some of the errors we seek to eliminate can be avoided only by foregoing entirely the activity that generates the risk of error. To put this more bluntly, one of the first things that I was told when I was doing the fieldwork for my book *Forgive and Remember: Managing Medical Failure* was: "You can lead a long life without deaths and complications, you just have to give up major surgery to do so."[1] A medical care system committed to desperate measures to save patients will experience miscalculations on occasion since the variety of unexpected developments is likely to exceed the capacity of medical professionals to assess situations that require time-pressured decisions.

So, if celebrated cases of medical error do not provide a platform for reasoned discussion or sound policy, what are they good for? In Levi-Strauss's memorable words, celebrated cases are "good to think with." But if the discussion is not reasoned, if the policies are not sound, how and why are celebrated cases "good to think with"? Typically, analysts of culture focus on public debates, contested domains, or crises in group life to discover the codes, vocabularies, collective representations, or socially structured and shared "frames" within which meaning is created from experience. The occurrence of the celebrated case forces stakeholders to articulate normally tacit assumptions about how the world works here in this social space. In speaking the normally unspoken, in making the latent manifest or the implicit explicit, the sentiments and beliefs that veil structures of authority and support inequalities become visible.

At a collective level, public debates function just as sociologist Harold Garfinkel's "breaching" experiments worked at the micro-interactional level to display the implicit rules upon which social order rests.[2] The questioning of the previously unquestioned brings into view the taken for granted assumptions so fundamental to public life that their existence is revealed only at those moments when that order appears to become unhinged, when, as Yeats says, the center fails to hold and mere anarchy is loosed upon the world. Celebrated cases of medical error have this property; the illusion of shared values and interests breaks apart as different stakeholders vie in public arenas to forward that version of events that best protects their interests.

But if this were all that made celebrated cases of medical error good to think with, then a close analysis of either the circumstances that permitted their occurrence or the discourse they generated would be, if not trivial, unnecessary. We did not need the transplant error case to inform us that medical care is risky and that when that risk materializes as error, the consequences are grave. We hardly need a surgeon of great public renown practicing at one of the world's leading academic medical centers to transplant organs of the wrong blood type into an adolescent immigrant to inform us that there are what Everett Hughes called "rough edges" of medical practice: places where the expectations, interests, and evaluation of treatment by hospital officials, medical staff, and patients diverge.[3] Nor do we need a second, ultimately futile, transplant to inform us that there are tensions around how limited resources are allocated in American society and that some of these tensions revolve around the "entitlements" of indigent immigrants who enter the country "illegally" to perform low-wage labor. We did not need the medical error that befell Jesica Santillan to create awareness of anti-immigrant sentiment. Nor was the first or second transplant necessary for bringing into focus the inequities, disparities, and indignities embedded in a system of care that ensnares patients in the "biotechnical embrace."[4]

Moreover, the contribution of celebrated cases like Jesica Santillan's toward bringing the normally hidden into view is far from complete. What the media coverage of the mismatched donor-recipient transplant kept from public view is as striking as what the coverage revealed. For example, the opposition of lifesaving miracle versus life-stealing mistake was used to organize many of the initial reports of the tragedy. As more than a few of the contributors to this volume point out, there is a certain facile disingenuousness to this opposition. It is neither entirely false nor completely true. The proper opposition would be certain death without the transplant versus a highly uncertain outcome with the transplant, which, even if successful, involves a life circumscribed by many restrictions, intruded upon by much medical surveillance, and extended by the ingestion of a staggering amount of pharmaceuticals, all of which have potential nasty side effects of their own. As Carolyn Rouse's essay in this volume points out, Jesica Santillan's status as an adolescent, a few months short of her majority, was also hidden from view by media accounts that depicted her as a "child" or an "angel." The fact of her status as an adolescent is not insignificant given the demands of the medical regime that she would have needed to follow in order for the transplant to succeed. Depiction of the burdens, restrictions, and uncertainties of living with a transplanted heart are rare; one exception is Michael Connelly's fictional depiction of FBI profiler Terry MaCaleb. Finally, the media kept the more controlling, lord of manor treatment that Mack Mahoney, Jessica's benefactor, visited upon the Santillan family out of view, favoring instead a narrative featuring him as a humble David facing down the medical Goliath, Duke, with no more than the slingshot of his moral outrage.[5]

Celebrated cases are not merely hooks on which various stray contentions of social life can be hung willy-nilly in neat little media packages, even though various stakeholders enlist them for this purpose, and even if, once enlisted, they are so useful for this purpose.[6] Celebrated cases are windows, prisms, or distorting mirrors that allow us an opportunity to interpret ourselves to ourselves. They are certainly useful for this purpose, provided that we remember to ask why this case so captured the public imagination and that we also remind ourselves that we hardly lack other opportunities for reflexive self-examination. A celebrated case such as Jesica Santillan's has another use as well: an analysis of where we choose to rest our inquiry into the case obscures or magnifies some of the internal contradictions that stakeholders must reconcile in order to preserve both the policies that claim to further the goal of patient safety and the worldviews, paradigms, gestalts, or belief systems upon which these policies rest.

For those interested in the issues that surround the domain of medical error and patient safety, the transplanting of mismatched organs into Jesica Santillan brings into focus some of the necessary fictions, self-delusions, and evasions of obdurate empirical reality that are necessary to sustain the belief that we know how to minimize risk, prevent error, and achieve safety in a domain as contingent, risky, technologically complex, resource-constrained, and organizationally varied as medical care in tertiary-care academic centers. In this essay, I use the case of Jesica Santillan to examine some of the social, legal, and cultural difficulties created when attempting to understand one celebrated case of medical error in the "systems" terms that policy reformers and system managers have favored since the release in fall 1999 of the Institute of Medicine's highly publicized report on medical error.[7] I focus on the difference between theoretical understandings of how errors are produced in systems and practical uses of the term "systems error" in public arenas. My analysis of the transplant error will not pay close attention to the patient's age, gender, ethnicity, citizenship, or insurance status as factors that contributed to the mistake. My concern is to understand how this mistake was understood at the time and to make sense of the steps taken by the Organ Procurement Organizations (OPOS) and Duke to reassure the public that "the causes" of this error had been discovered and fixed.

My analysis focuses on how certain words are used in interaction to serve organizational goals. At some point, especially in a social system undergoing a public relations crisis based on a human error that had a tragic outcome for an innocent child, organizational actors seeking to control events and the words used to describe them find those words appropriated by others who now shape them to fit their definition of the situation and their interests. The struggle to understand what happened, allocate responsibility, and fix blame is a highly charged one that is not played out on a level playing field. Duke's theoretical expertise, its organizational resources, and its community standing gave hospital officials greater access to the media, which, in turn, allowed them to take a fluid, amorphous set of possibilities and narrow them into an overly determined orderliness and clarity that made sense of just how a mistake of this magnitude could have happened. Further, the version of what happened that officials at Duke put forward aligns well with the latest thinking of policy experts on how errors are first avoided and then managed.

Three struggles over definition illustrate how the raw event of a horrible mistake was cooked into a pudding of public understanding that contained all the best policy options for minimizing the occurrence, and certainly the reoccurrence, of error. First is the set of difficulties inherent in defining a complexly coordinated system for the collection and distribution of organs for transplantation that spans multiple organizations across a broad geographic region, as well as in demarcating the boundaries of that system. Next are the issues involved in allocating responsibility and blame. Tensions are created by disjunctures between a systems perspective on the error, on the one hand, and a surgeon's understanding of professional responsibility, the workings of the malpractice system, and the cultural schemas of accountability, on the other. Lastly are the fictions we circulate to suggest that sources of error have been isolated and fixed, in particular, the idea that the performance of a root cause analysis identifies adequately the sources of the failure and provides the requisite wisdom to design procedures that assure such a mistake will not recur in the future.

In short, this celebrated case is "good to think with," not just because it reveals division among stakeholders with different positions and interests, but also because it reveals contradictions, inconsistencies, and gaps within the thinking of individual stakeholders—in this case, the hospital administrators at Duke—who claim pride in the way their institution has transformed such a terrible tragedy into a "learning opportunity." The fact that administrators make such claims is hardly surprising. However, the fact that we do not subject such claims to a more severe scrutiny is baffling. After a brief review of the basic elements of a "systems error" perspective for limiting the number of medical errors, or as they are now labeled, "preventable adverse events," the following provides a skeptical look at the claim that Duke's management of the error once it occurred was a model for other institutions to follow.

SYSTEMS THEORY: A NEW PARADIGM FOR
UNDERSTANDING AND REDUCING MEDICAL ERROR

The mismatched heart-lung transplant is commonly referred to as a "systems error." Such a characterization is, in part, descriptive and, in part, ideological. I do not mean to imply that "systems error" is an inaccurate descriptive term, a marker of a distorted or incorrect system of belief. Rather, I mean to emphasize that such a description has action implications. Systems errors require a set of policies that are different from those required if medical mistakes are understood as flowing from individual failures. Descriptive accuracy is not at issue here. One can build a case that all medical errors are systems errors. One can also build a case that all errors are the result of individuals making misjudgments. The choice between the terms "systems error" and "individual misjudgment" is as much political as it is empirical. Either term contains a metaphor about how the world is broken and how it is best fixed.[8]

Descriptively, the theory of systems error denotes one way that complex technological systems have "normal accidents" or errors built into the production process.[9] In this view, complex technologies are characterized by two features—tight-coupling and complexity. In such production systems, small deviations from normal performance standards that at the time go either unnoticed or are assumed innocent combine in unanticipated ways to produce disastrous error. No single deviation "caused" the problem; rather, it is the combination of small variations from standard operational norms that produces a negative outcome of unexpected magnitude, that when reviewed with all the wisdom that knowing the outcome provides, gets labeled as error.

Charles Perrow labels the accidents produced by tightly coupled production processes characterized by complex interactions as "normal" because such errors are built into the social organization of the production process itself. For Perrow, "normal" is a comment on inevitability—we know that production processes marked by tight coupling and complexity will produce stochastically a number of failures. What we cannot predict is either how frequently these normal errors will occur or how disastrous they will be when they do occur. Safety or warning systems that alert operators to impending disaster do not offer much hope for averting disaster in the operation of high-risk technological systems, according to Perrow. Warning systems simply add to the tight-coupling and complexity of the system; they are as likely as any other component of the system to malfunction, creating in the process a false sense of impending doom or reassurance.

A homely example of how warning systems fail to provide intended benefits is familiar to anyone with a kitchen on the first floor, a smoke detector on the second floor of a two-story house, and a fondness for cooking food in a wok. The very act of placing food in oil sufficiently hot for proper stir-frying generates enough smoke to create frequent false alarms. Aware of the frequency of false positives, system operators learn to ignore them. Skillful operators with foresight disable the smoke detectors before cooking. This work-around of an overly sensitive alarm system creates a new vulnerability. After the meal is consumed, the sated chef needs to remember to reconnect the smoke detector before going to bed. The problem cannot be solved by setting the tolerance for alarm higher. While a higher threshold for triggering alarm eliminates false positives, it also presumably misses some false negatives. False negatives or real causes for alarm are dangerous conditions that require a response.

Perrow is a thoroughgoing pessimist about human operators' ability to manage safely complex and risky technologies; for him, there are no limits to human imperfection; fail-safe or foolproof systems are unimaginable—the cleverness and ingenious perversity of fools easily outstrips the imaginative rationality of any system designer or engineer. However, there are a group of organizational theorists who believe that the tightly coupled, complex, technological work environments that Perrow describes can be safely operated. These researchers note that a number of high-risk technologies are operated without the baleful consequences that Perrow predicts. These researchers identify the characteristics of highly reliable organizations. Based upon observations on the flight deck of nuclear-powered aircraft carriers during training exercises, the characteristics these researchers identify include: task overlap and redundancy, a dense oral culture in which experienced personnel communicate dangers and pitfalls to neophytes through narratives of past accidents or close calls, and a command structure in which authority is dispersed and not dependent upon rank.[10]

Culture-of-safety advocates within medicine favor the optimism of high-reliability organizational theorists rather than the pessimism of Perrow's "normal accident" view of the world. This is not surprising. Perrow's is a counsel of despair. He suggests that the best we can do is possess the wisdom to reject those technologies whose potential for catastrophe is such that we should not accept risks of these sorts. Not only is this a counsel of despair, it has the further defect of being an unrealistic one. Perrow seems to ignore that the political mechanism through which risky technologies are rejected does not exist. He presumes further that the adoption of technology is a normative decision made through a political process rather than an economic one made in a private commercial organization.

That much said, there are a number of features of high-reliability theory that ought to temper the enthusiasm of safety advocates in medicine for this approach. First, high-reliability theorists observe the military, where, they note without irony, production costs are not a factor. They admit that their theories are silent when it comes to organizations where costs are a factor. Second, they note that their observations only apply to the situation of train-ing: "in the fog of war," all bets are off. The emergencies that characterize the tertiary-care academic center are more like those in "the fog of war" than those in a training exercise. Third, the theorists do not note, even though this is of more than trivial consequence, that the military has a device of social control that is not available in civil society—the court martial—for those of lower rank whose compliance with rules and procedures is spotty.

To say that the transplantation of mismatched organs was a "systems error" describes nicely an error that could have been averted had any actor in a long chain of actors asked at any time about blood compatibility. But the designation "systems error" is not merely descriptive; it signals as well a paradigm shift within medicine about the proper way to reduce adverse events and provide safe care. This paradigm shift is captured both in the subtitle of the Institute of Medicine's report on medical error, "*Building a Safer Health System,*" and the rhetoric of the report calling for policy change. The Institute of Medicine report seeks to reform a professional culture that deals with error in a dysfunctional manner. The report claims that inflated notions of individual responsibility that associate adverse outcomes with per-sonal shortcomings; responses to error that focus on naming, shaming, blaming individuals; and a working environment that refuses to discuss the underlying structural factors that contribute to mistaken action—all these are characteristics of the professional culture of medicine that require change.

Understanding preventable adverse events as "systems error" marks the change necessary to produce more productive responses to error. In a sys-tems perspective, error is not the result of individual negligence, incompe-tence, or momentary lapses: mistakes are viewed instead as a property of poorly designed systems that fail to anticipate sources of error and that fail to build in mechanisms for correction. As Cook and Woods have argued, human error is never the proper explanation or resting point of an inquiry that seeks to understand why a mishap occurred.[11] Rather, it serves only as a starting point, a place where discussion begins. We should seek to understand how a system was designed so that a competent, well-intended individual was permitted or not prevented from making a mistake. Finally, when actions go awry despite the best intentions of everyone involved, when individual slips, lapses, glitches, and loss of focus present openings for errors to occur, a well-designed system provides buffers to mitigate all-too-human fallibility. Well-designed systems that place a premium on safety and reliability are those that allow operators to "fail gracefully."

The term "systems error" not only describes how preventable adverse events occur; it also recommends a strategy for reducing these untoward outcomes. The first move in this strategic shift to a systems perspective is summarized by the renaming of errors as "preventable adverse events." In the longer, second term, there is an attempt to scrub from the language any suggestion of either culpability or agency: preventable by whom? The core of this strategy for error reduction is reducible to four propositions. The first we have already belabored: Errors are better understood as a traceable chain of multiple small missteps and miscalculations that add up to a large disastrous outcome rather than as the result of one actor's willful evil, carelessness, negligence, or incompetence. Even if actors are negligent or incompetent, error is never solely the result of individual agency. Properly designed systems anticipate the failings, predictable or not, occasional or recurrent, of individuals and create buffers that defend against ordinary human shortcomings. System designers recognize that "to err is human," and they design work processes accordingly.

Second, organizational cultures need to create conditions that reward the reporting of those latent defects that lead to error. What is needed is a "blame-free" environment that fosters supportive and corrective responses to error. A third element in the ideology of "systems error" is a faith in reporting systems with mandatory and voluntary elements. Only with full reporting of latent defects can systems make the continual adjustments that a culture of safety requires. The faith in robust reporting systems has a logical plausibility that elides the difficulties of designing a reporting system that works. Difficulties include decisions about what incidents to report, what form reports should take, who receives reporting data, how such data is aggregated, how the data is interpreted, and how the digested data is fed back to frontline workers. The difficulties are both theoretic and practical. In a resource-constrained work environment, how do we calculate the benefits of reporting systems against their cost in terms of effort that could provide direct care to patients?

Reporting systems that spot dangerous conditions before disaster occurs and nonpunitive environments go hand in hand. The final element in the ideology of "systems error" is a response to incidents that first demands a root cause analysis and then provides a set of proposals that typically include a triad of recommendations whose generality is as comforting to administrators in need of a concrete plan as it is maddening to clinical personnel who have to implement them. The triad of recommendations typically includes better administrative procedures, upgrades in the quality of personnel through more comprehensive training, and better technologies. Cook and Woods have pointed out that the danger exists that each response to error has the potential unintended consequence of creating a system that, rather than safer, is more rule-bound, less responsive to emerging, unanticipated contingencies, more brittle, and hence more vulnerable to threats.[12] While others might add or subtract a proposition from this short list of what I have labeled as the ideology of "systems error," the general point remains: "systems error" is more than a descriptive term; it is pregnant with policy implications—it advocates specific actions and suggests refraining from others.

SYSTEMS AND BOUNDARIES

The mismatched heart-lung transplant is quite accurately described as a systems error; but doing so creates as many problems as it solves. What is the system that produced the mismatched heart-lung transplant? System is an analytic construction—not what philosopher's call a naturally occurring "kind." In the heart-lung transplant mismatch, we have a number of interacting organizations that comprise a system of exchange: there is the institution from which the donated organ is procured, there is the organ procurement organization, and there is the recipient organization, in this case, Duke University. There are miscommunications at multiple points in the chain; there are multiple handoffs, always a point where muffs and miscues can occur. Yet almost all media accounts refer to the "Duke transplantation error" when describing what happened. If this was a systems error, why not refer to it as "Carolina Donor Services–Duke botched transplant"? After all, Richard Cook's reconstruction in this book of the chain of events that constituted the systems error reports that Carolina Donor Services, when calling UNOS to check on Jesica Santillan's status, reported her blood type incorrectly as A. The donated organs were transported in a container that was not marked as regulations require. The significance of this failure to comply with the rules that govern transfers was dismissed with a curious explanation—this was a rule that was so frequently breached that it was not a noteworthy breach of regulation.

This dismissal of the significance of the unmarked container and the more general silence about the misspelling of Jesica Santillan's name or the mis-reporting of her blood type by Carolina Donor Services raise issues about the way the transplant error both occurred and was understood to have occurred. First, performance studies of airline crews suggest that those teams that ignore small-rule breaches are precisely the ones that are most likely to commit serious and risky breaches of procedures. So in a medical community recently alerted to the omnipresence of systems error that has adopted the airlines as an industrial model for achieving safety, the dismissal of small breaches as insignificant is curious. Second, the conclusion that the failure to label the container had no impact upon the outcome of the event is surely correct, but it is not trivial on that account. The unlabeled container raises the issue of temporal sequencing in the error. In Cook's reconstruction, the chartered plane is sitting on a runway being de-iced as Jesica Santillan is being wheeled into an operating room to have her heart and lungs removed. At some point in the sequence, the unasked question about the blood type of the donor changed from a correctable omission into an irrevocable error. This moment when a latent system defect becomes manifest, causing irreversible error, is hard to pinpoint exactly. What seems more certain is that although the un-asked question was part of an interaction, responsibility for the omission does not rest equally on the parties in that interaction; by all accounts, it rests with the transplanting surgeon, Dr. Jaggers. While the transplant surgeon surely should have checked on compatibility at some point, the assumption that the heart and lungs would not be offered his patient unless there was a match was not unreasonable. Surely the miscommunication to UNOS by Carolina Donor Services and the failure to label the container did not provide the system an opportunity to recover from Dr. Jaggers's failure to perform the required check on compatibility. Moreover, all of these little gaffes, when taken together, indicate that considerable "practical drift" had occurred within the procedures and policies designed to produce safety and reliability.[13]

Despite the fact that multiple organizations collaborated in the failure, Carolina Donor Services drops out of accounts of the mistake quite quickly. The system is truncated and the mistake quickly becomes "the Duke trans-plant mismatch." Cook's essay suggests a number of reasons for this. There is intense competition among transplant centers and surgeons for scarce organs. Little is to be gained by Duke from drawing its local OPO into a debate about accountability. Institutional interests here suggest that the most prudent course is to shield Carolina Donor Services from criticism and accountability. Beyond the necessity of Duke sustaining its good relations with its local OPO, there is also some urgency to protect the reputation of the network of OPOS more generally. Any criticism of OPOS that suggest they contribute to the misallocation of organs has the very real possibility of making the acute shortage of organs suitable for transplantation worse by providing potential donors one more reason not to participate in organ donations.

The point here is that it is one thing to recognize that most, if not all, errors are systems errors and another thing to act on the implications of that knowledge. In addition, those implications are co-extensive with construction of the system and its boundaries. Systems can be constructed in constricted or expansive ways. The construction of the system and its boundaries determines accountability, has economic consequences when legal liability from error is at issue, and may reflect political realities as much as empirical ones. Since the boundaries of the system provide a shield from or exposure to accountability, labeling the care of Jesica Santillan the "botched Duke transplant case," thereby limiting the system (and consequently, the error) to Duke, speaks volumes about the politics of organ procurement and transplantation.

THE ALLOCATION OF BLAME

In the Institute of Medicine Report, systems error as the primary explanation for error is meant to displace inflated notions of individual, professional responsibility that are said to inhibit productive approaches for responding to mistakes. In the mismatched heart-lung transplant, there is considerable confusion about what it means to call an error a "systems problem." In the *Duke Med News* of February 17, Dr. William Fulkerson, the CEO of Duke hospital states, "This was a tragic error and we accept responsibility for our part." Two days later, he is quoted in the same publication as saying, "It is clear to us at Duke that we need to have more robust processes internally and a better understanding of all partners involved in the organ procurement process." There is, in this statement, a curious fatuousness. When a "preventable" error occurs, then, by definition, the policies and procedures in place were not robust enough to prevent it.

There is also a curious blindness. If the policies and procedures in place were not followed, as they were not in this case, then the failure can hardly be blamed on the regulatory framework. A set of policies and procedures that are not followed can never be robust. The failure to follow procedures is, from one point of view, a failure at the managerial level. However, Dr. Fulkerson does not say, "As CEO, I failed to convey to all at Duke the importance of following our policies and procedures in order for us to achieve our goal of creating a genuine culture of safety."

But Fulkerson is CEO of an institution that is facing unknown liability from a very public error, so he is not shy about laying responsibility at the transplant surgeon's feet. He told the local NBC affiliate that "one problem [leading to the error] was the assumption by the surgeon that when he gave the name to the agency to get the organs that there had been a confirmation of a match." Fulkerson goes on to state, in case anyone missed the point, that it was "the transplant surgeon's responsibility to verbally confirm that the organs were compatible and, in this case, this obviously did not happen." Fulkerson's operational definition of systems error appears quite limited. First, he states that Duke accepts its responsibility for the error. He then discharges that institutional responsibility by publicly blaming Dr. Jaggers for the mistake on every opportunity that presents itself. A month later on the CBS's *Sixty Minutes,* Dr. Jaggers's colleague Dr. Duane Davis answers a question about the nature of the error by stating that "absolutely" the error involved is one of both individual error and systems error. After this judgment, Dr. Davis repeats that checking blood compatibility should be "routine." He clearly faults Dr. Jaggers for not doing so. It becomes difficult to see exactly what the various representatives of Duke mean when they say the institution accepts its part in the error. There is some talk about a lack of redundancy, but this is quickly followed by pointing out Dr. Jaggers's omission of what ought to have been the most reflexive, automatic check.

For his part, Jaggers accepts the responsibility for the systems error that others keep thrusting upon him. It is not hard to see why he does so. His first public statement invokes the "captain of the ship doctrine." As the leader of the team, Dr. Jaggers believes that the responsibility for anything that happens to his patient is his responsibility. His entire training has ingrained in Jaggers the belief that what it means to be an honorable surgeon is to stand up and accept responsibility for mistakes.[14] In the narrative of the transplant error, viewed from the perspective of the collegium of physicians, Jaggers's statements are the most heartfelt and anguished. He describes the moment he is notified of the mistake as "like the experience of death." He describes going over and over events, trying to rework them, struggling to understand how he never asked about blood compatibility. His revisiting the event, his replaying of the disaster, has the feel of post-traumatic distress. Dr. Jaggers's revisiting the error over and over again to ask himself how this error occurred and how such errors can be avoided in the future is part of how surgeons are trained to think about unexpected negative outcomes. Improvement in performance is said to result from such reviews.

At issue here is not who is to blame, but where responsibility actually rests. In this case, there is more than enough blame to go around. In any case, the allocation of blame is more a political matter and less an objective one. The larger point here is how quickly a paradigm of error that claims mistakes are produced in systems and that correction and healthy responses lie in creating a blame-free environment crumbles when stressed. Even as administrators at Duke acknowledge that the transplantation of mismatched organs was a "systems error," they still place the blame on a single individual, Dr. Jaggers. At the very least, this recurrent pattern of explanation, labeling the problem a systems error while identifying an individual culprit indicates that a systems error perspective is easier to invoke than apply. But there is more involved than legal liability or an institutional responsibility. Also involved are cultural schemas that demand individual responsibility. If instead of a medical miracle what we have is medical murder, as the more anguished statements of representatives of the family suggest, then we need a guilty party to hang. This role falls to Jaggers for many reasons. Our cultural scripts require that individuals pay for the errors they commit. What is striking is how easily a commitment to the policies upon which a culture of safety are premised crumble when an organization is confronted with the pressures a celebrated case creates. As soon as policies prove to be costly or difficult to institute they are abandoned. Operationally, administrators at Duke claim to respond one way, praising their institution's response as a model for creating a culture of safety, but then they do not hesitate to "name, shame, and blame" Dr. Jaggers.

THE FICTION OF ROOT CAUSE ANALYSIS AND CORRECTIVE PROCEDURES

The administrators at Duke make the claim that the error occurred because the procedures of the institution were not "robust"; one indicia of this lack of robustness was inadequate redundancy. The official statements from the administration at Duke are reassuring: a root cause analysis has been preformed. The analysis uncovered not only the source of the error in the transplant but also the system defects that had the potential to cause error (although they had not yet done so). New procedures were adopted; these new procedures require both multiple confirmations of donor match by members of the care team before the transplantation begins and improved communications between the transplant team and the organ procurement organization. Additionally, the OPO network does not permit transplant surgeons to request organs for patients not listed as potential recipients.

There is some likelihood that these measures will appear to be successful. After all, a mismatched heart-lung transplant had not occurred at Duke before the Santillan case; repetition of the same rare mistake in a rare procedure in an institution on guard against the possibility of just this error is presumably remote. The absence of repetition of the same mistake, however, is not easily attributed to Duke's root cause analysis or the new procedures.

The term "root cause analysis" to describe the inquiry into the error is unfortunate. Any analysis is, of course, preferable to none. But calling an inquiry a "root cause analysis" suggests somehow that the investigation has gotten to the bottom of things. The designation of the analysis as having identified the "root cause" induces complacency about safety. It suggests that safety is produced and errors are avoided by rules and procedures rather than the constant vigilance and adjustments of operators in complex technological situations. Beyond this concern is another: the political structure of institutions surely impacts the scope of root cause analysis. There are presumably limits to the inquiry that all but the most socially inept recognize. Further, the announcement that Duke's attempt to achieve quality is guided by an industrial model known as *Six Sigma* that is used at General Motors and Ford Motor Company is hardly reassuring. It is somewhat mysterious why, at a time when the products of American automakers are said to be not competitive with their Japanese counterparts because of poor quality control, Duke administrators would call attention to their following the managerial lead of these companies.

Finally, there is some reason to be skeptical that the new procedures will fix the system problems that led to the transplant error. There were procedures in place when the mismatch took place; a variety of situational pressures led workers to evade these procedures. The new policies do not remove these situational pressures. In fact, to the degree that the new procedures take time and to the degree that time is a scarce resource that can ill afford to be wasted during transplantation, there is every reason to suspect that frontline workers will find ways to work around the new policies in order to complete tasks. It is possible that the new procedures increase safety. It is possible that they will serve to protect future transplant patients. However, it is equally possible that those afforded the most protection by the new policies are the administrators of Duke Hospital. Now, in the unlikely event that a transplant error recurs, administrators can point to the policies and procedures that were violated. These policies and procedures may have the consequence of making it impossible for workers to complete their tasks.

Larry Hirschorn indicates that this was the case in the nuclear power industry following the incident at Three Mile Island.[15] Scholar Scott Snook suggests that there is a "practical drift" in organizations as workers adapt to conditions on the ground and develop work-arounds that allow them to do their work while evading policies that make little sense in the environment in which work needs to be done.[16] In organizations that have multiple inter-linked components, the drift that occurs without communication or coordination sets the grounds for spectacular failures.

But these same new more muscular policies and procedures have the benefit of being a resource for upper-level management when mistakes occur. The leaders of the organization can simply point to the policies and procedures that were evaded and promise to deal harshly with workers who violated rules, all the while knowing that rule evasion is a necessity if work is to be done. At the end of the day, a culture of safety is created. Unfortunately, a culture of safety implemented in this manner protects administrators, not patients.

CELEBRATED ERROR AND THE RITUAL SYMBOLISM OF REFORM

This analysis suggests that the term "systems error" was deployed in the Santillan case in ways that are contradictory to behold. On the one hand, officials at Duke suggest that the mismatch occurred because policies and procedures were either evaded or lacked the robustness to prevent the error. On the other hand, whenever the opportunity presents itself, these same officials fault Dr. Jaggers for his failure to perform the most routine of checks —the systems error lay in the carelessness of a single individual operator. At the same time, Dr. Jaggers accepts the responsibility and blame being thrust upon him. Dr. Jaggers received his training before surgeons or physicians in any specialty were schooled in the language of systems errors. For Jaggers and his peers, the success or failure of the procedures they performed, the recovery or demise of their patients, was based solely on how they discharged their fiduciary responsibilities, on how much they were willing to sacrifice of themselves for their patients, and on how much they instilled in their team the same sense of duty that they possessed themselves. To lay failure at the feet of the system is, for surgeons schooled as Jaggers has been, unthinkable. To blame the system is the type of dishonorable behavior that causes a surgeon to lose the respect of peers.

So what we have is administrators claiming that the system is at fault while they name, blame, and shame the surgeon whose behavior is said to be the systems error—a repertoire of behaviors that model precisely that dysfunctional response to error that a system perspective seeks to remedy. This response that is so at odds with the systems error perspective is justified in terms of that model. The contradiction between what officials at Duke say they are doing and what they actually do is easy to overlook, if only because Dr. Jaggers's mistake is so obvious and blaming him is so consistent with cultural notions of accountability.

In a way, the confused, contradictory response of officials at Duke is understandable, for the choice between systems error and individual professional responsibility is the classic false dichotomy. The transplantation of mismatched organs is best understood as both a systems error and an individual error. But what are we to make of the claim that new policies and procedures will create a safer system and will protect against errors of this type in the future? Clearly, I do not share the same faith in rules and regulations that the officials at Duke or the policy experts who believe that system re-engineering creates safety possess.

In part, my skepticism rests on the fact that safety is not achieved by thickening the rule book. To achieve safety, given the complexity, resource constraints, chaotic diversity, and brittleness of a health care system forced to operate constantly at the very edge of its capacity, attitudes of humility, respect, and wisdom need to be cultivated among workers at all levels in the system. Arid proceduralism that fixes the last error and that closes the barn door after that horse has left the stable is unlikely to be productive. An overly detailed response to the rare error diverts attentional resources in ways that create new vulnerabilities and new opportunities for error. Beyond that, the place that I would anticipate new procedures to protect against just this error is among the transplant community at Duke. If they are capable of learning from experience, the lessons from this mistake are seared into their consciences and whatever there is of collective organizational memory. If they are incapable of learning from experience, then new policies or procedures, no matter how robust, are unlikely to have much impact. Further, creating overly specific procedures rather than modeling general principles does not guard against other forms of systems error, as officials at Duke learned when they discovered in late 2004 that equipment used in procedures involving approximately 3,800 patients had been washed in hydraulic fluid.

If this analysis is correct, if Duke was the last place in the world that we would expect a repetition of an error that involved not matching, then checking again in all the obsessive ways that we would expect the once burned to be twice cautious, how do we explain the fanfare with which new policies and procedures were announced? The detailed nature of the procedures and the public nature of their announcement serves as a symbolic way for the institution to demonstrate how seriously it takes its commitments to patient safety. The new policies and procedures have the look of an instrumental set of actions, but they have the feel of expressive behavior. By making public what they intend to do to make certain that no patient in the future suffers the same fate as Jesica Santillan, the officials at Duke are acting out a public ritual of apology, contrition, and remediation. The ritual of "putting on the hair shirt" that marked the private occupational ritual of the Mortality and Morbidity Conference has moved into a more public arena.[17] This somehow seems only fitting. As medical mistakes come into public view, the ritualized form of apology becomes a stylized public ritual as well. As in the Mortality and Morbidity Conference, in the new public ritual, actors accept responsibility for error, point out lessons this sad experience has taught them, and detail the steps necessary so that others are able to avoid just such errors in the future.

NOTES

1. Charles L. Bosk, *Forgive and Remember: Managing Medical Failure* (Chicago: University of Chicago Press, 2003).

2. Harold Garfinkel, *Studies in Ethnomethodology* (Englewood Cliffs, N.J.: Prentice-Hall, 1967).

3. Everett C. Hughes, "Mistakes at Work," in *The Sociological Eye: Selected Papers on Work, Self, and Society* (Chicago: Aldine-Atherton, 1971).

4. Mary-Jo Delvecchio Good, "The Biotechnical Embrace," *Culture, Medicine, and Psychiatry* 25 (4) (December 2001): 395–410.

5. Michael Connelly, *Blood Work* (New York, N.Y.: Warner Books, 1998); Michael Connelly, *The Narrows* (New York, N.Y.: Little, Brown, 2004).

6. Joel Best, *Threatened Children: Rhetoric and Concern about Child-Victims* (Chicago: University of Chicago Press, 1990); William A. Gamson and Andre Modigliani, "Media Discourse and Public Opinion on Nuclear Power: A Constructionist Approach," *American Journal of Sociology* 95 (July 1989): 1–37; Stephen Hilgartner and Charles L. Bosk, "The Rise and Fall of Social Problems: A Public Arenas Model," *American Journal of Sociology* 94 (July 1988): 53–78.

7. Linda T. Kohn, Janet M. Corrigan, and Molla S. Donaldson, eds., *To Err Is Human: Building a Safer Health System* (Washington D.C.: National Academy Press, 2000).

8. Clifford Geertz, "Ideology as a Cultural System," in *The Interpretation of Culture* (New York: Basic Books, 1977).

9. Charles Perrow, *Normal Accidents: Living with High Risk Technologies* (Princeton: Princeton University Press, 1984).

10. Karlene H. Roberts, "Some Characteristics of One Type of High Reliability Organization," *Organization Science* 1 (1990): 160–76; Karl E. Weick, "Organizational Culture as a Source of High Reliability," *California Management Review* 29 (1987): 112–27; Karl E. Weick and Karlene H. Roberts, "Collective Mind in Organizations: Heedful Interrelating on Flight Decks," *Administrative Science Quarterly* 38 (1993): 357–81.

11. Richard Cook and David Woods, "Operating at the Sharp End: The Complexity of Human Error," in *Human Error in Medicine*, ed. M. Bogner (Hillsdale, N.J.: Lawrence Erlbaum, 1994), 255–309.

12. Ibid.

13. Scott A. Snook, *Friendly Fire: The Accidental Shootdown of U.S. Black Hawks over Northern Iraq* (Princeton: Princeton University Press, 2000).

14. Charles L. Bosk, *Forgive and Remember: Managing Medical Failure* (Chicago: University of Chicago Press, 2003).

15. Larry Hirschorn, "Hierarchy vs. Bureaucracy: The Case of a Nuclear Reactor," in *New Challenges to Understanding Organization*, ed. by K. Roberts (Cambridge, Mass.: MIT Press, 1993), 137–49.

16. Snook, *Friendly Fire.*

17. Bosk, *Forgive and Remember*, 121–22.

JUSTICE AND SECOND CHANCES ACROSS THE BORDER

2

THE POLITICS OF SECOND CHANCES

WASTE, FUTILITY, AND THE DEBATE
OVER JESICA'S SECOND TRANSPLANT

KEITH WAILOO AND JULIE LIVINGSTON

In the days after the surgery, Jesica Santillan's second heart and lung transplant on February 21, 2003, became a flashpoint of controversy that helped generate a wide range of conflicting fictions, fantasies, and moral meanings. Two weeks after Jesica had received the first transplant with mismatched blood type organs, this second operation, much more than the first, marked a compelling turning point in the public discussion of the Santillan saga. As in so many transplant stories, her first operation had created enormous hope. How lucky she was to rise to the top of the list, suddenly to receive this long-awaited gift from another's misfortune. In the moments after that first operation, hope and anxiety turned to shock and despair. Within hours, the Santillan story was transformed into a case study in medical error—offering insight into a larger but often hidden problem in contemporary medicine. And then the second transplant occurred, and the meanings of the story compounded yet further. To many it seemed a risky proposition from the start, one that raised many questions—how were new organs found so quickly, was she really in a position to benefit from a second operation, and what were the priorities and methods for allocating resources in the transplant system that had made her so fortunate not once, but twice? The hastily arranged second transplant moved the Santillan story into ethically, socially, and politically problematic terrain for both professional and lay observers alike.

It was here, in the debates about the second transplant, that the moral fervor surrounding Jesica's story became elevated. For many observers, the second transplant brought the key issues of the case together: the problem of immigration, questions about the allocation of scarce resources, the proper remedies for medical error, the nature of malpractice and goals of tort reform, and the Janus-face of high-tech medicine. All these complex issues played off of one another as the public and professionals alike debated the second transplant.

It was not, of course, that second transplants were rare. Quite the contrary, life with a transplanted organ was unpredictable, and many transplant patients would experience second or sometimes even third or fourth transplants at some point down the line. Despite these realities of recurrent transplants, it is noteworthy that the fact of a second Santillan operation—coming so soon after the first—stirred intensely strong feelings. Implications of wrongdoing permeated the case. Were the surgeons or Duke (embarrassed by their mistake) responsible for getting Jesica special consideration, maneuvering her to the front of the queue so that she could obtain this second set of precious organs? Even in the transplant and ethics communities, there was debate about the wisdom of a second transplant. Did it represent Duke's commitment to do everything possible to save a patient? Or was it the epitome of scandalous double-dipping compounded by the extraordinary waste of a precious gift of life?[1]

The Santillan second transplant struck a nerve with many people, tapping into divisive views about American high-tech medicine. For many, the case was an irresistible opportunity to frame public and professional understanding about various crises in contemporary American medicine. Some portrayed the second transplant as futile, others as understandable and indeed justified given the gravity of the error, others as simply a waste of not one but three precious organs—a heart and two lungs. Many barely submerged concerns about the direction of American medicine and the commodification of body parts came to the surface of public debate. A story that had taken shape as one of "surgical expertise, undone by error" became a troubling tale about the waste of valuable resources in high-technology medicine, about the problem of futile interventions, and about fairness—who received, who gave, and who was locked out—in the allocation of putatively lifesaving organs.[2] Though these two operations followed one another in rapid succession, the meanings of the second transplant were dramatically different than those of the first; and it is instructive to ponder what these meanings tell us about the moral economy of modern health care.

ORGANS IN A ZERO-SUM SOCIETY

As one *Newsweek* article suggested shortly after Jesica's death, many Americans took an almost personal stake in the story. But it was the second transplant that generated particularly intense animus. "In Ontario, California," noted the article, "a 28-year-old woman named Luba Kobzeff watched the tragedy unfold in North Carolina with a distinct sense that Jesica may have gotten the second chance she [Kobzeff] deserved instead." Many Americans, both outside the transplant system and within it, saw little reason why Jesica should have had this "second chance." For Kobzeff, life on the organ waiting list with its own frustrations and fears gave the case special meaning. "I am waiting for a heart and two lungs," Kobzeff explained. "My doctors told me that I have a small chest and I would probably need organs from a child. I said, 'You know what? That could have been me. I've been waiting three years already.'"[3] This sense that someone else may have deserved the second organs that went to Jesica would become a lasting, resonant and all-too-common theme as the Santillan saga drew to a close. For many people, Jesica's gain was someone else's loss. The morality of the case, then, rested to a considerable degree on the idea of an organ shortage—on the fact that demand for transplants far outstripped the supply. In the wake of the Santillan tragedy, however, most commentators took the rising demand as a given; and few would examine how the proliferation of transplant centers, the rise of kidney dialysis, the increasing tendency of surgeons to place patients on waiting lists, and the idea of a transplant as a healthy second life shaped perceptions of a shortage. To what extent was Jesica's gain someone else's loss? As we shall see, the reality was far more complex than observers like Kobzeff suggested.

Like many Americans, Kobzeff understood Jesica's case within the abstract framework of a zero-sum game; but critics focused instead on the family's immigration status, characterizing the second transplant as a kind of high-tech grab. After Jesica's death and as the Santillan family pondered their legal options over the "botched transplant," one North Carolina woman (a registered organ donor) commented, "I definitely would not want them [my organs] to go to an illegal alien. . . . I don't think they should be able to come in here and take our hospital and take our medicine and turn around and sue us." For this sixty-five-year-old woman, the second transplant represented a case study in futility, and she voiced the righteous indignation of a citizen suspicious of immigrants misusing resources that could have saved the lives of deserving Americans. "This girl was likely to die anyway," she concluded casually. "She took the organs from two different people [that] could have perhaps saved a healthier child."[4] This notion that Jesica, who lay comatose the entire time, was an agentive subject who "took" valuable organs and usurped life from others, and (moreover) that her parents then acted ungratefully by pondering lawsuits revealed that the second transplant had an extraordinary ability to unearth powerful moralizing. Experts, too, debated the second transplant, some characterizing the decision in unflattering terms. "Heart-lung transplant, that's a big grab," noted one NYU transplant surgeon. "That's a very rare transplant. Someone needs a heart, someone needs lungs, you can transplant three people."[5] Such comments suggested that Jesica's second chance was nothing less than a "grab," robbing multiple patients of their single chance at new life.

As in so many high-profile cases (as essays by Barron Lerner and Charles Bosk point out), there was much in this public and professional commentary that was deeply problematic, uninformed, wildly speculative, or just plain wrong. For example, while many insisted that Jesica had already had her chance with the first operation, they ignored the obvious fact that any transplantation with organs of mismatched blood type was, in fact, not much of a chance at all.[6] It was a failure from the outset, and one that left her far worse off than she had been with her own, failing heart. Nevertheless, critics continued to insist that Jesica enjoyed not just one but an apparently unprecedented two chances at life, and they contrasted her good fortune in a span of ten days against the frustrations of others who waited years on transplant registries never to have even one shot at a transplant. As one author in *Newsweek* asked bluntly, "Should she have received a second set of organs after the first was rejected? After all, she had her chance with the first transplant."[7] In the face of such stark oversimplifications, at least one internist would counter, "I'd argue she never got the first transplant."[8] But this question of what constituted a "fair chance" in the face of medical error was not prominent; nor was the rareness of "second chances" ever questioned. Such complexities in how donor organs found their way to recipients remained beyond the scope of the public and professional debate in March 2003.

The media, the public at large, and a good part of the ethics and medical professions seemed unaware of the fact that second transplants were not altogether rare, and were often quite uncontroversial. Few would delve into the mundane reality of failed first transplants and the need for second transplants, perhaps because the notion that transplanted organs often failed after a time so thoroughly undercut the idea of a miracle cure. As early as 1983, one study of kidney transplants in thirty-nine institutions in the southeastern United States found, for example, that over the period of five years, and of 3,000 kidney transplants, 17 percent were second grafts, 3 percent were third grafts, and 0.4 percent were fourth grafts.[9] Such second transplants were significantly less common with hearts and lungs, since, as one 2000 Wisconsin-based study noted, "repeat heart transplantation has a significantly worse outcome when compared with primary (first-time) transplantation." Nevertheless, the authors' review collected 514 cases in which the "time from primary transplant to retransplantation ranged from 1 day to 15.5 years."[10] More than half the patients, they noted, suffered from chronic rejection. There were, of course, many political and economic reasons why the professionals at the center of this vast and burgeoning medical industry would play down these features which were so much at odds with the idea of a gift of life. For if transplants were not perceived as unambiguously lifesaving, would the urgency to donate be as strong?

Such findings highlight that livers, kidneys, and heart and lungs have a limited value to many recipients, and many recipients (days, months, or years later) are back onto the transplant registry lists waiting to obtain new organs. In many ways, Jesica's second transplant severely compressed into days a process that otherwise happened within years, or months, and occasionally days in the transplant arena. Organ transplant recipients often experienced organ failure. Jesica's life with her first set of transplanted organs was acutely compressed, but the fact that these organs were removed and replaced by another set was (in itself) hardly unusual. A life with transplanted organs is often but not always a precarious one. As one article noted in July 2001, "the most recent national liver transplant survival rates are 85 percent after one year and 73 percent after five years."[11] Many of the transplant patients died while waiting for a second transplant; the numbers of second-time transplants were small, but not inconsequential.

Understanding the broader reality of second transplants allows us therefore to see clearly what moral and imaginative issues were at work in making Jesica's second transplant so controversial. In a recent account, for example, a two-time transplant patient wrote of surviving for twenty years on the first kidney transplant; but eventually, he noted, "that two-decade kidney failed, and then another transplant failed in two years, and here I am again using hemodialysis." To him, "when a transplant works, it works spectacularly and instantly, as mine did." But transplants can also fail suddenly. He further noted, "My health had declined steadily for almost four years . . . and throughout the two years of the second transplant, which never really kicked in the way it should have."[12]

To be sure, other second transplants have been embroiled in controversy, but not for the same reasons as in the Santillan story. Into the 1990s, transplant surgeons, ethicists, and policymakers continued to debate whether retransplantation was an "appropriate use of scarce donor resources." While some reviews of the existing evidence suggested that survival rates for second transplants were lower, others suggested that rates were high enough to make restricting second transplants unethical.[13] Why then was the hasty transition from first transplant to second transplant in the Santillan case so fraught with controversy? Clearly, one must look to the broader cultural and political atmosphere surrounding the story—issues of "illegal immigration," public anxieties about access to health care, and preexisting debates over medical futility—to see why Jesica's second operation took on such heavy moral freight. The differences between the public view and the reality of second transplants is revealing—for much of the media saw the second transplant as an unusual and futile event, brokered by powerful if beneficent doctors and a high-profile institution that was seeking cover for its mistakes.

Another reason for the public portrayal of Jesica's second transplant relates to a broader mythic lay understanding of transplanted organs (perpetuated by donation networks and transplant professionals, to be sure)—that they are "healthy" organs that effectively and completely replace sick ones, thus fundamentally renewing the body. The reality of what it takes to treat and maintain transplanted organs and the commonplace fact of their steady deterioration are rarely mentioned. Ideals do not neatly mesh with the experiences of recipients and transplant insiders (see the essays by Tom Diflo and Richard Cook in this volume). Life as an organ transplant patient is in a sense more akin to living with a chronic illness, for like patients with HIV since the mid-1990s and people with juvenile diabetes, transplant recipients know that long-term clinical management is essential to survival. Integrating the parts of one person into the body of another is a complex and enduring immunological challenge.

Indeed, for at least one critic of Jesica's second transplant, surgeon Laszlo Fuzesi, it was the necessity of long-term postoperative care that raised key questions about the second transplant. In the wake of the "bungled transplant" and the second operation, Fuzesi (like so many others) spoke as if Jesica's family had no insurance and as if the costs of her long-term care would be borne by society at large. A heart transplant surgeon at Westchester Medical Center, he suggested that the long-term success of people without insurance was not good: "In general . . . that heart is not going to survive as long in that [poor or uninsured] patient as [in] another because they can't pay for the medication." Where foreigners were concerned, he noted, "they're going to leave the country where that heart can't be monitored—overall, as a transplant society, our goal is all these organs live as long as possible."[14] For this insider, then, it was the precariousness of life after transplantation that determined the long-term health of the transplanted organ. (Such questions, of course, created new moral tangles—and, indeed, since the early days of dialysis and transplantation, physicians and ethicists have sought to determine what role [if any] one's economic status, and one's capacity to care for the new organs, should have in determining eligibility. In 2003, the consensus in America was that privilege and poverty should have no place in determining eligibility for transplantation—and yet it also remained true that only patients with health insurance could qualify for transplantation.) This reality of long-term after-transplant care rarely made it into the news reports, which, by and large, focused on transplantation as a heroic and definitive second chance—a resurrection.

Though many observers, like Fuzesi and the prospective organ donor in North Carolina quoted above, saw the second transplant through the lens of immigration and citizenship, others were less troubled by the citizenship question than by the notion of "waste" that underlay Fuzesi's argument. For them, the most disturbing feature of the episode was the shadow of "futility" hanging heavy over the second transplant. Was Jesica "likely to die anyway"? Futility, of course, like beauty, depended on the beholder. Moreover, this problem of medical futility had a complex recent history, for it had become more widely discussed in medical ethics precisely as questions of cost began to shape medical decision-making, as insurance and managed care companies began to aggressively limit access to high-technology medicine, and as families continued to grapple with complex end-of-life decisions about when to withdraw life support. Arguments about what was futile medicine and what was worthwhile and, indeed, morally sanctioned risk-taking, then, did not emerge in a vacuum—they were part of a larger economic and social calculus weighing the pros and cons of access to high-technology resources. For those troubled by the inefficient use of resources and the careless distribution of scarce goods, Jesica's second transplant was part of a continuum of problems, an appealing object lesson. How much money, energy, time, and resources should be poured, they asked, into extended medical care at the end of life, or into aggressive treatments for sick individuals with little chance of survival?

In Jesica's case, however, the issue was not the dollars spent per se but a set of commodities (organs) that most Americans perceived as priceless, without monetary equivalence at least in the American system. (By contrast, essays by Thomas Diflo and Nancy Scheper-Hughes provide insight into the remarkable ways in which monetary payments and commodification come into play when Americans step outside their system.) Little wonder, then, that lay observers, philosophers and ethicists, and surgeons offered their own views about the second transplant. As a *Newsweek* writer asked bluntly, "Should someone have pointed out what, in retrospect, seems obvious: that her chances of surviving a second operation were almost nil?"[15] But was this, in fact, the case? Moreover, where some saw the second transplant as a pointless waste, Jesica's surgeon and her supporters insisted that the second transplant was a worthwhile, if long-shot, risk. For at least one observer, "the fact that she had two chances for a life-saving operation testifies to the compassion that one can find in the United States' health care system."[16] These conflicted meanings (across a spectrum from waste and futility to generosity and compassion) clung tightly to the public debate over Jesica's second transplant—even as the question of "second chances" took on vastly different meanings for patients situated elsewhere in the system.

VARIETIES OF ENTITLEMENT: AN AMERICAN PATIENT'S SECOND CHANCE

A few years before the Santillan debacle, another transplant controversy revolving around questions of fairness and deservedness, futility and scarce resources, took shape in Boston, in the plight of Belynda Dunn. Dunn was an HIV positive woman fighting to get her insurance company to pay for her liver transplant. Much of the story revolved around her struggle for a first transplant. In the end, she obtained not just one but two—separated by days, just as in Jesica's case. The first transplant had been problematic, though it does not appear to have entailed an egregious error, and Dunn (like Santillan) had not regained consciousness. In Dunn's case, however, the second transplant never became an issue, nor was it a topic of extended discussion. Indeed, it was portrayed as merely part of the continuum, a necessary step in her righteous struggle against a profit-making bureaucracy bent on denying her access to a lifesaving operation.

Belynda Dunn captured media and public attention in Boston and the region because of her struggles against her HMO. Dunn was forty-nine years old, and she had lived with hepatitis C for many years, a condition that had damaged her liver. From the HMO's perspective, however, the problem was that Dunn was HIV positive. She needed a liver transplant, and her brother was willing to donate a lobe of his own liver in order to save her life. But, as local news accounts noted, "the health maintenance organization has refused to pay for the surgery, saying that liver transplants, while common for generally health people, are considered experimental for people with HIV."[17] Where the debate around Jesica Santillan's transplant revolved around her tainted status as an "illegal immigrant," in the Dunn case it was her tainted status as HIV-positive that gave the case moral meaning. In these and other ways, Dunn had much in common with Santillan, especially in the early stages of their stories. Both were desperately ill people with limited resources, seeking a way into the health care system and its promise of lifesaving treatments, and dependent on benefactors and supporters to gain public attention and vital health services. Many saw Dunn's rejection by the HMO as unjust—"feels like discrimination to me," said the executive director of the AIDS Action Committee.[18]

That Dunn was a noted community AIDS activist meant, however, that she was part of an extended and well-developed advocacy system with significant lobbying resources. Indeed, by the time of Dunn's case, AIDS activists had become extraordinarily knowledgeable and successful in combating discrimination and compelling the NIH, the FDA, and other major health institutions to acknowledge their particular needs.[19] In Dunn's case, a live organ donor appeared (for portions of livers could be transplanted successfully—making these organs dramatically different commodities than hearts). Financial donors also emerged, and Dunn's story became (akin with the early stages of Jesica's case) a cause célèbre in the area. Boston's Mayor Menino and anonymous donors raised hundreds of thousands of dollars "in honor of a woman who taught thousands about AIDS prevention."[20] In this sense, the media and the broader community framed the story as one in which a community was giving back to someone who had done much to assist others.

Was this intervention—a liver transplant—to save the life of a person with HIV a futile treatment? Public ideas about futility in this case were in flux, as were the life chances of people with HIV at the time. Experts at the time pointed out that HIV was no longer necessarily a fatal infection and that as life expectancy had increased, the moral debate about organ transplants had also changed. "Somebody with HIV can live another 10 or 20 years . . . who knows how long," commented one scholar when asked about the Dunn case.[21] Although the HMO continued to resist (indeed, the money that was raised for Dunn, though topping $150,000, had been insufficient to cover the full costs), within a few months the state Medicaid program would order the insurer to pay the cost of such patients. The public media emphasized that, far from being a tainted recipient, Dunn was herself a by-product of modern medical advances, for "the prognosis for people with HIV has improved markedly since 1996 . . . [and] as a result many surgeons say it is not ethical to deny transplants to HIV patients."[22]

Another high-profile AIDS activist with HIV, Larry Kramer, was also in Dunn's position, and their stories were framed together in the local media as struggles waged by virtuous and articulate individuals against an unfair system. Their public appeals were in some ways simple and filled with a sense of entitlement—they were underdogs fighting an unfair system. Dunn insisted,

"You can't just go around telling people who is going to live and who is going to die. That is what these insurance companies are doing." Kramer framed his personal battle in more extreme terms. A "66-year-old novelist and playwright, AIDS activist and agitator," Kramer had struggled to be placed on the liver transplant list. He voiced a powerful sense of entitlement to scarce organs. For him, the problem with this system was not only the HMOs and the insurance companies (appealing targets for those challenging the moral economy of American medicine) but also those unwilling to donate their organs so that others might live. Stridently, he argued, "There has to be a revolution in this country . . . people should not be allowed to die and be buried with useful organs."[23]

These sentiments, among patients who after years of hopeful waiting saw their life chances slipping away (again), laid moral claim (based on utilitarian arguments) to the resources stingily held onto by others. Dunn and Kramer, building on their experiences of AIDS activism, believed that profits and crass commercial interests stood in the way of making people well again. In this view, America was not a zero-sum society at all but a place where profiteering and discrimination was rife. Kramer's comments took this a step further, suggesting that second chances and third chances could, in fact, become more commonplace if other people gave more of themselves—listing as organ donors—or if their organs were taken from them when they died.

For many Americans (only some of whom shared Kramer's extraordinary sense of entitlement to the organs of others), it was the fact that Jesica's mother allegedly refused to donate the young woman's organs that became emblematic of what was wrong with giving immigrants access to American organs. (Experts acknowledged, however, that her body, after days in a coma and suffused with powerful immunosuppressive drugs, was not in a condition to produce usable organs.) Yet the story of this irony became something of an urban legend. Commenting on the case during his television show, for example, conservative commentator Bill O'Reilly questioned ethicist George Annas about the failure of the family to donate Jesica's organs. Facing the combative O'Reilly, Annas responded, "But there was also some physicians who said they didn't think the organs were really usable. I just don't know the truth of the matter." But pressed by O'Reilly, he added, "If the organs were usable . . . and she didn't donate them, I think that's a problem." What sort of problem, he did not have time to say. O'Reilly quickly agreed, "That's the way I feel about it."[24] Many in the public would take aim at this last affront—her family's supposed unwillingness to donate. Kramer's views would reappear, then, in another guise—for such frustrated and entitled recipients would cast the Santillan story as part of a simple dichotomy—the stingy, undeserving, and ungrateful (read immigrant) versus the worthy, entitled, and beneficent (read American).[25]

In the wake of her own activism, Belynda Dunn's first transplant (and shortly thereafter, her second transplant) would be portrayed as part of the same narrative of virtuous struggle. In May 2002, Dunn received her first transplanted liver, but the transplant quickly failed. "The liver didn't work," said one official at the University of Pittsburgh Medical Center, where the operation had occurred. "We relisted her and got her retransplanted on Friday," noted the same official, "but she just never recovered. She was too far gone." The parallels and comparative silences with the Santillan story are striking, for nowhere in the public commentary was there discussion about the value and meaning of the second transplant. Blame was hard to locate. In Dunn's case, the first organ itself was to blame—it "didn't work." And to the end, Dunn was understood as the crusader who fought against her insurance company in order to gain this shot at life. A year later in North Carolina, by contrast, skeptical eyes came to rest on Jesica, on her status as an undeserving immigrant, on the question of whether her "second chance" had taken life from others, and on the problem of whether the so-called second transplant was a futile gesture.

TANGLED WEB: THE MORAL ECONOMY OF FUTILITY IN THE TRANSPLANT THEATER

While much of the attention concerned Jesica's "getting organs" that others deserved, many commentators also focused on the character of decision-making in the transplant arena and in the wake of errors—portraying the second transplant as a case study in futility. Even after the second transplant, when Jesica's parents' continued to hope and advocate for their daughter, their own struggle (in contrast to Dunn's) was portrayed as a losing battle. This was a portrait, of course, that transcended Jesica's case, for this problem of "not letting go" (and continuing to use resources to the very end of life) was one that had come to define the modern high-technology-oriented health care system increasingly in the 1990s.[26] In the years leading up to the Santillan story, the medical press was filled with new books on the topic of futility, with titles like *Wrong Medicine: Doctors, Patients, and Futile Treatment* (1995), *Medical Futility and the Evaluation of Life-Sustaining Interventions* (1997), and *When Doctors Say No: The Battleground of Medical Futility* (1998). Thus, where, for some, observations on the second transplant intersected with a politics of immigration and rights, for others, it fell squarely into the battleground over futility and over the complex terrain of physician-family relations at the end of life.

As physician Donald Murphy wrote in the 1997 book (echoing Kramer's argument over organs), the futility discussion was a debate about individualism versus communal thinking. "The futile intervention debate is one of the main arenas in which our society is experiencing a cultural shift," he insisted. "We need to make a transition . . . from the rugged individualism that formed our country to a more communitarian ethic that will help us survive . . . in the next century."[27] For such authors, the futility question in the Santillan case would be about the very future of the American health care system—a future in which individual rights, and the myth of individual self-sufficiency, would give way to a profound sense of interconnectedness. As Murphy concluded, "The futile intervention debate is not as much about actual dollars saved as it is about values."[28] And as Susan Rubin argued in *When Doctors Say No*, "Concerns about justice and allocation of scarce communal health care resources, and persistent calls for health care reform have also fueled the debate about futility."[29]

According to this emergent critique of individualism, doctors and patients simply did not know when to "pull the plug" and seemed incapable of thinking about this larger dimension of the problem. For some, doctors were less the problem than patients and family members hovering at the bedside, again reflecting a tension between the individual and the socially located patient. This problem of futility is all the more problematic in an age of scarce medical resources, for the overwhelming sentiment (as voiced by would-be organ recipients and medical ethicists) is that not knowing when to "pull the plug" has sweeping implications for others in line waiting to use those resources, that ICU bed, that ventilator, or those organs. The futility discussion is, in short, part of a larger discussion about the medical system's moral obligations to patients and families, and the role of doctors and insurers to manage resources and to imagine the larger world of health care consumers in line for those services.

Approaches to futility within a "transplant society" become more complex as futility and transplantation are intertwined in several key ways. On the one hand, the scarce medical resources at issue are organs procured from patients for whom further treatment is deemed futile. On the other hand, many of the costly technologies and intellectual resources that prompt debates over futility were developed as part of the emergent technologies of organ transplantation.[30] In this context, then, it becomes increasingly difficult to abstract and separate questions of futility for would-be donors from questions of futility for would-be recipients, as anthropologist Margaret Lock has cautioned:

> Among these patients [where questions of futility are at issue] are those marked as potential organ donors. The danger is very real that in the increasingly utilitarian climate of our times, we will all too readily define certain patients as having lives which are without meaning, especially if we perceive ways in which their bodies can be made "useful" to the medical enterprise, and thus indirectly to society. This is particularly likely to happen given the pressure to reduce expenditures that all medical systems are now under. A rationalization of procedures which free up hospital beds, and which serve at the same time to assist indirectly in "restoring" health to other patients, whose beds too will be liberated, can sound very persuasive in a climate where fiscal restraint is dominant.[31]

The Santillan story framed the question of futility in stark terms, facilitated by the anonymity of the donors in the U.S. transplant system and the oracular nature of the organ matching system (as described by Richard Cook in this volume). Were physicians at Duke double-dipping into the pool of available organs, thereby fulfilling a moral obligation to the Santillan family in the wake of the egregious first error? There was a powerful, if mistaken, impression permeating the media that strings had been pulled to jump Jesica to the head of the line. Did her doctors know full well that the effort would be futile? Did they truly believe that another intervention would work? Did Jesica's parents also really believe that a second set of organs could save their daughter's life?

But these rather stark questions on the public's mind oversimplified many complexities about organs, the people who donated them, the people who received them, and the logic of the system moving these commodities from one body to another. Perhaps the best public discussion of this vexing problem came months later after emotions had simmered down and the story left the front pages. In late July, Avery Comarow's story in the *U.S. News and World Report* devoted considerable attention to fears, myths, and realities about the way the matching system actually worked. "Suspicions about jumping the queue are raised whenever a critically ill celebrity—the late Yankee center fielder Mickey Mantle or Pennsylvania Gov. Robert Casey, for example—lands on the top of the list," Comarow noted.[32] Yet, he noted, in 2003 there were many restrictions on the information available to surgeons about organs, precisely because some transplant centers in the 1990s had learned how to manipulate the list "to favor their patients." Public skepticism about jumping the queue, then, was not totally unfounded.

But when patients waiting on transplant lists expressed their views that they, rather than Jesica, might have benefited from those organs, and that someone may have manipulated the system to benefit Jesica over them, they evinced a profound misunderstanding (and attendant frustration) about the ways in which the system worked. Patients like Luba Kobzeff in Ontario, California, were not, in fact, competing with Jesica for available organs. The rules that had existed since 1984 (when the National Organ Transplant Act gave UNOS authority over organ allocation policy) required that available donor organs be shared first locally and then within a larger region, and only then could it be offered nationally. There had long been criticism of this policy, for although it kept organs closer to home, it had helped to shape growing disparities in wait times across regions. In the 1990s, Secretary of Health and Human Services Donna Shalala and the Clinton administration, supported by an Institute of Medicine (IOM) report, pressed strenuously to revise the system for sharing organs—moving aggressively to create a "sickest-first" policy. Under the plan, the regional borders would disappear and the sickest person *in the country* would be first in line, and existing disparities in waiting times across the nation would be reduced. According to the critics of existing policy, there was no good reason for people in New York to wait longer for organs on average than people in Minnesota or Louisiana.[33]

Shalala did not count on the fact, however, that a variety of interests wished to preserve the regional borders of the system. As one 1999 article noted, "The proposal immediately touched off a fight between large and small transplant centers, with small centers insisting Dr. Shalala's rules would put them out of business by steering organs to big-city hospitals."[34] Before the dust had cleared, several states (Louisiana, Wisconsin, and Texas) had passed legislation "barring donated organs from crossing state borders" unless there was no medical match inside state lines.[35] In April 2000, the U.S. House of Representatives squelched Shalala's plan—to ensure that UNOS retained authority for allocating organs, and that the regional system stayed in place. Editorials in New York City and Pittsburgh (sites of large transplant centers with longer patient waiting lists) preached the virtues of a national system, decrying this "pathological parochialism" that meant that sicker, more deserving patients "across the [regional] border" would die; this was nothing more than a profound "unfairness to desperately ill patients who have the misfortune of residing outside the procurement area."[36] Surgeons and editorialists in Louisiana, Arkansas, and Alabama (states with small transplant centers) angrily disagreed.[37] Early in the debate, one editorial in Tampa, Florida, for example, insisted that "the sickest patients aren't always the best candidates for transplants" and another in Seattle, Washington, decried the "diminished local control" and the "intense special-interest lobbying by a few of the largest liver-transplant centers."[38] The IOM insisted that the fears of smaller centers losing business and anxieties about organs being exported from some regions into others was overblown. Yet the themes and imagery deployed in these debates highlighted the intense anxiety of Americans about these scarce resources and the powerful parochial interests already at play (shortly before Jesica Santillan's transplant took place) in the allocation of organs for transplantation.[39]

Border politics (in this case, moving organs across borders, serving parochial interests, and the economic needs of large and small transplant centers) had long been part of the organ transplant system. In the end, the Shalala reforms were severely compromised by the economic interests that sustained the existing system; the small centers and their political supporters succeeded in squelching the move to a "sickest-first" national policy. (Rhodes, in this volume, takes up these themes, analyzing the "sickest-first" policy, as well as the influence of small centers.) Among those opposing the effort, for example, were some state governors like Wisconsin's Tommy Thompson, who insisted, "In this state, we go out and aggressively encourage people to be donors, with me doing public service announcements. If I'm going to do that, I want those organs to stay in the state and take care of the patients that need it in Wisconsin."[40] Doctors, transplant centers, and patients continued to maneuver for best advantage within the constraints of the system. Frustrations with wait times remained an enduring part of the system. Severe sickness was, in itself, no guarantee of priority. Organs simply did not travel according to the logic that many Americans assumed that they did. Increasingly, given the constraints of the system, those with resources were finding ways around the system entirely, by being listed in regions in addition to their home region and by traveling abroad to purchase organs in other countries (as Scheper-Hughes and Diflo discuss in their essays).

Was there a queue for Jesica Santillan? Yes, but clearly it was not the queue that many commentators envisioned. In 2003, writer Avery Comarow noted that one of the few ways for a patient to make it to the top of the list was "to get sicker"—and this is one factor that moved Jesica up the list after the first transplant. Another was for her surgeon to accept organs that others "might find iffy" or less than optimal. (Indeed, some eight months before Jesica's first transplant, Jaggers had rejected such "iffy" organs for Jesica, suggesting that they "were marginal in the first place.") "The true story," Comarow concluded, "is that her second set of organs came through the usual conduit";

they were the heart and lungs of a a middle-aged woman who smoked and had "a touch of emphysema."[41] They were "not ideal," the surgeon Jaggers explained to the reporter. Not enough information was published at the time, or has been since, to determine with any certainty just how sick Jesica was before these organs were offered, but clearly there is a fine line between futility and movement to the front of the line.

But whatever the politics of the rules and guidelines, weren't second transplants more problematic? As we noted above, the surgical evidence was (at best) conflicted on this point; however, the moral dynamics of the surgeon-patient relationship clearly tilted toward second transplants. Writing in the mid-1990s, ethicists recognized that questions of futility in the transplantation arena were a different and more complex affair than in other areas. Offering a useful insight into the dynamics of the Santillan story, Lawrence Schneiderman and Nancy Jecker noted in their book, *Wrong Medicine*, "post-transplant care involves the most sophisticated weapons in the technological arsenal, and can be an emotional roller coaster, with miraculous survival waiting at one end and death buried within tubes and machinery in an isolated, laminar flow room at the others."[42] Their comment captures nicely the intense compression of potential outcomes, different emotional trajectories, and moral meanings—all tangled into a single moment. For them, the sharp polarities, the highly charged atmosphere, and the drama and rapid momentum of transplant medicine dictated that desperate and futile measures would be the norm. "Physicians, patients and their families become locked in a mutual dependency," they wrote, "relentlessly pursuing more and more desperate and futile measures to keep the patient alive—including even repeated efforts at transplantation—because of the momentum that developed." In this rapidly evolving therapeutic arena, they suggested, facts, deliberation, and larger considerations about the distribution of resources have little practical value. Thus, the Duke team's ongoing commitment to Jesica was not unusual (in fact, it is the type of commitment most patients hope to find from their doctors); and their powerful feelings of responsibility toward Jesica in the aftermath of the error surely must have grown. In such settings, the individual mores and roles of the physician conflict with (and supplant) any broader public policy goals of organ distribution. It is precisely for this reason that in the transplant arena, surgeons, patients, and families became "locked in mutual dependency"—seizing on slim chances, gambling on positive outcomes with the emotional stakes high.

Futility aside, however, there was another important factor driving the second transplant in Jesica's case: the powerful fact that the second operation was crucial for repairing the moral agency of the surgeon and the hospital. Unquestionably, the "bungled" first transplant severely compromised the ability of the institution to act within the sphere of health and healing as a moral agent. The error damaged Jesica, the surgeon, and the hospital. The second transplant was necessary, then, to recast the surgeon (the expert, the lifesaver) from an agent of harm back into a healer. The larger moral economy of medicine (and transplantation) depended upon this repair, for it meant that Americans could see Jaggers and Duke again as morally unambiguous and beneficent forces striving to improve the health of their patients. With Duke's ability to receive moral approval severely damaged after the error, the second transplant repaired the damage—even if it meant exposing other fracture lines in the moral economy of patient care. And the institution would portray the second transplant as a heroic sign of its boundless commitment to patient care.

Could second transplants, as a group, be considered futile? Considering the problem in the abstract, the authors of *Wrong Medicine* in 1995 had answered yes, noting that "if a first heart or liver or lung transplant fails, a second effort in the wake of the failure has a much poorer chance of success. Others waiting desperately for their first chance at such organs would almost certainly do better."[43] Such skepticism, then, did not originate with the Santillan case—but undoubtedly the nationally publicized story communicated these paradoxes far more widely. Yet, as Schneiderman and Jecker suggested, futility was not a concept that penetrated easily into this world. It was perhaps too much (given the structure of this system) to expect surgeons to behave and think differently in this intensely family-centered, high-technology arena, sitting on the brink of many different possibilities. The authors noted that "when asked about the irrationality of performing repeat organ transplant operations despite sharply reduced odds of success, surgeons will almost always point out how emotionally difficult it is to 'abandon' a patient once the process has begun."[44] Yet, for many Americans (whether they were standing outside this system or on the periphery, envisioning organs in a zero-sum society, or troubled by immigration questions), it seems that abandoning Jesica was the best course.[45]

THE MYTHOS AND ETHOS OF SECOND CHANCES

The Santillan story, then, brought a range of complex and puzzling issues into the open, if only for a short time. One emergent theme was an American myth about entitlement and second chances; another was the transplant

ethos itself and its internal contradictions to do everything possible for patients while at the same time not wasting organs in futile operations. In the
immediate aftermath of the second transplant, these complexities were
slowly unearthed and opened to various kinds of cultural analysis and critique. Lessons were offered—among them that second chances were not so
unusual after all; that Jesica's "first chance" was no chance at all; that futility
in the transplant arena was a tangled web of moral conundrums and commitments; that surgical gaming of the system certainly had been done in the
recent past, but it was not responsible for Jesica's second transplant. These
lessons could reassure the public, for they offered a positive image of the
transplant system. Yet these lessons competed at every turn with powerful
and widespread myths about Jesica's unwarranted second chance.

Jesica Santillan had become a lightening rod, a focal point for those with a
claim to resources, a frustrated sense of entitlement, and a gripe about their
own accommodations within the American health care system. For them,
Jesica was far more appealing as a topic of political and cultural commentary
than, say, Belynda Dunn. In critiquing Jesica, many Americans voiced their
various displeasures with society while simultaneously preserving their cherished myths about the system—about transplantation as a second chance at a
new life, about the queue that would deliver that opportunity, about the
interest that stood between them and a better life. Many would almost will-
fully ignore the complex web of realities colliding against these myths. Mistaken notions and powerful sentiments about second chances (earned and
undeserved) swirled around Jesica's case. "That could have been me," commented Luba Kobzeff. "I've been waiting three years already." This, for many
with strong investments in the myth, would become the lasting memory and
moral meaning of Jesica's second transplant.

What drew people to use the Santillan case to voice these opinions? What
made Jesica Santillan's second transplant fair game for moralizing and reflection? As Leo Chavez and Beatrix Hoffman point out elsewhere in this volume, it was the fact of her status as an undocumented immigrant without
entitlements that drew hostility from many Americans. But as Lesley Sharp
and Carolyn Rouse also note, there were many other controversies buried in
this tangled web of a case. Something about her liminal status as both noncitizen and comatose adolescent allowed others to feel that they could speak
about her and, to some extent, accuse her of "taking" organs from others.

To move beyond these moralizing struggles (she got what was rightfully
mine) at the heart of the transplant system, some would have us embrace a
greater communitarian ethos, others suggest financial and other incentives

for donors, and yet others propose a variety of mechanisms for moving beyond the zero-sum sensibility. The hope is that such administrative, financial, and technical innovations could increase the supply of organs, and (thereby) lead us out of a world where Jesica's gain is seen as Luba's loss. Such innovations, however, would inevitably create new moral problems—as they already are. (See the Scheper-Hughes and Diflo essays.) Far more challenging is the problem of moving Americans beyond their mythos of entitlement and their beliefs about second chances; equally challenging, too, is the problem of rethinking the ethos of transplant medicine—a field in which waste is reviled but where the line between hope and futility is an extraordinary blur. (See Nancy King's essay in this volume.) Coping with these challenges should rightly be the legacy of Jesica's second transplant.

NOTES

1. As a March 5, 2003, story on *CBS News* noted, "Some have questioned whether the second transplant was proper and whether the organs could have saved the life of another patient. Others question why an illegal immigrant received such high-intensity medical care," <http://www.cbsnews.com/stories/2003/02/18/health/main5409 07.shtml>.

2. "Surgical Expertise, Undone by Error," *Washington Post*, February 24, 2003; see also Kher Unmesh, "A Miracle Denied," *Time*, March 3, 2003.

3. Jerry Adler, "A Tragic Error," *Newsweek*, March 2, 2003, 20.

4. Christina Headrick and Vicki Cheng, "Some Link Citizenship, Transplants," *Raleigh News and Observer* (March 4, 2003), A1.

5. Quote is attributed to Lewis Teperman, director of transplantation at New York University in Adler, "Tragic Error," 20.

6. There has been some experimentation with transplanting organs of a different blood type in infants—some of it successful. But the state of knowledge and technology at the time of Jesica's transplant was such that a mismatched pediatric heart and lung transplant was certain to leave the patient in even worse health than before the operation.

7. Adler, "Tragic Error," 20. On this topic, ethicist Robert Veatch has noted in his book *Transplantation Ethics*, that "the UNOS Ethics Committee, when it considered retransplant, came to the reasonable conclusion that when people are in organ failure the crucial issue is not whether one has had a previous graft. The other variables that go into organ allocation—factors such as HLA-match, medical urgency, PRA, or time on the waiting list depending on the organ—are what is morally relevant, not whether one has received a previous graft. . . . Being a candidate for a repeat transplant does not count against the individual in the allocation of organs" (Robert M. Veatch, *Transplantation Ethics* [Washington, D.C.: Georgetown University Press, 2000], 332).

8. Sheryl Gay Stolberg and Lawrence K. Altman, "An Ethical Dilemma with Few Precedents," *New York Times*, February 21, 2003, 23.

9. E. K. Spees, W. K. Vaughn, J. C. McDonald, R. R. Bollinger, G. M. Williams, F. P. Sanfilippo, P. Adams, G. Mendez-Picon, and G. Niblack, "Why Do Secondary Cadaver Renal Transplants Succeed? Results of the South-Eastern Organ Procurement Foundation Prospective Study," *Journal of Urology* 129 (3) (March 1983): 484–88. "From June 1977 to March 1982," the authors wrote, "3,215 cadaver kidney transplants were performed at 39 institutions. There were 2,535 first, 564 second, 103 third and 13 fourth grafts."

10. R. Srivastava, B. M. Keck, L. E. Bennett, and J. D. Hosenpud, "The Results of Cardiac Retransplantation: An Analysis of the Joint International Society for Heart and Lung Transplantation/United Network for Organ Sharing Thoracic Registry," *Transplantation* 70 (4) (August 27, 2000): 606–12.

11. Michael Lasalandra, "HIV Doesn't Override Rights, Say Ethicists," *Boston Herald*, July 21, 2001, 6.

12. Lawrence Henry, "Am I On Life Support?" *American Spectator*, April 1, 2005.

13. For kidney transplants, for example, one 1984 study suggested that "the poor second graft survival rates have not improved since the introduction of cyclosporine A in 1984" and pointed to a "higher rate of immunological failures in the first 3 months" (A. Yanagiya and J. M. Cecka, "Second Transplants," *Clinical Transplants* [1989]: 397–405). A later study in 1994 at Massachusetts General Hospital, however, argued that the hospital's own second-transplant survival rates were quite good and "not significantly different from the survival rates of primary allografts at this center." They concluded that "because excellent second-renal allograft survival is attainable and comparable to primary-renal allograft survival and because the costs are comparable, restricting suitable patients to subsequent lifelong dialysis becomes unethical" (F. L. Delmonico, N. Tolkoff-Rubin, H. Auchincloss Jr., M. L. Farrell, D. M. Fitzpatrick, S. Saidman, J. T. Herrin, A. B. Cosimi, "Second Renal Transplantations: Ethical Issues Clarified by Outcome; Outcome Enhanced by a Reliable Crossmatch," *Archives of Surgery* 129 [4] [April 1994]: 354–60). A third study in Minnesota found that "short-term outcome for primary and retransplant recipients has been similar; however, long-term outcome seems worse for retransplant recipients" (A. Moss, J. S. Najarian, D. E. Sutherland, W. D. Payne, R. W. Gruessner, A. Humar, R. Kandaswamy, K. J. Gillingham, D. L. Dunn, A. J. Matas, "5,000 Kidney Transplants—A Single-Center Study," *Clinical Transplants* [2000]: 159–71). For heart transplants, one study by a pediatric transplant team in Atlanta argued that "cardiac retransplantation can be performed in children with results comparable with those for primary transplantation" (K. R. Kanter, R. N. Vincent, A. M. Berg, W. T. Mahle, J. M. Forbess, and P. M. Kirshbom, "Cardiac Retransplantation in Children," *Annals of Thoracic Surgery* 78 [2] [August 2004]: 644–49). These questions were not confined to the American surgical community. For a cautiously positive endorsement of liver retransplantation in a French institution, see D. Azouly, M. M. Linhares, E. Huguet, V. Delvart, D. Castaing,

R. Adam, P. Ichai, F. Saliba, A. Lemoine, D. Samuel, and H. Bismuth, "Decision for Retransplantation of the Liver: An Experience- and Cost-Based Analysis," *Annals of Surgery* 236 (6) (December 2002): 713–21.

14. "Unresolved Problem: Interview with Heart Transplant Surgeon Laszlo Fuzesi and Ethicist George Annas, Boston University," Fox News Network, *The O'Reilly Factor*, February 25, 2003.

15. Adler, "Tragic Error," 20.

16. David Resnick, "The Jesica Santillan Tragedy: Lessons Learned," *Hastings Center Report* 33 (4) (2003): 15–20. Resnick points out as well that "patients frequently get second and third chances at organ transplants in the United States. Indeed, any patient that receives a heart transplant at a relatively early age will probably need a second heart before he or she dies."

17. "Agency to Rule on HIV Case Transplant," *Boston Globe*, July 19, 2001.

18. "On Her Own: Panel Denies Transplant for AIDS Activist," *Boston Herald*, July 20, 2001.

19. Stephen Epstein, *Impure Science: AIDS, Activism, and the Politics of Knowledge* (Berkeley: University of California Press, 1996).

20. "Wish Come True: HMO, Donors to Fund Transplant," *Boston Herald*, July 21, 2001.

21. "HIV Patients Get Fresh Hopes for Donor Organs," *New York Times*, December 11, 2001.

22. Ibid.

23. Ibid.

24. "Unresolved Problem."

25. To those who asked why someone in the country illegally was eligible to obtain a transplant in America, some media reports noted that "the United Network for Organ Sharing, which oversees the distribution of organs nationwide, allows up to 5 percent of recipients to be from other countries. 'Part of the rationale is that it may be hypocritical to accept donors who are not U.S. citizens, but not allow them to be transplant recipients,' said Joel Newman, UNOS spokesman." *CBS News*, March 5, 2003. For discussions of UNOS and transplant criteria, see essays by Jed Adam Gross, Rosamond Rhodes, and Eric Meslin in this volume.

26. Over the past decades, of course, this saga of Americans, technology, futility, and end-of-life care has taken many turns. The problem has been dramatized in a series of high-profile controversies. First was the Karen Ann Quinlan story and the emergence of the "right to die" discussion in the mid-1970s in the famous New Jersey case. To be sure the Barney Clark–Jarvik 7 heart experiments in the early 1980s in Utah gave the public yet another view of the complex entanglements between technology, futility, and end-of-life care. More recently, the story of Terri Schiavo in Florida in 2005 has brought these issues again into the public view—this time with another set of political and religious concerns about the "culture of life" animating the discussion. The 2003 story of Jesica Santillan rightly figures prominently as a key part of this

ongoing controversy. See also Susan Lederer's discussion of the Bruce Tucker transplant case in this volume.

27. Donald Murphy, "The Economics of Futile Interventions," in *Medical Futility and the Evaluation of Life-Sustaining Interventions*, ed. Marjorie Zucker and Howard Zucker (Cambridge University Press, 1997), 123.

28. Ibid., 130.

29. Susan Rubin, *When Doctors Say No: The Battleground of Medical Futility* (Bloomington: Indiana University Press, 1998), 37.

30. Margaret Lock, *Twice Dead: Organ Transplants and the Reinvention of Death* (Berkeley: University of California Press, 2002).

31. Margaret Lock, "The Quest for Human Organs and the Violence of Zeal," in *Violence and Subjectivity*, ed. Veena Das, Arthur Kleinman, Mamphela Ramphele, and Pamela Reynolds (Berkeley: University of California Press, 2000), 273–74.

32. Avery Comarow, "Jesica's Story," *U.S. News and World Report*, July 28, 2003, 51.

33. One Minneapolis story used the case of football star Walter Payton, ill and in need of a liver transplant, to highlight the variations nationwide. "Unless his case qualifies for rush status," the article in the *Minneapolis Star Tribune* noted, "he's likely to wait 100 to 200 days for a liver. . . . The typical wait has been longer than two years in some regions. Minnesotans exceed the national average in donating organs, and that's one reason the wait is shorter here" (Sharon Schmickle, "Wait Time for Organ Donations: Is it Fair? Walter Payton's Need for a Liver Transplant Has Put a Spotlight on a Controversy in the Allocation System," *Minneapolis Star Tribune*, February 4, 1999, 1A).

34. Sheryl Gay Stolberg, "Agreement on Plan to Revamp Organ Distribution," *New York Times*, November 12, 1999, A1.

35. Bruce Alpert, "House OKs Bill to Repeal Law Giving Organs to Sickest First," *New Orleans Times-Picayune*, April 5, 2000, 8A.

36. The *Pittsburgh Post-Gazette* noted, "If it weren't for the politics of protecting small transplant centers, organs would be distributed nationally based on a sickest-first policy. It is the most efficient use of these scarce and precious resources, and it is the only fair way to do it. But UNOS has been distributing organs geographically. . . . That means that less sick patients may get an organ, while a patient across the border dies waiting. It's not only absurd but also offensive" (Editorial, "Pathological Parochialism: Regional Organ Centers Get their Way in the House," *Pittsburgh Post-Gazette*, April 6, 2000, p. A-24). See also Editorial, "Transplant Politics," *New York Times*, April 6, 2000.

37. In 1999, for example, the *New Orleans Times-Picayune* reported that "the argument over who controls the limited supply of organs continues. . . . It pits the representatives of states with large transplant hospitals, like Pennsylvania, Texas, and California, against lawmakers from states like Louisiana, Arkansas and Alabama, where smaller transplant centers fear losing locally donated organs to the major transplant centers with longer patient waiting lists" (Bill Walsh, "Donor Organ Plan Is Again on Hot Seat," *New Orleans Times-Picayune*, October 21, 1999, A1).

38. Editorial, "Washington Should Not Take over the Organ Distribution Process," *Tampa Tribune*, August 9, 1999, 8; Editorial, "Organ Transplant Use Should Remain Local," *Seattle Times*, August 4, 1999.

39. The chronology of this political conflict over borders, fairness, organs, and transplant centers goes roughly as follows. In 1984, the National Organ Transplant Act created the modern organ allocation system, giving UNOS the contract for running this system. In 1998, Shalala, Secretary of Health and Human Services, proposed new rules to overhaul the system in favor of a national, "sickest-first" system of organ allocation. Between 1998 and 1999, a few states like Texas, Louisiana, and Wisconsin responded with laws barring the movement of organs out of state if local matches were available. Congress imposed a moratorium on the new HHS regulations and requested an Institute of Medicine study. In July 1999, the IOM report (looking at liver transplantation) suggested breaking the nation up into regions of 9 million each (instead of the widely varying population regions in the UNOS system). In November 1999, Shalala worked with Congress to enact the new national, sickest-first system. It was still opposed bitterly by many in Congress. In April 2000, the House voted to strip HHS of authority—to ensure that all authority remained with UNOS.

40. Sheryl Gay Stolberg, "States Fight Federal Government Transplant Policy," *New York Times*, March 11, 1999, 10A.

41. Comarow, "Jesica's Story," 51.

42. Lawrence Schneiderman and Nancy Jecker, *Wrong Medicine: Doctors, Patients, and Futile Treatment* (Baltimore: Johns Hopkins University Press, 1995).

43. Ibid.

44. Ibid.

45. But after the second transplant, as Jesica's hold on life grew more fragile, her most vocal supporter, Mack Mahoney, would argue that the new organs seemed to be functioning quite well, it was the tangled web of machinery, the aptly named "life support" that was killing Jesica. "Life support ruins kidneys, it ruins brains, it ruins all the organs of the body," he insisted. See "Botched Transplants Lead to Brain Damage," *Windsor Star*, February 22, 2003. Mahoney further insisted that Duke's delay in admitting the error and taking responsibility had doomed Jesica: "What we've done is played with that little girl's life, trying to make a decision on whether they was going to fess up." Elsewhere he argued, "Had she not spent this much time on these machines it would not be a problem. Even if she did have to have another heart, if they had gone ahead and fessed up in time for us to find another one in time this would not be a problem" ("Girl Has Brain Swelling after Transplant," *United Press International*, February 21, 2003).

TUCKER'S HEART

RACIAL POLITICS AND

HEART TRANSPLANTATION IN AMERICA

SUSAN E. LEDERER

Organ transplantation, especially moving the heart from one body to another, exemplifies American investment in high-tech medicine. Although the first human heart transplant was performed in a South African, rather than American, hospital, by surgeon Christiaan Barnard, the 1967 exploit was made possible only by the training he received in transplant surgery programs in the United States. By the time Jesica Santillan underwent her consecutive heart-lung transplants in 2003, American transplant programs remained a destination for individuals and their families seeking such high-tech interventions.

As in Jesica Santillan's story, the early American experience with heart transplantation was haunted by the specter of exploitation and inequality, dogged by questions of who should receive the "gift of life," and colored by ethnic politics. In Santillan's case, much of the debate revolved around the recipient. Her status as a Mexican immigrant disqualified her, in the eyes of some observers, for a scarce national resource, an American heart. Although Mexican labor was critical to the success of American farming and other economic endeavors, Mexicans were not welcome to reap the full benefits of citizenship. Four decades earlier, a similarly revealing controversy flared in the nascent field of organ transplantation—focusing principally on the donor side of the transplant equation. American racial politics provided a potent backdrop. African Americans had yet to secure their full rights as American citizens and as American patients. Until the enforcement of the Civil Rights Act of 1964, hospitals in the American South remained segregated. In Arkansas and Louisiana, blood banks were required by law to label blood by the race of the donor ("Caucasoid," "Negroid," and "Mongoloid") and to obtain explicit written permission from the recipient for crossing the color line in transfusion.[1] In 1968, only four years after the passage of historic civil rights legislation, race remained a critical issue in American medicine. The harvest of a heart from an African American man named Bruce Tucker and its transplantation into a white recipient sparked controversy over who would benefit from this new kind of high-tech medicine and whose bodies would make it possible for them to do so.

AN AMERICAN TRANSPLANT TRAGEDY

In May 1968 surgeons at the Medical College of Virginia (MCV) performed the tenth heart transplant in the United States. Surgeons removed the heart from the body of a severely brain-damaged fifty-four-year-old man and placed it in the chest of a fifty-three-year-old man. Amid the intense media interest in heart transplantation, officials from MCV did not initially identify either the donor or the recipient.[2] But on May 28, 1968, a reporter from the *Washington Post* labeled the MCV surgery as the first American interracial transplant: a Virginia "white" received a "Negro's heart" in a Richmond hospital.[3] Although Joseph Klett, the retired white businessman who received Bruce Tucker's heart, lived only seven days before he succumbed to massive rejection of the transplanted organ, the story surrounding Tucker's heart lived on. It became the focus of a lawsuit, an eventual judicial decision about the nature and determination of brain death, and a spur to legislatures to craft new statutes for defining death.[4] As the first legal case in the United States to challenge the conventional "definition of death" in the context of heart transplantation, citations to *Tucker v. Lower* appeared (and continue to appear) frequently in the bioethics literature.[5] But a curious thing happened in many of these discussions; the issue of race disappeared.[6] Yet the fact that the heart of an African American man was removed and placed into the chest of a white man was not incidental in 1968, in Richmond, and to members of Bruce Tucker's family. From the outset, organ transplantation has entangled questions of race with debates over the meanings of transplantation, the commodification of body parts, and the ethical implications of the political economy of high-tech medicine.

Before Christiaan Barnard performed the first human-to-human heart transplant in December 1967, he had spent three months at MCV, working with transplant pioneer David Hume. During his stay in Richmond, Barnard assisted in kidney transplants and learned how to manage the postoperative care for transplant recipients, including the study of rejection and the use of drugs to suppress the immune system. When he returned to Capetown, Barnard began preparations for human heart transplantation. In December 1967 he transplanted the heart of a young woman, extensively brain damaged in an automobile accident, into the body of Louis Washkansky. The recipient lived for eighteen days before he succumbed to pneumonia. Barnard's success ignited a media frenzy; it also spurred American surgeons to join the transplant enterprise.[7]

Within days of the Capetown transplant, New York surgeon Adrian Kantrowitz performed the second human-to-human heart transplant.[8] On December 6, 1967, he transplanted the heart of an anencephalic infant into another infant (eighteen days old), but the child lived for only six hours with the new organ. One month later, Stanford surgeon Norman Shumway performed the world's fourth heart transplant; his patient, Mike Kasperak, lived fifteen days before he died. In Texas, surgeon Denton Cooley joined the transplant race in May 1968 (Cooley transplanted hearts into seventeen patients in the remaining months of 1968, including a sheep-to-human heart transplant). In Richmond, the surgeons were eager for their opportunity to take part in this emergent transplant enterprise. (Indeed, MCV surgeon Richard Lower [who was also Shumway's first resident at Stanford] believed that Barnard became interested in heart transplants when he visited MCV, and witnessed the relative simplicity of the procedure.[9]) MCV surgeons had a potential candidate for a heart transplant—Joseph Klett, a retired executive with ongoing heart problems. But where would they get the necessary heart?

They located the organ in the body of Bruce O. Tucker, a fifty-four-year-old African American man and a longtime employee at a Richmond egg-packing plant. After a severe fall onto concrete, Tucker was brought by ambulance to MCV. He was unconscious, and alone. At MCV, he underwent a craniotomy to relieve the pressure in his brain. He was placed on a respirator, which kept him "mechanically alive." The following afternoon, Tucker was evaluated by a neurologist, who offered the opinion that it was "very likely" that Tucker's condition was "irreversible." He received both anesthesia and oxygen to maintain his organs. When he was removed from the respirator, the surgeons waited for his breathing to stop. They called for the medical examiner to pronounce him available for organ "harvesting," the term widely used to describe surgical retrieval from donors. Both his heart and kidneys were removed for transplant into other patients.[10]

Tucker had been declared "unclaimed dead," which would have made his body, under Virginia state law, available for medical use after twenty-four hours. Many of the facts of what happened remain in dispute, but it appears that no attempt was made by the hospital to contact his family. The members of Bruce Tucker's family were not consulted about the decision to remove his heart and kidneys. The family was not informed that Tucker had been declared one of the "unclaimed dead." Tucker's brothers, William and Grover Tucker, had called the hospital three times seeking information, and only later did they discover their brother's role in transplant history from the undertaker, who received the body for burial. The surviving Tuckers were especially distressed not only by the identification of their loved one as "unclaimed" but by how quickly his status mutated from dead person to "unclaimed dead." African Americans had long-standing and well-justified fears about the medical appropriation of black corpses. In fact, Virginia law required a twenty-four-hour waiting period for family or friends to come forward to claim a deceased loved one before he or she could be declared unclaimed. Amid the exigencies of the transplant race, however, surgeons disregarded the waiting period because such a delay would have made Tucker's organs unusable for transplant. Within one hour of the state medical examiner's pronouncement that he was "unclaimed dead," surgeons made the incision into his chest to remove his heart.[11] Angered by these events, William Tucker retained a young African American lawyer, L. Douglas Wilder, and brought two lawsuits. One lawsuit sought $100,000 from the three MCV surgeons, Richard Lower, David Hume, and David Sewell, and the Virginia state medical examiner, Dr. Abdullah Fatteh, on the grounds of "wrongful death, deprivation of property rights, insubstantial due process and 'mutilation' of the body without consent." The other, a federal suit made possible by recent 1960s legislation, sought $900,000 dollars in the U.S. District Court for deprivation of civil rights.[12]

Attorney Douglas Wilder explicitly identified race as a critical issue in the MCV heart transplant. A person accorded higher status in the community, charged Wilder, would not have been treated in the manner accorded Bruce Tucker. The hospital "pulled the plug because he was poor and black, a representative of the faceless masses."[13] Against the backdrop of Virginia race politics, before the case came to trial, Wilder, who also served as the first black state senator in Virginia since Reconstruction, successfully opposed a bill in the 1970 Virginia state legislature that would have legalized the removal of organs for transplantation without permission from the family of the deceased. Wilder called on long-standing African American popular beliefs about so-called night doctors who abducted black children for use in medical experiments, noting, "They're not going to be taking the hearts of any white mayors. You know whose hearts they're going to be taking. If this bill passes, its going to be so that black mothers will tell their children, 'Don't go walkin' down by the Medical College at night or the student doctor's gonna get you.'"[14]

Despite Wilder and his client's claims, MCV surgeons maintained that race played no role in the decision to take Tucker's heart; the transplant, they insisted, would have proceeded in an identical fashion if a middle-class white man had been brought to the hospital in a similar brain-damaged state. Moreover, MCV chair of surgery David Hume suggested that giving people "free" care in a state institution should shield MCV doctors from such charges. "Look," he told a reporter, "this [MCV] is a state-run institution and a large proportion of our patients are black. We've done some 235 organ grafts here, and none of the recipients has ever been charged doctors' fees or hospital costs. We should be the last ones to be picked on over racial matters."[15] Tucker did not prevail in his lawsuit; an all-white, all-male jury deliberated little over an hour before they absolved the surgeons of wrongdoing and accepted a novel medical definition of death based on the loss of brain function.[16]

Race relations, after playing this prominent role in the establishment of new medical criteria for determining death, certainly seem to have played a role in the subsequent heart transplants undertaken at MCV. On August 25, 1968, Richard Lower and his surgical team at MCV performed another heart transplant. Initially reticent to release the details in order "to protect the privacy of the organ donors and their families," the hospital announced that a forty-three-year-old man had received the heart of a seventeen-year-old gunshot victim.[17] But, unlike the Tucker transplant, both the donor and recipient in the August transplant were African American. In subsequent news reports, the recipient was identified as Louis B. Russell Jr., an elementary school teacher from Indianapolis. Russell became the thirty-fourth transplant recipient when he received the heart of Clarence Robert Brown, who had been shot in the back of the head with a small-caliber pistol following an argument in a Virginia restaurant.[18] A Richmond radio station broke the news of the identity of the donor.[19] Although newspapers outside the Richmond area did not identify the donor's race, a front-page story in the *Richmond Times-Dispatch* described the gunshot victim as "Brown, a Negro."[20] When the parents of the boy expressed the desire to meet Russell, MCV arranged transportation for the family to the Richmond hospital where Russell was convalescing.[21] Russell went on to become one of the longest surviving heart transplant patients in the early cohort of recipients; he survived six years with the transplanted heart. After his death in November 1974, the American Heart Association created the Louis B. Russell Jr. Memorial Award in 1976 to encourage greater outreach to minority and low-income communities.[22]

What difference did race make in the early years of heart transplantation? Was Tucker's race material to his selection as a heart source? Is it significant that Russell's race was not initially identified in news reports (and Brown's only rarely identified in print)? How did Russell's status as the "longest living American heart recipient" influence the role of race in heart transplantation? How did the racial politics of heart transplantation comport with similar issues of access and success in kidney transplantation? How did the lawsuit brought by the Tucker family influence the selection of subsequent donors?

Certainly the Tucker case resonated with the specter of racial selection already excited by Christiaan Barnard's South African heart transplants. Even before he electrified the world in December 1967 when he performed the first human heart transplant, Barnard's surgeries in apartheid South Africa rippled with disturbing racial undercurrents. In October 1967, when he performed the first kidney transplants in Capetown, Barnard acknowledged the "overtones of racial integration in a limited physiological arena" when his white patient, Mrs. Edith Black, received the kidney of "a colored youth." The world press could not resist such headlines as "Mrs. Black Receives Black Kidney."[23] Positioned like many white South African doctors between a desire for recognition by the international medical community and the racial politics and privilege that facilitated his practice, Barnard claimed to have hoped that his first heart transplant recipient would be "a Bantu with cardiomyopathy" but that a South African colleague told him, "Our first patient will never be black or colored because overseas they will say that we are experimenting on nonwhites."[24]

Perhaps in an effort to downplay the racial overtones, Barnard's first heart-transplant patient, a white, Jewish man named Louis Washkansky, received the heart taken from the body of a twenty-two-year-old white woman, Denise Darvall. In the blaze of media attention, reporters also noted how one of her kidneys was transplanted into a "colored boy" (or "mulatto" in some news reports).[25] But in January 1968, Barnard decisively crossed the cardiac color line. The heart recipient was Philip Blaiberg, a fifty-eight-year-old white, Jewish dentist. The source of the transplanted heart was Clive Haupt, identified as "Cape Colored," according to the South African racial caste system codified under apartheid.[26] Amid the hubbub of the interracial transplant and the perception that black bodies were providing the raw materials for transplant, Barnard announced that a "black African" would receive a heart in a transplant operation. As he offered this news, Barnard also informed reporters that his "black African" candidate "was not mentally stable so he might not be suitable for the operation." He went on to explain that this patient would not be likely to comply with the demanding post-transplant regimen. "So if the next patient is an African," Barnard concluded, "we will probably make some facilities available to keep him around for a few years."[27] Despite Barnard's announcement, however, his next recipient was a "white former policeman" in South Africa who received the heart of a "pregnant black," whose family, much like Bruce Tucker's, reportedly learned about the transplant only after they learned of her death.[28] After criticism in the press about the use of "black donor hearts" and the "harmful" reporting of transplants in the media, Barnard announced in 1975 that his hospital would stop using blacks as donors.[29]

This organ integration excited tremendous discussion in South Africa, America, and around the world. Some of it was piqued by the persistent notion that more than the tissue itself was transplanted. In the United States, for example, it was reported that Clive Haupt's widow could detect the personality traits of her late husband in the heart recipient, Philip Blaiberg.[30] In South Africa, some white South Africans apparently believed that the transplant represented "miscegenation of sorts."[31] At least one South African diplomat reassured the public that Philip Blaiberg's possession of a "colored" heart would not alter his legal status as a white man.[32]

Some American commentators welcomed the news of the Haupt donation: "The acceptance of the heart of a colored donor by a white patient, or the heart of a woman by a man, is a lesson in ethics as well as physiology. . . . The dying South African accepted the heart of a colored man as eagerly as he would have the heart of a white man, and not even the most bigoted Afrikaners said a word."[33] Africans in South Africa had few international outlets to voice their protest over the racial undertones of the transplant enterprise. But African Americans in print questioned Barnard's policies. In a letter to the *New York Times*, for example, Ellen Holly called for Barnard to use the organs of a white man to save a black man's life, noting, "All I know is that, as a black, if I lived in South Africa, I would be terrified at the prospect of going into a white South African hospital with a major illness. I also know that because of the inadequacies of the bush hospitals I might have no other choice."[34] The editors of *Ebony* magazine noted the rich irony of how the transplant would enable the Cape colored man's heart to go places that Haupt himself had not been permitted to enter: "Haupt's heart will ride in the uncrowded train coaches 'For Whites Only' instead of in the crowded ones reserved for blacks. It will pump extra hard to circulate the blood needed in a game of tennis where the only blacks are those who might tend the heavy rollers to smooth the courts. It will enter fine restaurants, attend theaters and concerts and live in a decent home instead of the tough slums where Haupt grew up."[35] But the editors cautioned that the use of a black person's organs to save a dying white man in South Africa also raised fears that the practice would not remain in South Africa. "Many black people today in both the United States and South

Africa," the editors noted, "fear hospitals because they believe that white doctors use black patients only for experimentation." This fear, they added, would lead families of potential black donors to refuse to authorize organ donation, because they believed that the doctors would "hurry a death" in order to finish a transplant.[36]

This fear was not limited to blacks. In Houston, a major center of heart transplantation, the media called attention to the fact that dying Mexican patients were transferred to Houston hospitals where patients awaited heart donors—much the way dying Africans and coloreds would have been transferred into otherwise segregated hospitals to facilitate Barnard's work. In 1968, Maria Acosta, a thirty-eight-year-old Mexican woman with a severe brain hemorrhage, was transferred in an ambulance from a hospital in Yuma, Arizona, to St. Luke's Hospital, where surgeon Denton Cooley ran a major heart transplant program. "No one says that Mrs. Acosta was actually taken from her Yuma hospital to St. Luke's for the specific purpose of being a heart donor," a reporter for the *Nation* wrote. "But this is certain: there are at present more than thirty potential heart recipients in St. Luke's; and some have been waiting as long as three months for a donor. Was someone playing God with Mrs. Acosta's life?"[37] In February 1969 Mrs. Guadalupe Montez, the widow of a Mexican American heart donor, filed a million dollar lawsuit against Cook County Hospital in Chicago alleging that her husband died as a result of "careless and negligent acts" in order to hurry a transplant operation.[38]

The Tucker lawsuit represented a transitional moment in the history of organ transplantation and the determination of death by new criteria involving the brain. But it also resonated with traditional medical practices involving low-income and minority patients. William Tucker was convinced that the MCV surgeons killed his brother in order to take his heart. His attorney made reference to the undue haste with which the medical examiner declared Bruce Tucker to be "unclaimed dead." As Douglas Wilder emphasized in his closing arguments, because Bruce Tucker was black and poorly dressed (and also because he had, according to various accounts, injured himself while drinking), he was declared "unclaimed."[39] Wilder also angrily pointed out that the chief medical examiner of Virginia, Dr. Geoffrey T. Mann, had reassured him that his (Wilder's) body would never be declared "unclaimed," "presumably because [Wilder] was plainly well dressed."[40] The determination that his brother's body was unclaimed particularly inflamed William Tucker. As the judge noted, when Bruce Tucker entered the hospital, his wallet contained a business card with the address of his brother's store (located within fifteen blocks of the hospital). Moreover, William Tucker had visited the hospital three times seeking news of his brother with no success. Despite William's efforts and the information on Tucker's person, his body was identified "unclaimed dead."

The Tucker case, a critical milestone in the history of brain death, also draws attention to Bruce Tucker's status as "socially dead" before he was pronounced dead by the medical examiner. Ethnographer David Sudnow used the term "social death" to refer to the state in which a hospital patient "is treated essentially as a corpse, though perhaps still 'clinically' and 'biologically' alive."[41] Bruce Tucker entered the hospital without friends or family members. Even worse in terms of medical decision making about his "terminality" as a patient, he entered the hospital with alcohol on his breath and on his clothes. "The alcoholic patient," Sudnow observed during his study of public hospitals in the late 1960s, "is treated by hospital physicians, not only when the status of his body as alive or dead is at stake, but throughout the whole course of medical treatment, as one for whom the concern to treat can properly operate somewhat weakly."[42] In the case of Bruce Tucker, physicians' level of concern about his recovery was colored by views of his race, by his socioeconomic class, and by his alcohol use.

The controversy over Bruce Tucker's bodily remains reverberated in American popular culture, and remained focused on the expropriation of black bodies, rather than the need for increased minority access to the benefits of American high-tech medicine. In 1969 the black comedian Dick Gregory played Carnegie Hall in New York City. In addition to riffs on the draft, Vice President Spiro Agnew, President Nixon, and the police, Gregory joked about interracial heart transplants. The heart that ran the longest, he noted, "was a black heart transferred into a white patient. That heart would be goin' yet," Gregory continued, "if he'd eaten a little soul food." Warning the audience, comprised of mostly young, white people, that blacks were not "goin' to be your spare parts," he called for transplants that could not be hidden: "I'd like to see a white cat get a black foot. Next summer, let him take that to the beach with him: Hey! They'd be yelling at him, 'take off your sneaker and come into the water.' "[43]

Gregory was not the only one to satirize the cultural possibilities of medical miscegenation. In the 1969 film Change of Mind, the brain of a white liberal lawyer dying of cancer is transplanted into the body of a recently dead black man. The black man finds that both his mother and his wife cannot accept his transformation, so he seeks solace in the arms of the widow of the man who furnished the body for brain transplant. Lawrence Louis Goldman's novel The Heart Merchants, published in 1970, featured a transplant surgeon faced with choosing which of two patients—an old, rich, white man or a young, poor, black man—will receive a donor heart. Complicating the issue of the transplant is the donor's father, who says that his son's heart won't be "goin' in no nigger body!"[44] In the end, the young black man receives the heart transplant, but the heart does not function.

How did racial attitudes, anxieties, and relations influence the practice of heart transplantation in the late 1960s and early 1970s? The information regarding race in both the medical and popular press was sketchy and inconsistent. Clearly there were anxieties about the unequal burdens of transplantation. In 1968, when the American College of Chest Physicians Committee on Heart Transplantation recommended greater responsibility in media reporting of heart transplants, including that all donors remain anonymous, W. Montague Cobb, editor of the *Journal of the National Medical Association*, insisted that their endorsement of anonymity was premature. Cobb cited the practice of declaring some dead persons as "unclaimed" as a particular area of concern. "Minority and impoverished groups," Cobb explained, "would be the most likely to be affected by the policy of anonymity. Therefore, any approval of such a policy should be withheld until all aspects of the situation have been publicly explored in depth."[45] In 1970, Dennis Cokkinos, a resident in cardiology at St. Luke's Hospital in Houston, cited in a *Journal of the National Medical Association* article a report from the American Civil Liberties Union's ad hoc committee on civil liberties and organ transplantation, which claimed that, among the first 100 heart transplants, there were sixty-four black donors but only one black recipient.[46]

The registry of heart transplants maintained by the American College of Surgeons–National Institutes of Health offered a somewhat different picture. In 1970, the ACS-NIH compiled a list of heart transplants by the race of the donor and the recipient over the previous few years. Whites served as donors in 110 cases, and 113 white patients received hearts. Hearts were obtained from 7 black donors, 1 "Oriental," and 4 individuals identified as "other." Nine blacks received a heart, as did one "Oriental." Only one "other" patient received a heart transplant.[47]

In the United States, the number of black heart transplant recipients seemed quite limited. The first woman and the first African American to receive a heart transplant was Ester Matthews, a forty-one-year-old Dallas housewife. In June 1968, she received the heart removed from the body of a twenty-six-year-old white man. Doctors at Parkland Memorial Hospital had hoped to transplant the heart of a woman into Matthews, but the woman's father refused permission for the transplant.[48] Houston surgeon Denton

Cooley reported in September 1968 a case in which a two-month-old "Negro girl" received the heart of a one-day-old white anencephalic infant.[49] At MCV, following the Tucker transplant, surgeon Richard Lower and his colleagues transplanted the heart from a young black man into Louis Russell, a black schoolteacher, who survived six years with the new heart until he succumbed to rejection. In October 1968, Lower transplanted the heart of a young black man (killed by a gunshot wound in the head) into a nineteen-year-old African American woman. One week later, Lower's team transplanted the heart from a white Norfolk policeman into a former Alexandrian police officer (also white). Lower did not cross the color line in cardiac transplantation after the Tucker controversy.

TUCKER'S HEART

Comedian Dick Gregory joked that black people were not willing to supply the spare parts needed for white people. But for some black Americans, this was not a laughing matter. In 1974, Sandra Haggerty explained that most blacks did not approve of transplants because of their distrust of doctors, who decide when you are dead. She quoted from an informal poll the range of black views about transplantation:

> "You notice the heart transplants have all been from blacks to whites. I'd like to see a little reciprocation before I get on the bandwagon!"
> "No way! A brother's likely to go in the hospital with a cold and come out without a heart."
> "I just can't trust the Man. He's made it purrfectly [sic] clear whose life he values. No sense in me volunteering."[50]

Distrust of the white medical establishment has also been cited by Howard University transplant surgeon Clive Callendar as one of the factors responsible for the lower rates of organ donation among African Americans. Yet these donation rates need to be viewed in relation to equally low transplantation rates among blacks. When he testified before the House Commerce Committee Subcommittee on Health and Environment in 1998, Callendar reminded members of Congress that African Americans continued to wait twice as long as other Americans for kidney transplants. (In 2002 the waiting time for a cadaveric kidney is almost twice as long for an African American as it is for whites. Moreover, African Americans are less likely to have living donors.)[51] He pointed to a history of inequitable organ allocation, distrust of the medical establishment, and fear that signing an organ donor card would lead to erroneous or premature declarations of death. Thirty years after Bruce Tucker's heart was removed, questions of race and identity continue to shape the politics and therefore practices of organ transplantation—for both donors and recipients, as in the Jesica Santillan story.

The cultural complexity of donation was largely invisible in the Santillan drama, but it remains a prominent and potent theme in contemporary debates over organ transplantation. In 2002, the Hollywood film *John Q* featured actor Denzel Washington as a hard-working man engaged in a desperate struggle to ensure that his son will receive the heart transplant necessary to save his life. Many American filmgoers reportedly identified with Washington's character as he confronted the harsh realities of managed health care. Although the film generally received only tepid reviews, some reviewers praised the film for not exploiting "the race card." Still, in the film all the doctors and hospital administrators are white; the hero and his family are black. Although the issue is not the topic of explicit discussion in the film, the film's skepticism about the medical establishment and its provision of care resonates with experiences like the Tucker family's and the lingering resentment about differential treatment (or lack of treatment). As Nation of Islam minister Louis Farrakhan has caustically claimed, the failure of white society to control black-on-black violence provides a steady supply of organs: "When you're killing each other, they can't wait for you to die," Farrakhan announced at a rally. "You're good for parts."[52] Bruce Tucker proved good for parts, more useful as a source of an organ than as a patient.

Unlike Bruce Tucker, Jesica Santillan—characterized as an unworthy recipient by many—was not good for parts. She represented a drain on American resources. Relying on financial resources from the community, she was able to obtain scarce organs intended for American citizens, not illegal immigrants. Still, the response to the Santillan story reveals many parallels between the two cases, for it was part of a long history of troubling concerns that have shadowed the transplantation system from its early years—concerns about equity, about the role of money and the purchasing of privileged access, about the process by which one person's "parts" becomes another person's "gift of life," and about who gives and who receives.

NOTES

1. Susan E. Lederer, *Flesh and Blood: A Cultural History of Transplantation and Transfusion* (New York: Oxford University Press, forthcoming).

2. See "College Sets Report on Transplant," *Washington Post*, May 31, 1968, B9.

3. Victor Cohn, "Va. White Got Negro's Heart," *Washington Post*, May 28, 1968, B1.

4. There is an extensive literature on brain death; see, for example, Margaret Lock, *Twice Dead: Organ Transplants and the Reinvention of Death* (Berkeley: University of California Press, 2002); Stuart Youngner, Robert Arnold, and Renie Schapiro, eds., *The Definition of Death: Contemporary Controversies* (Baltimore: Johns Hopkins University Press, 1999); and Peter McCullagh, *Brain Dead, Brain Absent, Brain Donors: Human Subjects or Human Objects* (New York: Wiley, 1993). See also Martin Pernick, "Brain Death in a Cultural Context—The Reconstruction of Death, 1967–1981," in *The Definition of Death—Contemporary Controversies*, ed. Stuart J. Youngner, Robert M. Arnold, and Renie Shapiro (Baltimore: Johns Hopkins University Press, 1999); Gary S. Belkin, "Brain Death and the Historical Understanding of Bioethics," *Journal of the History of Medicine and Allied Sciences* 58 (2003): 325–61; and Mita Giacomini, "A Change of Heart and a Change of Mind? Technology and the Redefinition of Death in 1968," *Social Science and Medicine* 44 (1997): 1465–82.

5. See *Tucker v. Lower*, No. 2381 (Richmond, Virginia, Law & Equity Court, May 23, 1972).

6. Sarah D. Barber, "The Tell-Tale Heart: Ethical and Legal Implications of In Situ Organ Preservation in the Non-Heart-Beating Cadaver Donor," *Health Matrix* 6 (1996): 471. In both editions of the *Encyclopedia of Bioethics*, the entries for brain death (each written by Alexander Capron) mentions *Tucker v. Lower* but does not mention race. Margaret Lock discusses the Tucker lawsuit in "Inventing a New Death and Making it Believable," *Anthropology and Medicine* 9 (2002): 97–115, but does not mention race. There are exceptions, however. Robert Veatch, for example, discusses race in his accounts of the Tucker case. See Robert M. Veatch, *Death, Dying, and the Biological Revolution* (New Haven: Yale University Press, 1976), 21–25; and Veatch, *Transplantation Ethics* (Washington, D.C.: Georgetown University Press, 2000), 43–44.

7. Christiaan Barnard and Curtis Bill Pepper, *One Life* (Toronto: Macmillan, 1969).

8. This enumeration counts surgeon James D. Hardy's chimp-to-human heart transplant in 1964 as the first heart transplant . Different accounts assign the Virginia human-to-human transplant a different number in the heart transplant chronology. There are several popular histories of the heart transplants, including Tony Stark, *Knife to the Heart: The Story of Transplant Surgery* (London: Macmillan, 1996), and Nicholas L. Tilney, *Transplant: From Myth to Reality* (New Haven: Yale University Press, 2003).

9. Sara J. Shumway and Norman E. Shumway, eds. *Thoracic Transplantation* (Cambridge, Mass.: Blackwell Science, 1995), xi–xii.

10. Abdullah Fatteh, "A Lawsuit that Led to the Redefinition of Death," *Journal of Legal Medicine* 1 (July/August 1973): 30–34.

11. Veatch, *Transplantation Ethics*, 43–44.

12. "Seeks $1 Million in Mixed Heart Transplant Case," *Jet*, June 11, 1970, 15.

13. "Civil Rights Questions Nag after Transplant Death Trial," *Medical World News*, June 16, 1972.

14. "Heart Snatch Case," *Richmond Afro-American*, June 3, 1972, 1–2. For "night

doctors," see Patricia A. Turner, *I Heard It Through the Grapevine: Rumor in African-American Culture* (Berkeley: University of California Press, 1993), 67–70.

15. See "Civil Rights Questions."

16. "Jury Rules in Favor of the Heart Team," (Richmond) *Journal and Guide*, June 3, 1972, 16.

17. "Man, 43, Receives a Heart Transplant at Virginia College," *New York Times*, August 25, 1968, 50.

18. See "Heart Donor's Killer Sought by Police," *Washington Post*, August 29, 1968, E18, which does not include mention of race. For identification of Russell by name (but not race) the following day, see "Latest Heart Patient, 43, Fed Day after Transplant," *New York Times*, August 26, 1968, 8.

19. "34th Heart Transplant Aired," *Washington Post*, August 25, 1968, C2.

20. Beverley Orndorff, "Heart Transplant Performed at MCV," *Richmond Times-Dispatch*, August 25, 1968, 1. In the numerous articles that appeared subsequently about Russell's successful transplant, the race of the donor was not mentioned. The only place where the race of Russell's donor was identified was in the *Times-Dispatch* article. My thanks to Jodi Koste for helping to locate this item.

21. "Teacher with Transplanted Heart Returns to Classroom," *Jet*, February 27, 1969, 46–52.

22. Diana Christopulos, *Time, Feeling and Focus: A Newly Designed Culture: The Evolution of the American Heart Association, 1975–1997* (American Heart Association, 2000). The first recipient of the award was a black nurse from Los Angeles, Winifred Ray Carnegie, 1977. See Press Release, American Heart Association, January 28, 1977, AHA materials.

23. Barnard and Pepper, *One Life*, 249.

24. Ibid., 251.

25. See ibid., 279, for Darvall's father's description of the kidney recipient. For reference to the "coloured boy" who received Darvall's kidney, see also "Two from One," *Chicago Defender*, December 16–22, 1967, 28. Barnard, of course, received his transplant training in the United States; he participated in American conferences regarding heart transplantation. Given this background and training, the idea that the first transplant was a South African breakthrough and Barnard's decision to go first clearly disturbed American heart surgeons. For more on Barnard and American surgeons, see Donald S. Fredrickson Papers, 1910–2002 (bulk 1960–99), in Modern Manuscripts Collection, History of Medicine Division, National Library of Medicine, Bethesda, Maryland, MS C 526.

26. In a front-page story, the *Washington Post* explained that Cape Coloreds are usually a "mixture of European, Hottentot, Asian, and Black African Stock." See "Another Heart Transplant: White South African Receives Cape Colored Man's Heart," *Washington Post*, January 3, 1968, 1, and Philip Blaiberg, *Looking at My Heart* (Portsmouth, N.H.: Heinemann, 1969). Long before the current heyday of reality TV, the NBC network sought to capitalize on intense interest in transplants; the network

paid Philip Blaiberg $50,000 for exclusive rights to film his operation and successfully sued when a photographer posing as a medical student sold photographs of the operation. See W. David Gardner, "The Heart is a Lonely Hunter," *Ramparts* 7 (June 1969): 34–38.

27. "Black African Due to Get Next Heart," *New York Times*, January 9, 1968, 29.

28. See "A Pregnant Black Was Heart Donor," *New York Times*, September 8, 1968, 34; and "Heart Donor Was Unknown," *Washington Post*, September 12, 1968, A3.

29. "Barnard Stops Using Black Donor Hearts," *Chicago Tribune*, February 3, 1975, 4.

30. See Brewer, "Cardiac Transplantation," *Journal of the American Medical Association* 205 (1968): 691.

31. "Showbiz in Operating Room," *New York Times*, January 7, 1968, E9.

32. "No Legal Significance," *New York Times*, January 3, 1968, 32.

33. "Surgical Show Biz," *The Nation* 206 (January 22, 1968): 100.

34. Ellen Holly, "Transplant Abuse," *New York Times*, September 29, 1968, p. E11.

35. "The Telltale Heart," *Ebony*, March 1968, 118.

36. Ibid.

37. Desmond Smith, "Someone Playing God," *The Nation* 207 (December 30, 1968): 719–21.

38. Charles Carroll, "The Ethics of Heart Transplantation," *Journal of the National Medical Association* 62 (1970): 14–20. See "Heart Donor's Widow Sues," *New York Times*, February 9, 1969, 16.

39. There is no information about whether Tucker's drinking arose during the trial. The judge published a lengthy analysis of Tucker but did not mention drinking as a precipitating factor. See A. Christian Compton, "Telling the Time of Human Death by Statute: An Essential and Progressive Trend," *Washington and Lee Law Review* 31 (1974): 521–43. The ur-source for Tucker's drinking seems to be Lawrence Mosher, "When Does Life End?" *The National Observer*, June 3, 1972. Several of the contemporary accounts, and recent popular and historical accounts, continue to mention Tucker's drinking as a precipitating factor. See, for example, Peter G. Filene, *In the Arms of Others: A Cultural History of the Right-to-Die in America* (Chicago: I. R. Dee, 1998), 56–57.

40. Victor Cohn, " 'Brain Death' Upheld in Heart Transplant," *Washington Post*, May 26, 1972, A1.

41. David Sudnow, *Passing On: The Social Organization of Dying* (Englewood Cliffs, N.J.: Prentice-Hall, 1967), 74.

42. Ibid., 104.

43. McCandlish Phillips, "Dick Gregory in an Hour at Carnegie," *New York Times*, November 27, 1969, 51.

44. Lawrence L. Goldman, *The Heart Merchants* (New York: Paperback Library, 1970), 245.

45. "Withholding Names of Organ Transplant Donors," *Journal of the National Medical Association* 60 (1968): 523.

46. Dennis Cokkinos, "Human Cardiac Transplantation: Experience and Results with 21 Cases," *Journal of the National Medical Association* 62 (1970): 8–13, 24; in the same issue, Charles Carroll, "The Ethics of Heart Transplantation," 14–20, 24.

47. Registry Data, Richard Lower Papers, Box 6, folder: Transplant Registry, Archives, Tompkins-McGaw Library, Medical College of Virginia, VCU, Richmond, Virginia.

48. "Texas Negro Woman Dies after Implant," *Los Angeles Times*, June 8, 1968, 6.

49. Denton Cooley et al., "Human Heart Transplantation: Experience with Twelve Cases," *American Journal of Cardiology* 12 (1968): 804–10, quotation on 806.

50. Sandra Haggerty, "Blacks' Attitudes about Heart Transplants," *Los Angeles Times*, January 22, 1974, A7.

51. Joint Hearing of the House Commerce Committee Subcommittee on Health and Environment, June 18, 1998, <http://www.med.howard.edu/ethics/handouts/joint—hearing—of.htm>.

52. Trevor Corson, "Organ Rejection: Why Do Blacks Fear Organ Donation?" *American Prospect*, May 20, 2002, 27–28.

JUSTICE IN ORGAN ALLOCATION

ROSAMOND RHODES

As a philosopher and medical educator, I teach a broad range of topics in medical ethics with medical students, house staff, and faculty. It is not surprising that issues related to transplantation frequently arise in my teaching because my home institution, Mount Sinai, is a major transplant center that has had its own share of controversy. Nevertheless, I was somewhat surprised when the Santillan case was mentioned twice on a recent morning, first in a teaching session with residents from orthopedics and second during surgery teaching rounds. A resident in orthopedics mentioned Santillan in the context of comparing the Duke administration's handling of their tragedy with the response of the Mount Sinai administration to a particular incident at the hospital. A surgery resident mentioned the case in the context of a discussion about whether patients should be told that a new material for hernia repair is produced from cadaveric tissue. The resident remarked that when advocates were clamoring for a second set of organs for Jesica, no one seemed to notice that they came from a cadaver. These are a few of the many interesting points raised by the case.

In what follows, I discuss the case's central ethical issue, the question of whether transplant organs were allocated justly. Specifically, I argue that organ allocation should be governed by a distinct set of principles that are a small subset of the considerations of justice. As I see it, there are certain factors that are important and appropriate in the allocation of resources in a variety of social interactions. For example, "equality" is an appropriate principle for the distribution of Monopoly money at the start of a game. "Worthiness" is an important consideration in hiring job applicants. Expectation of "future contribution to society" is relevant in awarding research grants. "Past contributions" are significant in bestowing honors. "Personal relationships" are important for issuing invitations to a dinner party. Head Start early childhood education programs provide children with "fair equality of opportunity." Emission standards and sanitation measures are imposed for their "utility," since the clean environment that they yield provides the greatest benefit to the greatest number.

In medicine, however, we do not expect clinicians to give equal amounts of resources to all patients, but to allocate their time, energy, equipment, and technology according to patient "need" and the "urgency" of their need. We do not want doctors sorting patients according to who they might count as worthy, nice, or useful; we expect clinicians to avoid making such distinctions and to treat each patient with "caring" and "respect." And when there are not enough resources to save all of those who need saving (for example, in the aftermath of a mass casualty event), we expect medical professionals to make the difficult choices rather than yielding to the pull of sympathy and drama or the desire to give the most to those who are nearest and dearest. We count on doctors to make decisions based on "medical triage" or "efficacy," to focus their efforts on those who are most likely to survive, in order to minimize losses.

These differences between ordinary concepts of justice and the considerations that are appropriate for the allocation of medical resources indicate that principles of "clinical justice" are frequently radically different from those of justice in other contexts. This distinction suggests that it is important to examine allocation principles in terms of the context in which they are being used. In this discussion, I argue that principles imported from other social domains are inappropriate in the allocation of transplant organs and that organ allocation policy should be governed exclusively by principles of clinical justice.

THE CASE

Seventeen-year-old Jesica Santillan was an illegal immigrant from Mexico who had been smuggled into the United States by her parents in hopes of getting treatment for her failing heart. Her age made Jesica a good candidate for heart transplantation, and in January 2002, she was listed for a cadaveric heart with the United Network for Organ Sharing (UNOS). As she waited for an organ, her lungs deteriorated, and by May 2002, she was listed for a combined transplant of heart and lung. Ultimately, Jesica received two heart-lung transplants at Duke University Hospital, the first on February 7, 2003, the second on February 20, 2003. Suffering acute rejection after the first transplant of organs with the wrong blood type, she was sustained on life support until she was allocated new compatible transplant organs. Unfortunately, neither transplant was able to save her life, and she died on February 22, days after her second transplant.

The transplant organs that Jesica Santillan received were allocated to her according to UNOS policies. This essay focuses solely on the issue of whether UNOS policies for the allocation of scarce transplant organs reflect an appropriate conception of justice. I review some of the history that set the stage for UNOS policy and then discuss some of the most recent developments in UNOS policy, namely the Model for End-Stage Liver Disease (MELD) systems for the allocation of cadaveric livers.

HISTORICAL BACKGROUND

Albert R. Jonsen, author of *The Birth of Bioethics* and organizer of the 1992 Seattle conference by that name, argues that the American bioethics movement began with the creation of the Admissions and Policy Committee, which has become known as the "God Committee." The committee determined the way in which kidney dialysis treatment, which was extraordinarily scarce at the time would be allocated at the King's Count Medical Society's Seattle Artificial Kidney Center. The committee, appointed by the institution's board of trustees, began its work in 1962 and continued to function until 1972. Its seven anonymous members were a minister, a lawyer, a homemaker, a business man, a labor leader, and two physicians who were not nephrologists. They began their work with a case-by-case review of candidates for dialysis, examining "extensive personal, social, psychological, and economic information on the candidates."[1] Using that information, over time they developed a set of selection criteria. First they established that Washington residency was a necessary criterion for treatment because the initial dialysis research had been funded by Washington taxpayers. Their list of "social worth criteria" for selection eventually included "age, gender, marital status and number of dependents, income, educational background, occupation, past performance, and future potential."

Shana Alexander's *Life* magazine article, "They Decide Who Lives, Who Dies," about the committee and their selection process sparked national interest followed by active debate about the process.[2] Theologians, philosophers, sociologists, and legal theorists began to write about the issue. Public attention finally produced legislative changes in the Social Security Act providing federal funding for disease management under the End-Stage Renal Disease Amendment (1972).

The dialogue pointed to one remarkable feature of the allocation of medical treatment: that decisions were left largely in the hands of nonphysicians. The debates were fought in terms of the ethics of everyday life, and arguments about social worth, egalitarianism, and utilitarianism took center stage. These debates and others about medical ethics also took on a political cast with the creation (starting in 1980) of a series of National Presidential Commissions focused on problems of ethics in medicine, in which the membership reflected the political perspective of the appointing U.S. president.

Over the same period, as techniques for managing organ rejection (primarily the introduction of cyclosporine) and for identifying histocompatibility developed, kidney transplantation became an alternative to dialysis and transplantation became a treatment for other organ failure. With these technological advances, the debate about the allocation of scarce life-preserving therapy, which had once revolved around dialysis, extended to the domain of organ transplantation. When the debate began there was no centralized network to increase the utilization of scarce donated organs and no criteria to govern organ allocation. There was, however, concern that wealthy citizens of foreign countries were coming to the United States to take advantage of transplantation technology and using scarce transplant organs that should be allocated to terminally ill U.S. residents.

Several important milestones in the development of U.S. organ allocation policy reflected these concerns:

1968

The Uniform Anatomical Gift Act (adopted in some form by every state by 1973) enabled individuals to legally declare that their bodily parts may be used for transplantation after their death. If the wishes of the deceased are not known, the next of kin are assigned the right to make this decision.

1972

The End-Stage Renal Disease (ESRD) Program, established through an amendment to the Social Security Act, made people with ESRD eligible for Medicare coverage. The costs covered by this program include renal dialysis, renal transplantation, organ procurement costs, and expenses of the Organ Procurement Organizations (OPOS).

1984

The National Organ Transplant Act created the National Organ Procurement and Transplantation Network (OPTN), a federally funded agency to act as the public's agent in matters of organ allocation with authority to set and enforce rules controlling OPO membership and organ allocation at both the local and the interagency level. It provided that only member agencies of OPTN could procure organs and only member hospitals could transplant organs.

1986

The U.S. Department of Health and Human Services awarded a one-year contract to a private organization, the United Network for Organ Sharing, for the development and implementation of the national network. The entire system went into effect October 1, 1987. All clinical transplant centers, organ procurement organizations, and tissue-typing laboratories in the United States belong to and participate in UNOS. UNOS has developed membership criteria (based on the education, training, and experience of medical personnel) and performance standards and policies, and it monitors compliance. It maintains a national waiting list of all patients in the country waiting for solid organ transplantation and matches organs with recipients. UNOS operates as the OPTN under contract with the U.S. Department of Health and Human Services and submits to department oversight, providing extensive information to the department for its review regarding OPTN policies. The OPTN/UNOS Board and committee members are primarily physicians and health care workers. Out of the 415 total members, approximately seven of the twelve lay members are not health care professionals.[3]

1990s

Under President Clinton, Secretary of Health and Human Services Donna Shalala, became actively involved in the organ allocation debate and promulgated rules to minimize region as an allocation factor because geographical location does not reflect the urgency of a patient's need.

These policy developments reflect the success of transplantation. Successful transplants have encouraged new patients to turn to transplantation to extend their lives, have allowed previous patients to outlive the viability of their transplanted organs so that they return for retransplantation, and have encouraged doctors to offer transplantation as an effective treatment for an increasing array of lethal medical conditions. These new uses of cadaveric organs, in turn, increased the demand for transplant organs. Although the rate of organ donation is on the rise, and in spite of national and local efforts to increase organ donation, it is not rising fast enough to meet the growing demand. About 6,000 Americans die each year for lack of a transplant organ.[4] This severe shortage of human organs for transplantation has created competition for the cadaveric organs that are donated and has made allocation policies highly controversial. In turn, the organ shortage has pressed the transplantation community to develop allocation mechanisms that can hold up to public scrutiny.

Families that donate the organs of deceased loved ones do so out of appreciation for the great good that transplanted organs provide and out of trust that their gifts will be allocated justly. They expect that all those in need of organs will be treated equitably and that cadaveric organs will be allocated according to principles that reasonable people could endorse. Transplant surgery, transplant centers, and institutions responsible for organ retrieval and allocation all exist because our society acknowledges the great benefit that transplantation provides for those with end-stage organ failure and because society intends the equitable allocation of its scarce transplant organs. In general, society expects that the focus on the good of the patient is the central moral goal of medicine, and in transplantation, society expects that the commitment to the good of individual patients and the good of the pool of potential transplant recipients is the guiding principle in the establishment of organ transplant programs and the design of equitable organ allocation policies.

In what follows, and with the Santillan case as a background consideration, I critically evaluate the principles that should support a just system of organ allocation.

CLINICAL JUSTICE

In making their decisions, the "God Committees" of the early 1960s that were formed to allocate use of scarce dialysis equipment scrutinized the lives of individuals with end-stage kidney failure to determine which candidates were most worthy of the lifesaving treatment.[5] Committee members, upstanding members of their communities, brought a range of guiding principles and commitments to their considerations. They considered individuals' past contribution to society, possible future contributions, family relationships, community involvement, age, behaviors that may have contributed to their current situation, how badly off one person was relative to others, etc.

Such considerations are very appropriate to many decisions that we make every day about the distribution of limited resources. As I already noted, people's past contributions are relevant when we choose who to honor. We consider the likelihood of future contributions in awarding grants. Relationships and friendships are important considerations when we choose who to invite to dinner at our homes. Community involvement may be a factor in electing public officials. Age may matter when purchasing movie tickets, where children and seniors are offered discounted admission, or in allocating nurturance and respect. Being the one who breaks or forgets an umbrella could leave you wet in the rain; on the other hand, being worse off than others in not having enough food to feed your family could entitle you to the charity of others. In other words, an array of principles of distributive justice are invoked in various contexts of human interaction.

Similarly, consider the deliberation of the several Presidential Commissions on ethics and medicine. Historically, commissioners have invoked their favorite philosophic and political perspectives and attempted to mold policy according to their own conceptions of the good and their own priorities. Some draw on utilitarianism, others refer to deontic rules of ethics (that is, ethics relating to rules and obligations), some invoke liberal values, others draw libertarian lines, and recently in the political arena some have decided that it is appropriate to be guided by their personal religious traditions.

Nevertheless, whether you were sympathetic to President Clinton's National Bioethics Advisory Commission or President Bush's President's Council on Bioethics, when it comes to setting organ allocation policy, it is easy to imagine that you might prefer to have health care professionals, rather than commissioners, council members, or the God Committee, craft the organ allocation rules. The difference between decisions made by a committee of good citizens from the community and those made by a committee of health care professionals is more than a difference in knowledge. For good reason, the thought of having such community groups set the agenda for medical policies, including organ allocation policy, would strike many people with horror and trepidation.

If we imagine a doctor in a crowded hospital emergency room, we immediately recognize that the range of appropriate principles for allocating the doctor's finite supply of energy, skills, time, and medical supplies is drastically restricted. For the most part, we expect doctors to treat first those whose condition is most urgent, then to allocate the resources that they command according to need. In situations of extreme scarcity, such as the aftermath of a cataclysmic disaster or on a battlefield, we accept that doctors will also consider efficacy. When faced with acutely insufficient resources, doctors are supposed to triage patients. They identify those who are most likely to require a significant investment of medical assets and least likely to derive significant benefit and they ration resources by assigning that group the lowest treatment priority with the expectation that many of them will not survive. In the face of a drastic shortage, we actually expect doctors to withhold treatment from a few patients in order to avoid the worst outcome for the entire pool of patients. We do not want doctors to stop before providing needed treatment to first assess a patient's worthiness of their attention. We do not want doctors to choose whether to treat or not to treat based on how much they value each patient. To the contrary, we expect that doctors are committed to the nonjudgmental regard of every patient and to a caring attitude toward each.

In sum, only a few of a standard array of allocation considerations are appropriate for medical decisions. Medicine recognizes only urgency, need, efficacy, and equality as appropriate principles for what I call "clinical justice." For the most part, there is such a general agreement on these principles that we can claim that an overlapping consensus of those in our society accept the view that allocations of medical resources according to those criteria are equitable. That acceptance also means that we expect doctors and other health care professionals to limit their allocation decisions to those constraints.[6]

In most cases, comparative appraisals of patients that go beyond considerations of clinical justice are illegitimate for the allocation of medical resources. Clinical justice eschews comparative judgments of patients' worthiness even when such distinctions might best promote the interests of some group that other citizens or theorists would give allocation priority, such as the richest, the most famous, or the least advantaged. In the most dire circumstances, clinical justice even sometimes requires clinicians to implement "medical triage" in order to avoid the worst overall outcome, and to eschew the emotional pull of the "rule of rescue," which would instead direct tremendous and scarce resources to a dramatic attempt at saving a victim with dismal prospects for survival but whose case tugs at the public's heart strings.

UNOS ALLOCATION POLICY

For the most part, UNOS policy can be seen as an attempt to allocate transplant organs by prioritizing potential organ recipients based only on medically relevant differences so that transplant candidates can be treated "equitably." The system's stated aim is to establish instruments for making uniform measurements for urgency of need (that is, how *soon* someone will die without the transplant and how *badly off* someone will be without it) so that patients who are listed for transplantation at different centers can be fairly assessed and compared, allowing similar cases to be treated similarly.[7] Although arguments persist about how much weight should be assigned to each consideration, the criteria that quantify severity of disease are intended to reflect differences in urgency and need that can be validated with clinical

Table 1. Child-Turcotte-Pugh (CTP) Scoring System to Assess Severity of Liver Disease

Points	1	2	3
Encephalopathy	None	1–2	3–4
Ascites	Absent	Slight (or controlled by diuretics)	At least moderate despite diuretic treatment
Bilirubin (mg/dl)	<2	2–3	>3
Albumin (g/dl)	>3.5	2.8–3.5	<2.8
INR	<1.7	1.7–2.3	>2.3

Source: UNOS, <www.unos.org>, September 4, 2001

data and adjusted to reflect an evidence-based refined understanding. While the specific criteria and standards vary somewhat from organ to organ, because of immunological sensitivities and features specific to the survival of particular organs, these assessment instruments are supposed to quantify medical differences and rank them based exclusively on medical considerations. Beyond the relatively objective UNOS criteria, allocation priority is left to fairness as approximated by a rule of first come, first served.

Controversy in the field of liver transplantation has prodded policy refinements in this area, so I take it as my illustrative example. The Child-Pugh score, the primary instrument for listing and ranking liver transplant candidates until 2002, assigns points for symptoms and biological markers of disease (table 1). It was used to approximate an objective standard for assessing the seriousness of need and the urgency of liver transplantation. Patients with liver disease had to have seven points to be listed for transplantation. Then, depending on the number of points their condition merited and factors about their disease, they were assigned to a category of urgency (for example, 1, 2A, 2B, 3) (table 2). Theoretically, those with the most urgent need were given priority for receiving an organ.[8] Organs were also matched to recipients based on biological factors, such as size and tissue compatibility, so as to minimize harm and to maximize benefit.

POLICY DEVELOPMENT

As I have noted elsewhere, original UNOS policies, crafted by an assortment of stakeholders, left us with the injustice of local priority, preferential treatment for small transplant centers, and discriminatory waiting period

Table 2. Adult Donor Liver Allocation Algorithm

Local

1. Status 1 patients in descending point order

Regional

2. Status 1 patients in descending point order

Local

3. Status 2A patients in descending point order

4. Status 2B patients in descending point order

5. Status 3 patients in descending point order

Regional

6. Status 2A patients in descending point order

7. Status 2B patients in descending point order

8. Status 3 patients in descending point order

National

9. Status 1 patients in descending point order

10. Status 2A patients in descending point order

11. Status 2B patients in descending point order

12. Status 3 patients in descending point order

Source: Table 1, UNOS Policy 3.6 Allocation of Livers (June 16, 2000), <www.unos.org>.

rules for past users of alcohol and narcotics.[9] (See also essays in this volume by Gross and Wailoo and Livingston.) In contrast, the Model for End-Stage Liver Disease plan, which went into effect on February 27, 2002, and replaced the Child-Pugh system, was developed by doctors. The MELD system assigns points to different evidence-based indicators of serious liver disease and thus provides a number to represent each potential recipient's urgency of need.[10] By more accurately predicting just how long a patient with liver failure can survive, it makes the assessment of urgency more objective than the previous Child-Pugh scoring system and allows those in most urgent need to have priority. Waiting time, which had previously played a significant role in allocation, is now given a diminished role because doctors recognized that time on the list largely reflects social and economic differences related to access to care. Medical reasons for deviating from MELD point allocation, as well as treatment innovations, are studied and treated as potential rules to be incorporated into revised MELD policy.[11] Based on this line of reasoning, the accumulating evidence that patients with very high MELD scores have a significantly lower likelihood of survival than other candidates, should, in the future, move clinicians to accept an efficacy-based numerical cap on eligibility. (In order to maintain transparency, all of these policies and supporting data are posted on the national UNOS Web site.[12])

DISPARATE WAITING TIMES AND THE
INFLUENCE OF SMALL CENTERS: A STRIKING
FEATURE OF CURRENT TRANSPLANT POLICY

In her June 1, 1998, letter to Congress, Donna Shalala, then secretary of Heath and Human Services, discussed a significant problem in the way organs were allocated for transplantation in the United States. Describing the effects of the UNOS policy, she explained that "the median waiting times for the two major liver transplant centers in Kentucky were vastly different—38 days at one center, 226 at the other. Similarly, in Louisiana, the median waiting time at one center was reported to be 18 days, while at another it was 262 days. In Michigan, the numbers were 161 days and 401 days. Although these numbers do not tell the whole story, they certainly reflect that unacceptable disparities in waiting times exist, even within states."[13]

While many disparities in what people have and get are unavoidable, other disparities can be averted, and while many disparities are ethically unproblematic, others signal serious problems of injustice. Social policies are just when they provide for equal treatment of all who are similarly situated and attend to relevant and important common human concerns. Policies are unjust when they give priority to extraneous concerns and irrelevant differences and thereby give people in relevantly similar situations inequitable treatment. For people who need an organ transplant to live or to live without significant disability, their primary concern is receiving a successful transplant. For people charged with equitably allocating transplant organs, the most appropriate considerations for distinguishing between potential recipients should be the urgency of patient need and the likelihood for success. Beyond those medical standards, patients should be treated equally.[14]

Yet a careful examination of UNOS allocation policies reveals that additional agendas inform its positions and practices. While UNOS policies are supposed to provide for the just allocation of cadaveric transplant organs, and while they take significant steps in that direction, the disparities in waiting times suggest that UNOS policies still have some way to go in achieving justice. Current policies that provide for local priority contribute directly to waiting disparities.[15] Furthermore, changes in UNOS policy that ultimately determine allocation are decided by a vote of the UNOS members. Yet this system itself influences outcomes because only one vote is allotted to each transplant center regardless of how many different transplant programs the center includes and regardless of how few transplants the center actually performs. In this way, current UNOS membership rules and voting policies allow small transplant centers to protect their own interests. The consequent disproportionate voting power of small centers promotes maintaining small programs and their interests rather than improving patient and organ survival, even though it is the larger centers that have the adequate resources for doing the job well and demonstrated excellence in outcomes.[16] Policies that favor center interests over considerations of equity and efficacy in organ allocation oppose clinical justice, whereas policies that focus on equity and efficacy lead us closer to clinical justice. These allocation policy issues are particularly relevant to the story of Jesica Santillan.

EQUITY

Transplantation policies do not and should not treat all people equally: It isn't possible to give everyone equal access to organs for transplantation (for example, one per person). Transplant organs are reserved only for those who need them. Principles for the just distribution of scarce organs aim at achieving equity (rather than equality) by establishing a uniform method for grappling with relevant differences among transplant candidates. While there are many differences among such patients, the crucial policy problem becomes specifying which differences are relevant, and then assigning relative values to those differences in order to create a system of prioritization. When a policy gives irrelevant differences significant weight or when an allocation policy results in unequal treatment of similarly situated transplant candidates, the policy is, on its face, unjust.

So far, transplant programs have treated nonmedical judgments about patients as irrelevant differences and have, for the most part, resisted the impulse to make blatant personal or relative judgments about recipient worthiness.[17] This attitude reflects medicine's general commitments to a nonjudgmental regard of every patient and a caring attitude toward each. These are professional commitments because they have an essential role in promoting the community's trust. We all want our doctors not to judge us harshly and to take good care of us regardless of our social standing and what we have done. For example, in wartime, doctors have a professional responsibility to treat all medically needy soldiers alike, those from their own army as well as enemy soldiers. Medicine's implicit attachment to these principles of nonjudgmental regard and caring for all encourages patients to go to doctors so that they can receive the benefits that medicine has to offer. These professional positions on the appropriate physician attitude toward patients have translated into the transplant community's reluctance to judge a recipient's worthiness, behavior that may have contributed to a patient's present need, a recipient's age, or even the share of good life that the patient has already enjoyed.[18]

JESICA AND EQUITY

In general, society expects that the good of patients is the central moral goal of medicine. As we see in transplantation, society also expects that the commitment to the good of the pool of potential patients is the guiding agenda in the establishment of medical programs and the design of equitable allocation policies. My guess is that most people would, therefore, put greater trust in medicine's goals, commitments, and judgments than they would grant to a group of stakeholders making decisions based on their own personal, economic, religious, or political values. The narrow range of principles of "clinical justice," namely, urgency, need, equity, and efficacy should, therefore, constitute the relevant considerations for organ allocation policy.

These conclusions have significant implications for considering the case of Jesica Santillan. After several years as a U.S. resident and because of her medical need, it was appropriate for Jesica to be listed for a transplant with cadaveric organs. When the first set of organs was allocated to her, the transplant was consistent with principles of clinical justice. That she was an immigrant or an illegal alien resident should not be factors in clinical justice, so those facts should not have been held against her. That she was young and attractive, or that her case pulled at the heart strings of parents in the community, should not be factors in clinical justice, so those facts should not have counted in her favor.

Some of the media reports echoed views expressed by people in the community and revealed values that were considerably at odds with principles of clinical justice. Newspaper columns and TV talk show hosts expressed their disapproval of Jesica being in America, repeatedly referring to her being "smuggled" into the country. They argued that illegal immigrants took more organs than they donated. They also charged that treating illegal immigrants such as Jesica dearly cost deserving Americans, in terms of both organs allocated to the undeserving and higher medical costs that are passed along to worthy citizens as increased health insurance premiums. We heard such community attitudes in the comments of Peter Brimelow, who wrote, "Wait a minute! What about equal protection? Aren't ordinary Americans eligible for these 'additional support services' too?"[19]

Others in the press presented the image of a sympathetic would-be movie star, a heroic angel in a situation of desperate need. "Over the past few weeks, Ms. Santillan, 5 foot 2, 80 pounds, has become like a saint in Durham," reported the *New York Times*. "Her image hangs in homes, restaurants and churches. Her brown eyes sparkle from every newspaper box. People pray for her each night." They described her hard-working devoted parents who took the jobs that no one else in North Carolina would do. They described the supportive Latino and Durham, North Carolina, communities that became committed to saving Jesica. They chronicled the story of Jesica's "quest for a new heart since shortly after she arrived" and told the gripping story of "Mack Mahoney, a 55-year-old Texas home builder, [who] got things started. Mr. Mahoney was so moved when he read a newspaper article about the sick girl, who lived in a trailer with no windows, that he founded a charity to build houses for free to raise money for her surgery. He called it Jesica's Hope Chest and got Ms. Santillan on an organ donation list."[20]

For the most part, we recognize that language that promotes derision and discrimination is divisive and dangerous to a multicultural democratic society. Giving voice to such inclinations undermines our national spirit of cooperative mutual support for our fellows in times of need. It encourages prejudice and bigotry that is anathema to justice in allocation, and it thwarts the goodwill of those good Samaritans who donate organs out of love for their neighbors, even those who don't hail from North Carolina.

Generally, we also recognize that preference for those who are especially appealing, near, or dear is sometimes appropriate. Yet the usual rule for when it is morally acceptable to acknowledge such priority is that other reasonable people could not object to the preferential treatment (for example, the priority we accept for family and close friends).[21] Clearly, the controversy over organ allocation is not a place where society accepts preferential treatment based on people's attractiveness or on how gripping their stories are.

Both sides of the colloquial discussion about whether Jesica was deserving of the organs expressed positions that are incompatible with principles for medical resource allocation. Neither side in the public debate approximated the values of clinical justice that governed the first organ allocation decision.

Aside from urgency of need, medical professionals who are engaged in the allocation of scarce medical resources accept the appropriateness of medical triage. In situations of critical resource scarcity, when life is on the line, doctors pointedly deny treatment to some patients in order to avoid the worst overall outcome; that is, they accept the inevitable deaths of some patients who are least likely to survive regardless of medical investment and put their efforts into those who have a better chance of living in order to avert a greater loss of life. Triage is a well-accepted principle of clinical justice that is invoked on the battlefield, in intensive care units and emergency departments, and in planning the medical response to mass casualty events. Those of us outside of medicine, who cannot know whether we or our loved ones will be among the unsalvageable who are set aside without treatment or among those who are helped, would be likely to endorse triage policies because they would give us or our loved ones the best chance for surviving. The extreme shortage of transplant organs and the extreme need of patients who will die without transplantation make triage an appropriate principle for organ allocation.

UNOS listing criteria appear to accept and address the importance of efficacy in organ allocation by including standards for determining the likelihood of a transplant candidate's survival. UNOS also tracks outcome data, again suggesting an interest in efficacy. Policies for organ distribution take the limitations of cold ischemic time into account in order to maximize organ viability. And when a potential recipient becomes so ill that the likelihood of survival is significantly diminished, the patient is not listed for transplantation or is made inactive on the UNOS organ recipient list (for example, status 7 for liver transplantation).

Patients are also evaluated with respect to the likelihood that they will adhere to rigorous post-transplant protocols so that the transplanted organ will not be lost to rejection. Typically, when a patient's history raises questions about the likelihood of adherence to a schedule of antirejection medications and post-transplantation medical monitoring, the patient is further examined and assessed by a psychiatrist or a social worker. Adherence and efficacy are reasonable and relevant medical considerations for the evaluation of individual patients. Moreover, cadaveric organs should be allocated not only to achieve the greatest benefit but also to avoid the worst outcome—that is, allocating them to patients who will die soon regardless of the transplant while patients who could have survived for a significantly longer period with a transplant die for lack of an organ.

While small differences in efficacy may not be significant enough to justify drawing lines between those who may receive an organ and those who may not, policy should attend to significant differences in likely survival. Those who have a significantly worse chance of living for several years after a transplant should be triaged off the list of eligible recipients so that patients who are much more likely to do well have a better chance of receiving an organ.

Differentiation in listing, prioritization, or allocation of organs without an adequate basis of evidence should be looked upon with suspicion because drawing distinctions based on unsupported assumptions about efficacy creates injustice. For that reason, transplant policy distinctions that rest on claims about the efficacy of transplantation for groups of patients (for example, alcoholics) must be supported by compelling evidence.

Commitments have costs. Medicine's commitment to principles of clinical justice requires that clinicians pay the price of not yielding to the psychological pull of the "rule of rescue" in the allocation of scare and crucial resources such as transplant organs. Triage decisions are difficult enough in the face of a mass casualty event. Imagine how much more difficult they are when large numbers of victims are not spread out before you. Doctors' standard commitment to serve the interests of their patients, coupled with their natural reluctance to exclude the neediest patients who are also least likely to survive because of organ allocation eligibility, can explain the absence of any policy to limit the allocation of transplant organs based on low efficacy. But, even though some transplant surgeons, particularly those at small centers, may not see large numbers of patients who are dying for lack of an organ, surgeons in large centers do see such patients and the data reports them all. This irrefutable evidence of critical scarcity demands the implementation of new policies that draw lines at significant differences in efficacy.

A transplant organ allocation policy that takes efficacy into account can and should leave considerations of need and urgency in place. Doing so would simply require that a triage line be drawn when an ill patient becomes significantly less likely than similarly ill patients to have a good outcome from a transplant organ. In liver transplantation, for example, it could mean classifying patients with MELD scores over 38 as status 7, or temporarily inactive. Currently, by focusing allocation exclusively on how close to death a transplant candidate is, patients with the highest MELD scores are allocated organs, but those tend to be the patients who are least likely to do well. Adding triage considerations into current policy would still allocate organs first to those who are sickest but also allow for the acknowledgment of sad reality.

By the time of her second transplant, Jesica's doctors observed that her condition had deteriorated to the point of her having no better than a 50 percent chance of survival. That estimate was likely to have been shaded with optimism and influenced by the underlying guilt and embarrassment of the transplant error. Most heart recipients at the time of transplant have about an 86 percent chance of surviving for one year. Most heart retransplant recipients have about a 78 percent chance of surviving for that period. The figures for most lung recipients are 79 percent and 62 percent, respectively. Most heart-lung transplant recipients have about a 67 percent chance of one-year survival at the time of transplant. According to the data listed on the UNOS Web site as of June 24, 2005, the number of patients who have received heart-lung retransplantation was too small for computing percentages. No data is given for one-year survival; one patient in the United States survived for three years; and two have survived five years.[22] The low likelihood that a heart-lung retransplantation patient will survive is likely to account for there being so few cases of heart-lung retransplantation. In some cases and with other organs, retransplantation has a predicted success rate that is close to the success rate for primary transplantation. In terms of clinical justice, in cases where the prospect for a good outcome is not significantly worse for retransplantation than it would be for transplantation, there is no reason for distinguishing between candidates for primary transplantation and candidates for retransplantation. Clearly, however, there would have been a significant difference in expected outcome (67 percent versus less than 50 percent chance of survival) if the heart and lungs that Jesica received were allocated to some other candidate who was near death and waiting for those transplant organs.

On the basis of the poor expectation for a good outcome, the second set of organs should not have been allocated to Jesica for retransplantation. Regardless of who was responsible for the original mistake and regardless of the public attention, the sadness, and the sense of responsibility that the transplant community shared, and because others on the list would have had a far better chance of surviving, medical triage, justified by low efficacy and extreme organ scarcity, should have determined the decision about retransplantation.

After the tissue typing error led to Jesica Santillan's bungled transplant, the media accounts were full of blame, recriminations, and detailed analyses of who was at fault. The media conveyed public sentiment in stories that were full of desperation and remorse. According to a story in the *New York Times*, Ms. Santillan gasped in Spanish to Mack Mahoney, a North Carolina building contractor who became her leading advocate, "Help me, Mack, I can't believe I'm dying," during a brief moment of consciousness after her first surgery.[23] Dr. Jaggers, Jesica's surgeon, reportedly said, "I am heartbroken about what happened to Jesica. My focus has been on providing her with the heart and lungs she needs so she could lead a normal life."[24] Another news item reported that Jesica's mother, Magdalena Santillan, said, "Right now my daughter is between life and death. She could die at any moment. . . . My daughter needs a transplant of a heart and lungs to survive. It's the only hope that we have because the doctors made an error."[25] And Mack Mahoney was quoted as saying, "If she dies, they murdered her."[26] Such sentiments, however powerful they are in social debate, must remain separate considerations for those concerned about efficacy and clinical justice.

INCENTIVES OPPOSED TO EFFICACY

Although UNOS shows some concern for efficacy as a feature of a just allocation system, the MELD system and other organ allocation policies actually compromise the efficacy of organ allocation. These policies give urgently ill patients transplant priority. None of these policies incorporates rules or incentives to encourage programs to triage out the patients who are least likely to derive a significant benefit from a transplant. Without agreement across the transplant community on restricting organ allocation based on lack of efficacy, and without a strictly enforced policy to monitor center compliance, each center continues to draw its own line at low efficacy. So long as the system validates the practice of allocation to those who are most ill, individual transplant teams are not likely to limit access of their own patients to organs, even when those patients have a low likelihood of long-term survival. Two factors account for this practice: 1) Because UNOS allocates organs to the sickest patients, individual programs that draw a line at efficacy when other programs do not will receive far fewer cadaveric organs for transplant than they otherwise would. The result would be detrimental to programs that employ a principle of triage. 2) Each program is committed to providing significant medical benefits for its patients. Except for the most markedly poor transplant candidates who are actually more likely to be harmed by transplantation than benefited, centers are encouraged to transplant very sick patients with poor prospects because doing otherwise would be treating their own patients worse than other centers treat theirs.

According to current practice and policy, no allocation rules were violated in Jesica Santillan's retransplantation. Yet public policy should provide incentives to promote the behavior that the public values and to discourage the behavior that the public wants avoided. Allocation policy that focuses on urgency without also attending to efficacy is likely to provide less long-term overall benefit. We want transplant programs to try hard to provide benefits to all patients who have a similarly good chance of benefiting from transplantation and not to restrict the procedure to only those who will be easiest to manage or who have the greatest likelihood for survival (for example, everyone with at least a 75 percent chance for long-term survival and not just those with a 95 percent chance of survival). But we also want programs to avoid allocations to those who have a significantly diminished chance for long-term survival (for example, those with less than a 60 percent chance).

Without adding some mechanism for efficacy accountability, current policies promote wasting organs. Without a policy designed by cool, calm medical professionals based on principles of clinical justice, individual transplant teams will continue to yield to their own feelings of guilt and remorse, bend to public sentiment, do what is best for the program, and conform to the public relations agendas of their home institutions. Jesica Santillan's second heart-lung transplant illustrates both the inevitability of such outcomes and the painful costs of yielding to such temptation because one or two other patients may have needlessly died owing to this organ allocation indulgence.

Individuals have their own unique conceptions of what is good. Nevertheless, because human beings have common needs, there is a significant overlap in their views of what counts as good. It is reasonable to presume that anyone who is a candidate for an organ transplant sees life, the ability to function, the enjoyment of liberty and pleasure, and the avoidance of disability as good.[27] Since policies are just when they attend to people equally with respect to their most important human concerns, policies that govern allocation of vital organs for transplantation must address what is most important to potential recipients. If receiving a transplant is necessary for a patient's enjoyment of all of the most important goods, the primary good that a just policy must provide is a transplant organ. In the face of the current shortage of transplant organs, policies should promote the goal of increasing the likelihood that a transplant candidate will receive an organ, and benefit from a successful transplant, while allowing each organ transplant candidate a fair chance at receiving the organs that they need.

This is not to say that other matters related to transplantation are not important as well. Transplant candidates will want programs to provide respectful treatment, caring attention, honest and clear communication, clean and attractive surroundings, and convenience. These considerations will have different priorities for different individuals; some factors will be significant to some patients and trivial to others. Yet it is hard to imagine that having a fair chance of receiving an organ in a successful transplant is not the *first* priority of organ transplant candidates with respect to transplant programs and policies. Indeed, when patients understand the differences among transplant centers and have the option, they flock to the programs with a proven track record of success, as Jesica Santillan's family did, or they travel to regions where they are more likely to receive an organ.[28] In life, when different options offer opportunities for satisfying different preferences, people make choices and they triage their values so they can achieve what is most important to them. Various considerations have different weight in different contexts and what is less important is sacrificed for the sake of achieving what is most crucial.

Because of the priority that most patients in need of organ transplantation would accord to receiving an organ and having a successful transplant, reasonable transplant candidates would be likely to endorse policies that tend to increase organ availability and to improve the likelihood of transplant success over policies that provide greater sympathy for dramatic stories and urgent need, particularly if yielding to pity should cost organs.

The tragic story of Jesica Santillan's bungled heart-lung transplants offers important lessons for organ allocation and medical policy. Many of the array of considerations that upstanding members of the community may want to introduce into these decisions are irrelevant to the allocation of scarce medical resources, and medicine is called upon to steadfastly hold the line at considerations of clinical justice. In general, medicine must maintain its nonjudgmental regard of patients and, without giving priority to "appealing" patients or shortchanging unappealing ones, aim at distributing medical resources equitably according to need and urgency. Transplant organs and other severely limited medical resources must be carefully parceled out according to principles of medical triage in order to fulfill medicine's duty of avoiding the worst outcome. Scarce medical resources should be allocated in strict accordance with principles of clinical justice. Thus, in addition to partaking in the glory of saving lives, medicine has to muster the courage to refuse to try to save patients when the cost is too great for the system to bare.

NOTES

1. Albert R. Jonsen, *The Birth of Bioethics* (New York: Oxford University Press, 1998), 212.

2. Shana Alexander, "They Decide Who Lives, Who Dies," *Life* 53 (1962): 1002–25.

3. This estimate is based on the author's review of the membership.

4. See, for example, "Death Removals by UNOS Status by Year," at <http://www.optn.org/latestData/rptData.asp>.

5. Alexander, "They Decide Who Lives," 1002–25.

6. R. Rhodes, "Justice in Medicine and Public Health." *Cambridge Quarterly of Healthcare Ethics* 14 (1) (2005): 13–26.

7. F. M. Kamm, *Morality, Mortality*, vol. 1 (New York: Oxford University Press, 1993), 234.

8. The 1996 rule change that gave priority to Status 1 patients over Status 2A patients raises questions of evidence and justice. The argument for the change was that patients with chronic illness had a lower chance of surviving than patients with acute liver failure who had otherwise been healthy and, therefore, had a better chance of surviving. The implicit justification was that the change in policy would allow more people to benefit from transplantation. See J. Showstack, P. P. Katz, J. R. Lake, R. S. Brown Jr., R. A. Dudley, S. Belle, R. H. Wiesner, R. K. Zetterman, and J. Everhart, "Resource Utilization in Liver Transplantation: Effects of Patient Characteristics and Clinical Practice," *Journal of the American Medical Association* 281 (15) (April 21, 1999): 1381–86. Opponents of the change have argued that the data does not support the distinction and therefore that the change in policy unjustly puts those with chronic illness at a disadvantage.

9. Rosamond Rhodes, "Justice in Transplant Organ Allocation Policy," in *Medicine and Social Justice: Essays on the Distribution of Health Care*, ed. R. Rhodes, M. P. Battin, and A. Silvers, 345–61 (New York: Oxford University Press, 2002).

10. United Network for Organ Sharing (UNOS), 2003 Annual Report to the U.S. Scientific Registry of Transplant Recipients and the Organ Procurement and Transplantation Network, <http://www.optn.org/AR2003>; Questions and Answers for Patients and Families about MELD and PELD, <http://www.unos.org/data.htm> (both accessed March 11, 2004).

11. UNOS Policy 3.6 Allocation of Livers, June 16, 2000, <http://www.unos.org/frame—Default.asp?Category=About>.

12. Organ Procurement and Transplantation Network, All Kaplan-Meier Graft Survival Rates for Transplants Performed: 1995–2002 (based on OPTN data as of May 13, 2005).

13. D. Shalala, Letter from Secretary of Health and Human Services to Members of Congress, online February 26, 1998, <http://www/unos.org/Newsroom/archive—other—022698—shalala.htm>.

14. R. Rhodes, C. Miller, and M. Schwartz, "Transplant Recipient Selection: Peacetime vs. Wartime Triage," *Cambridge Quarterly of Health Care Ethics* 1 (4) (1992): 327–31.

15. Institute of Medicine (IOM), *Organ Procurement and Transplantation: Assessing Current Policies and the Potential Impact of the DHHS Final Rule* (Washington, D.C.: National Academy Press, 1999).

16. Rhodes, "Justice in Transplant Organ Allocation Policy."

17. The transplantation stand is in opposition to the earlier stand of committees that rationed access to dialysis machines in the early 1960s according to "social worth criteria" (Jonsen, *Birth of Bioethics*, 211–17). Criticism of those criteria have led to the adoption of medical criteria that focus instead on urgency of need and equity.

18. On this last consideration, Kamm (*Morality, Mortality*) and others argue for the opposite view, that considerations such as age are relevant and should be taken into account in organ allocation policy.

19. Peter Brimelow. "That Santillan Saga: Lies, Damned Lies, Immigration Enthusiasts and Neosocialist Health Bureaucrats," May 31, 2003, <http://www.vdare.com/pb/santillan.htm>.

20. Jeffrey Gettleman and Lawrence K. Altman, "Grave Diagnosis After 2nd Transplant." *New York Times*, February 22, 2003, A11.

21. T. M. Scanlon, *What We Owe to Each Other* (Cambridge, Mass.: The Belknap Press of Harvard University Press, 1998), 158–71.

22. UNOS 2003 Annual Report; United Network for Organ Sharing, UNOS Critical Data, October 18, 2005, <http://www.unos.org/data.htm> and <http://www.unos.org/data/data—resources.asp>.

23. Randal C. Archibold, "Benefactor Championed an Immigrant Girl's Cause." *New York Times*, February 26, 2003, A18.

24. "Review of Blood Type Mismatch for Jesica Santillan Continues," *Duke Med News*, February 16, 2003.

25. *The Gazette* (Montreal, Quebec), February 19, 2003,

26. "Botched Transplants Lead to Brain Damage," *Windsor Star*, February 22, 2003.

27. Bernard Gert, K. Danner Clouser, and Charles Culver, *Bioethics: A Return to Fundamentals* (New York: Oxford University Press, 1998).

28. UPMC News Bureau Release, November 18, 1997, "Data Analysis Supports Idea of Broad Sharing of Donor Livers," <http://www.upmc.edu/NewsBureau/consad.htm> (accessed December 4, 1998).

PLAYING WITH MATCHES
WITHOUT GETTING BURNED

PUBLIC CONFIDENCE IN
ORGAN ALLOCATION

JED ADAM GROSS

The great desiderata *are public and private confidence. No country in the world can do without them. . . . The circulation of confidence is better than the circulation of money.*—James Madison, Ratifying Convention for U.S. Constitution, 1788

According to one journalist, Jesica Santillan "died after a botched heart and lung transplant that shook the nation's confidence in the organ donation system."[1] Even before Jesica Santillan became a household name, members of America's transplant establishment recognized that public controversy over a range of issues could undermine confidence in the transplant enterprise. These flashpoints included determining when transplant surgery was medically and morally justifiable, foreign patients' access to donated organs, and disparities in medical care along lines of race and wealth. In the aftermath of Santillan's death, the United Network for Organ Sharing (UNOS), the nonprofit organization that oversees the country's organ allocation network, reaffirmed its commitment to "ensur[ing] public confidence in the transplant system."[2] This chapter first examines why public confidence is a paramount priority for transplant policymakers and why it is so difficult to sustain. It then traces how competing constructions of public confidence have shaped the flow of organs through American medical institutions.

PUBLIC CONFIDENCE AND QUESTIONS OF TRUST

The immediate explanation for this sensitivity to matters of public confidence is straightforward enough. In a democratic society, the use of transplantable organs is subject to the consent of the public. More specifically, state legislation establishing an opt-in system of organ procurement necessitates not merely passive acquiescence but the express consent of individual donors to sustain the transplant enterprise. At the same time, because Congress has prohibited the sale of organs, advocates of organ donation must appeal to motives other than monetary gain. Further, transplant surgery is costly, and its costs must be borne by members of the public, whether through tax payments, insurance premiums, or some other mechanism. Thus, public confidence is constructed in two ways: by persuading individuals and families to donate organs, and by building collective political and economic support for the transplant enterprise.

The media, Congress, medical centers, and religious organizations are among the institutions in which public confidence is solidified or weakened. Within these institutional arrangements, the actual task of building public confidence has a circular quality: while the ability to allocate organs to needy patients depends on the public's willingness to donate, the public's willingness to donate also depends on how the organs are allocated. Thus, for nearly as long as organ allocation policies have been subject to human choice, the people setting the policies have endeavored to ensure that they will promote a virtuous cycle and not a vicious spiral.

The organizational forms that the American transplant project took were not foreordained by transplantation's technical requirements. Whereas the American system relies on voluntary, uncompensated donors, other liberal democracies obtain organs by presumed consent or allow valuable compensation to organ providers. Whereas American allocation policies center on the nation-state, many continental European countries participate in a multinational Eurotransplant network. Nor can one simply conclude that such fundamental design decisions reflect Americans' general policy preferences in matters of political economy. In 1984, Congress effectively established a single, national organ distribution system that would restrict nonresident aliens' access to transplants, but such regulatory interventions in vital sectors were hardly characteristic of the Reagan era. Indeed, certain aspects of the American organ transfer system—the use of genetic criteria for allocating organs and the instrumentalization of ethnic loyalties to recruit donors—could be quite offensive in another national context. As Richard Cook notes in another chapter of this book, organ allocation and transplantation are a "socio-technical" process. Understanding why public confidence demanded a particular architecture for organ distribution requires an appreciation of some peculiar technical features of transplantation in the United States and why these features were particularly of concern for much of American society.

THE SPECIAL STATUS OF TRANSPLANTATION IN THE UNITED STATES

Transplantation is unusual because it forces members of our affluent society to confront dire scarcity and the rivalries scarcity engenders. These rivalries include both conflicts of values and competition for material resources. Cultural observers from Alexis de Tocqueville to twentieth-century historian David Potter have proposed that the abundance of the American continent bolstered Americans' commitments to liberty and equality, enabling us to define the two ideals in terms of "freedom to grasp opportunity."[3] For transplant patients, this freedom to grasp opportunity is debased as a currency because there are precious few opportunities to grasp. Further, transplantation implicates a degree of dependence that challenges American culture's mythic commitment to rugged individualism. The transplant candidate can only "make something of himself" by assimilating others' parts, whereas the archetypal self-reliant individual can afford to be completely self-absorbed.[4] This combination of scarcity and dependence also means that when one patient receives an organ, other patients in the queue have lost an opportunity to utilize the same organ. Multiple transplants compound the zero-sum nature of allocation (see the essay by Wailoo and Livingston in this volume); indeed, one volatile aspect of the Jesica Santillan story was the fact that the six organs Jesica received theoretically could have gone to six different individuals.

And then, as is discussed in the concluding sections of this essay, there is a third novel social dilemma implicit in the problem of matching—for the diversity and distribution of tissue types across the population (discussed by Cook in this volume) plays an important role in shaping the allocation of organs and the flow of these resources, and therefore intersects with existing problems of equality and disparities in America.

THE AMERICAN DREAM AND AN AWAKENED PUBLIC

In some societies, transplant medicine has encountered resistance because the physical process of dispersing organs from brain dead individuals runs up against deeply held cultural beliefs, such as taboos against bodily mutilation.[5] In contrast, transplant politics in the United States have focused less on surgical techniques than on the rules, principles, and ideals guiding how the organs are allocated. As noted, transplantation challenges some widely shared American norms, assumptions, and expectations head-on. In the process, it obliquely challenges "the American way of life" by pitting cherished values, which ordinarily seem quite compatible, against each other.

"The American way" has always been a delicate balance of incommensurables: majority rule and equal citizenship, personal autonomy and democratic governance, laissez-faire and nationalism.[6] And plausible principles for allocating organs—equality of opportunity, medical need, therapeutic efficacy, ability to pay, putative social worth—can likewise conflict with each other. American society, however, has developed (or stumbled upon) effective ways of managing the contradictory impulses within our culture *in ordinary circumstances*. Frederick Jackson Turner famously proposed that, at least within a relatively "homogenous" pioneer community, the material conditions of the American frontier helped to sustain a characteristic liberal political culture in which "[d]emocracy and capitalistic development did not seem antagonistic."[7] More recently, legal scholar Amy Chua has added an ideological commitment to self-reliance, constitutional constraints on the appropriation of personal property, and material redistribution to the long list of devices on hand for "mediat[ing] the paradox of free market democracy."[8] Market capitalism and democracy are not the only rivalrous ideals American society has managed to reconcile, of course, but their harmonization is emblematic of the negotiated compromises at the heart of our political culture.

Many of these posited mediating devices—homogeneity, ample resources to distribute and redistribute, individual self-reliance, and reliable legal rules —are precisely what the frontiers of transplantation lacked. Competing notions of distributive justice contain the seeds of social conflict. Scarcity, dependence (often on strangers), and unpredictability supply fertile ground for these seeds. Organ allocation involves "tragic choices" because no mechanism or criterion can fully satisfy the panoply of rivalrous values at stake, including equality of opportunity, democratic governance, individual choice, compassion for the least fortunate, nationalism, and capitalistic entrepreneurship.[9]

Further, any allocation formula can be said to favor some transplant candidates over others. (See, for example, the essay by Rhodes in this volume.) An organ transfer system developed through majoritarian political processes is likely to disadvantage those without political franchise, such as undocumented immigrants. The public may perceive a system based on genetic compatibility as creating disadvantage for members of ethnic groups with low donation rates and high rates of organ failure. A laissez-faire approach to organ allocation would likely result in worse access to transplants as one moves down the socioeconomic ladder. Because, as has been noted, the distribution of scarce resources implicates cherished values, the politics of organ allocation cannot be reduced to material interests. But material considerations and high ideals often converge so as to give critiques of organ transfer policies a standard, stylized form: allegations that some group of patients is unfairly or improperly receiving "privileged access" to the nation's organs. On a higher level of abstraction, critics will contend that an allocation protocol violates some tenet of "the American way"—without acknowledging the extraordinary difficulty of reconciling these tenets in the transplant context.

Even against this contentious backdrop, Jesica Santillan's transplants were remarkable in that they summoned up virtually every major flashpoint in our organ allocation politics: foreigners' access to organs, the role of money and political connections, racial disparities, medical error, futility, individual campaigning for transplants, and, ultimately, notoriety. The remainder of this essay examines the long history of how American society grappled with such concerns before the Santillan case reenergized them, and how issues of public confidence were continually central to the evolving organ transfer system.

THE CULTURAL-TECHNICAL ORGANIZATION OF MATCHING

In the early years of transplantation, there was no formal allocation "system" to speak of, and public hope and confidence in the emerging, experimental system was linked to the specifics of whose organs were matched with whom. (The Tucker case and numerous others discussed in the essay by Lederer in this volume provide examples of this tendency.) Solid organ transplants first became a viable clinical option in the 1950s, but generally only between identical twins.[10] Allocating organs according to genetic identity left little room for value judgments. From the start, transplanters pushed the bounds of this narrow conception of the acceptable match. Genetically distinct skin and renal grafts occasionally worked as bridges until patients regenerated their own skin or a faltering native kidney began functioning again. Nonetheless, the element of luck or fate in finding a suitable match seized the public imagination. Thus, a 1955 article in *Time* magazine about a skin transplant recounted this hospital conversation: " 'It was *unfortunate*,' the chief surgeon remarked, that patient Rodney Madeira 'did not have an identical twin, since only skin from the patient's own body or from such a twin would do for a permanent graft.' Replied Madeira, 'I have one.' " A year earlier, an airman had recovered from severe burns because "he *chanced* to spot his twin brother wandering around the hospital corridor."[11] Surgeon Francis D.

Moore asserted that so "[m]any coincidences were necessary" for the success-ful first twin transplant that it initially struck doctors as "a medical freak."[12]

As immunosuppressive therapy and antigen matching technologies devel-oped in tandem, they synergistically expanded the number of patients who could hope for long-term graft survival. Even so, technological constraints practically necessitated a reliance on living donors in solid organ transplanta-tion's early years, and people invested in this project spoke of their "hopes" for it, rather than their "confidence" in it. Before the introduction of mechan-ical ventilators in the late 1950s and the medical endorsement of brain death in the late 1960s, organs could not be supplied with blood in the donor's body and removed at the moment of need.[13] Until dialysis machines became widely accessible, end-stage renal patients could not wait long until a cadaver kidney became available. Only with the development of effective techniques for preserving organs outside the body in the late 1960s did the cadaveric kidney transplant become "elective" surgery rather than "an emergency pro-cedure."[14] Thus, even as the genetic compatibility requirement began to loosen, organ allocation remained contingent on coincidences of time and location in the lives of donors and recipients.

As a technical matter, some Americans questioned how well transplanta-tion would work. A California homemaker, responding to a 1968 Gallup poll on public attitudes toward organ donation, remarked, "These transplants will perhaps stall death a week or a month, but I don't believe they'll ever be able to get a man back on his feet again."[15] Yet even here, the criterion for evaluat-ing therapeutic success was not purely technical. The problems transplanta-tion posed for the preexisting cultural trope of "standing on one's own two feet" may help explain why variations on this theme were frequently invoked in public discussion of transplants. A more recent news article, focusing on attitudes toward donation among ethnic minorities, quoted an African Amer-ican donor recalling, "I remember my mother saying, 'I was born with two legs, let me die with two legs.' "[16] As these examples suggest, Americans did not evaluate transplantation as a matter of abstract logic; rather, they assessed the new type of surgery in light of personal experiences, cultural traditions, and collective memories, which may or may not have been widely shared in society at large. At a minimum, organ donation was inconsistent with some conventional notions about respectful treatment of bodies. "Are organ do-nors weirdoes?" asked one publication as late as 1974.[17]

Within the legal academy, cadaveric organ donation as a donative transfer opened another line of discussion; it became a province of trusts and estates law, a branch traditionally concerned with the establishment of wills and trusts. The Uniform Anatomical Gift Act (UAGA) of 1968, written by members of the National Conference of Commissioners on Uniform State Laws to clarify and standardize procedures for donating organs and tissue, enshrined the conception of organ donation as the bestowal of a gift. The original UAGA's conception of an anatomical gift was detailed and quite literal: not only did the "donee" have a right to "reject the gift," but the donee could also "transfer his ownership to another person."[18] This model legislation was quickly adopted in forty-one states.[19] The UAGA's respect for donor autonomy in the face of scarcity thus parted ways with the utilitarian, statist thrust of much public health policy by allowing salvageable organs to be buried for want of authorization to remove them. Libertarian traditions within the legal profession[20] were not the only consideration favoring this gradualist, consensual approach to organ procurement, though. The need to build *public* support for transplantation in a majoritarian democracy also powerfully cautioned against rushing to impose a more aggressive opt-out procurement regime on an ambivalent public.[21]

ENLISTING THE PUBLIC BUT NOT THE PUBLIC AS A WHOLE

Early efforts to promote organ donation, which were oriented toward building majority support for donation, similarly emphasized the goal of rapidly expanding the scope of transplantation over the goal of serving all segments of American society equally well. While this essay can only touch on the topic, doctrines and imagery familiar to the major Western religious traditions, and especially Christianity, have long informed broader discussions of public confidence, trust, and matching. As early as 1970, a *Michigan Law Review* article by a prominent trusts and estates scholar identified several specific religious doctrines, associated with diverse faiths, that could hamper donation: "A fundamentalist Christian might consider organ removal inconsistent with the principle of bodily resurrection. A Jehovah's Witness might object to the shedding of blood. Many orthodox rabbis have opposed autopsies, invoking a principle of Judaism that the body must not be violated."[22]

In a predominantly Christian society, however, public discussions of organ transplantation frequently invoked (vaguely or explicitly) Christian imagery, and a majoritarian objective—securing the support of mainstream Christians —was more easily achieved than the egalitarian correlative—reconciling transplantation with America's myriad religious traditions. This religious orientation was largely a result of individual commentators' drawing on widely shared religious and cultural resources, rather than conscious policy choices. "What if one beloved child could resurrect another?" asks *Newsweek* editor Anna Quindlen, employing the theme of bodily resurrection to promote donation.[23] Such Christian imagery does not end with the theme of resurrection: the transplant waiting list is described in the *New York Times* as "purgatory."[24] While such metaphors may help many Americans (including non-Christians) make sense of the unknown, their appeal is not necessarily universal. The ubiquitous slogan, "Don't take your organs to heaven . . . Heaven knows we need them here," speaks to a particular set of religious concerns, but transplantation may raise a different set of concerns for a religious tradition holding that "[k]arma is encoded in . . . the body."[25]

This majoritarian approach to donor recruitment, though, represented a more general pattern in how transplant policymakers initially confronted tensions between the pressing societal need for an organ transfer system and America's commitment to egalitarianism. Much as the availability of transplantable organs in a predominantly Christian society depended on the willingness of Christians to donate organs, the availability of organs in a predominantly English-speaking society depended on the support of donors who could comprehend English-language public service announcements. In contrast, transplant professionals' attempts to understand and address the concerns of minority demographic groups got off to a clumsy start. In a 1996 newspaper interview, a leading heart transplant surgeon called Jewish law "mysterious" and "difficult to understand" but elaborated upon the low donation rate among Orthodox Jews by remarking that they "behave sociologically like lower-class Asians, Blacks, and Hispanics."[26] Recognizing such a pattern, however, is but a first step toward understanding the beliefs, anxieties, and motivations that influence willingness to donate among specific demographic groups. The moral and therapeutic hazard of this majoritarian bias— whether with respect to race, language, or religion—is not merely possible disadvantage to minority patients in the short run but also the potential alienation of minority donors (or potential donors) in the long run.[27]

The refinement of tissue typing and the widespread adoption of the UAGA facilitated the development of organ sharing networks, institutionalizing the need for public confidence in transplantation. In the United States, seven West Coast transplant centers established a common computer-based system for matching organs and patients in 1968.[28] In 1969, a transplant surgeon from the Medical College of Virginia and a Duke University immunologist initiated the South-Eastern Regional Organ Procurement Program. The program, which quickly entered a contractual agreement to link nine transplant centers between Baltimore and Atlanta, was incorporated as the nonprofit

South-Eastern Organ Procurement Foundation (SEOPF) in 1975. SEOPF's board took the lead in creating a national network by introducing UNOS, originally a computerized matching system, in 1977, and establishing a "round-the-clock" kidney placement support center in 1982. The network that emerged from this process of consolidation in 1985 was organized into nine regions consistent with "previous organ sharing patterns between transplant centers."[29]

As to concerns about equality in organ allocation, for the moment, the glaring answer to "who was providing organs?" remained "not enough people." And if the recipients represented a privileged elite, everything about transplantation was extraordinary. Christiaan Barnard's transplantation of blacks' hearts into white bodies in apartheid South Africa, widely covered by the American media, did draw scrutiny during the civil rights era. A 1968 letter to the *New York Times* questioned these transplants "in a country where one variety of human life is so clearly placed at a higher value than another"; the letter's attention to the circumstances in which the hearts were procured suggested that public anxieties about transplantation focused less on how the organs were allocated than on the potential abuse of donors. As "interracial" transplants captured the public's imagination, however, suspicions of racial disparities on both the supply and allocation sides of the U.S. system meshed with new doubts about the system's trustworthiness stemming from aggressive organ procurement (see the essay by Lederer in this volume).

THE POLITICS AND ECONOMICS OF ORGAN ALLOCATION

As better immunosuppressive drugs improved unrelated-donor transplant outcomes, the politics and economics of organ allocation were thrust into the public consciousness—shaping new understandings of the system. In October 1983, North Carolina senator Jesse Helms carried a jaundiced eight-month-old into a "packed" room for Senate committee hearings on proposed legislation to establish a national organ sharing network. "Josh is now first on the . . . waiting list at the University of Minnesota Hospital," the senator declared. Governor James Hunt Jr., who was running against Helms in the 1984 election, "said North Carolina had recently amended its insurance program to cover transplant surgery, which in Josh's case would cost about $200,000."[30]

Within a decentralized, loosely coordinated institutional matrix, personal resourcefulness, regional boosterism, and political patronage facilitated the development of transplant surgery and influenced the allocation of organs.

Tissue typers' work in uniting regional kidney transplant centers into expansive organ sharing networks was just one example of this sort of individual and institutional initiative.[31] Perhaps nowhere was the role of local enterprise more apparent than in the emergence of the University of Pittsburgh's Presbyterian Hospital as an international transplant hub. Pioneering liver transplanter Thomas Starzl, reportedly "tired of chasing research grants" as surgery chair at the University of Denver, in 1980 "agreed with a handshake to set up a liver transplant program" in Pittsburgh. The city's location—within an hour's flight from 70 percent of the American population—was ideal for time-sensitive organ procurement, and by 1984, "Presby" surgeons were performing half of all liver transplants in the United States.[32] Multiple institutions and constituencies were part of the action as the growth of the city's health care sector partially offset manufacturing job losses. The *Pittsburgh Press* surveyed "30 prominent Pittsburgh people" to see how many held organ donor cards.[33] In 1985, the *New York Times* described Pittsburgh as "a prime goal for surgeons, who compete for slots," noting that the Presbyterian "name on a resume [could] make a big difference in fees and status."[34] Transplant Recipients International Organization (TRIO) made its home where so many patients had gotten their new lease on life.[35]

As transplantation became a realistic clinical option for more patients, one aspect of America's diffuse, informal organ transfer system greatly frustrated transplant families and troubled onlookers: access to transplant surgery depended on factors far removed from technical considerations, and many of these factors seemed needlessly unfair to individual patients. The role of politicians in pressuring state health insurance programs to pay for operations "case-by-case,"[36] and the Reagan administration's efforts to publicize individual patients' need for organs, in particular, struck critics as partial fixes to systematic and comprehensive gaps in organ procurement and allocation.[37] Some complained about the unpredictability and capriciousness of decisions determining patients' access to transplants. "These things can't be left to chance," said one hospital administrator. Massachusetts Blue Cross had first agreed to cover the administrator's daughter's liver transplant, then reversed its position, and finally restored coverage after the state House Speaker and the media took an interest in the case.[38] Others emphasized the biases inherent in this system of allocation. The *Washington Post* noted legislators' frustration with a "system that provides new organs to those who are savvy enough to go to the White House, resourceful enough to get themselves on television or lucky enough to live in the right state."[39]

For transplant centers, too, this lack of settled, consistent allocation rules consumed time and energy. UCLA's medical director explained how his institution haggled with out-of-state Medicaid programs over the cost of transplants: "Someone will say they're not going to pay, and we'll say, 'Well, we can't do it.' Then they'll come up with a little money and we'll lower our price a bit. . . . The stress on the patient and our institution is very great."[40] One result is that even relatively well-off transplant families—perhaps especially the well-off—felt they could not clear the process's hurdles with their dignity intact. "After working my whole life, [Massachusetts Medicaid] made a panhandler out of me," protested "affluent businessman" Myron Teicholtz. "Here we were, a family draining every resource, and these people were playing with us like chips on a chess board. Today yes, tomorrow no."[41]

All these complaints took on a new sense of urgency, however, when the private sector offered a remedy that many Americans found unpalatable—the purchase of organs domestically or abroad for sale in America. Congressman Al Gore reportedly added a provision banning organ sales to pending legislation "after being sent a brochure from a New England company that offered to register donors, offering them the potential of a $10,000 payment if one of their organs was used in a transplant." In 1983, de-licensed Virginia physician H. Barry Jacobs contacted the Food and Drug Administration to "inquir[e] whether he needed a license to import organs"; Jacobs claimed that hospitals had "expressed interest in removing kidneys" from paid donors he would "solicit." Both the supply and demand sides of the proposal generated objections: it would advantage economically privileged kidney patients over those who were not wealthy, and it would exploit desperate organ sellers. In a country burdened by the historical subordination of some human beings into the category of property, this new kind of commodification was quickly condemned as akin to slavery.[42] A Red Cross official who previously headed the American Association of Tissue Banks called the plan "immensely damaging."[43] It threatened not only the status and reputation of transplant professionals but also America's image in the world. As bioethicist Samuel Gorovitz asserted, "At a time when we urgently need to nurture good relations with the nations of the third world, our international credibility would be dealt a severe blow by our tolerance of a plan according to which the poor in underdeveloped countries were exploited as a source of spare parts for rich Americans. Our antagonists behind the iron curtain would love such a public relations windfall—and they would be right."[44]

In the U.S. House, Representative Gore spearheaded the National Organ Transplant Act (NOTA), legislation that would prohibit organ sales, require state Medicaid programs to formalize and standardize transplant financing, establish a national organ sharing network to be managed by a private contractor, and commission a national task force on transplant policy. In congressional hearings, bioethicist Roger Evans warned that, with the introduction of the powerful immunosuppressive drug cyclosporine, "the lack of two vital resources—money and donor organs" was "likely to limit the number of persons who will benefit from organ transplantation."[45] Rather than directly confronting difficult allocation decisions, however, much of the NOTA commentary focused on the easy targets of waste and poor coordination in the existing system. Gore himself alleged that in Pittsburgh, "There were 300 livers that could not be used and were disposed of principally because . . . the transplant teams were otherwise occupied when the liver became available, or they were exhausted. . . . [T]here was great difficulty in getting them to the right place in the proper time."[46] A witness alleged, "[E]ven though [pediatric liver patient Ashley Bailey] was on the Minnesota University Hospital priority list, and had two previous mentions by the president of the United States, [she] was not included on one of the main computer donor lists until just about 2 weeks ago."[47] Some of the testimony emphasized the difficulty any one patient or family would have collecting all the pieces necessary for a successful transplant—funding for hospitalization, funding for immunosuppression, the surgery itself. Congressman Dan Glickman suggested a "bill to direct the NIH to establish within a set timeframe at least a Federal information network along the lines of what Congress directed the Justice Department to do with regard to missing children,"[48] reinforcing the notion that organs were being lost.

By this point, then, the question of public confidence in the system was fully engaged. The public's stake in making more kidney transplants possible was clear; but so too was the public stake in portraying a system whose rules and parameters meshed neatly with mainstream American values and notions of fairness and equality.

Increasingly, the questions of the cost and savings associated with transplantation became part of this public discussion. Since 1972, Medicare's End-Stage Renal Disease (ESRD) program was providing nearly universal coverage of kidney dialysis costs; ten years later, the program covered 70,000 dialysis patients at an annual cost of $2 billion.[49] Although the initial cost of a kidney transplant was about $30,000,[50] Oscar Salvatierra, president of the American Society of Transplant Surgeons, estimated that 10,000 kidney transplants would save $500 million over four years.[51] The anticipated savings did not merely reflect the difference between the cost of immunosuppression and the cost of maintaining dialysis patients' health; research indicated that 39 percent of kidney transplant recipients collected income support from the federal government, as compared to "60 percent of the dialysis patients."[52]

As other organ transplants became more effective, patients pressured federal, state, and private insurers to cover the cost of extrarenal transplantation, and these developments drew attention to problems of equal opportunity. At the same time, however, a lack of initiative stifled organ procurement and sharing. Until liver transplantation became larger in scale and more lucrative for transplant professionals, there were few incentives to build a UNOS-type network for allocating livers, and without such a network, there was no feasible way to enlarge the scale of liver transplantation. NOTA did not create an ESRD-model insurance program for other types of organ failure, but it did provide for the creation of a multi-organ network, removing a major obstacle for patients in need of extrarenal transplants. Patient organizations, organized around a common medical condition rather than economic class interests, adamantly opposed the sale of organs themselves, which threatened to divide these associations' constituencies, although they did not necessarily share a common philosophy of allocation. "What happened to equal opportunity, when the rich can live and the poor must die?" asked Gail Rempell of the American Liver Foundation.[53] David Ogden of the National Kidney Foundation discussed the foundation's support for a system that distributed organs "based on medical need and criteria without discrimination based on race, sex, social, or economic status."[54] To the extent that participants in the 1984 NOTA hearings recognized a tension between equal opportunity and therapeutic efficacy, there remained a hope that this tension could be reduced by eliminating waste and addressing collective action problems to increase the supply of organs and make the most of tax dollars. "Two things happened to the patient mix once the government became involved in treating end-stage renal disease," Gore observed. "First, the availability of care became more equitable. This is demonstrated by a patient mix that more closely parallels the incidence of kidney disease within the general population. Second, doctors abandoned the use of medical practice standards that . . . had been in place prior to government intervention. . . . [P]atients who were once medically deemed unsuitable for this type of treatment were now being treated."[55]

How to recover more organs, of course, was a central predicament of the NOTA debate. With such issues as equal opportunity and government intervention now part of the discussion, and given the unprecedented nature of the problem and the potent symbolism of organ extraction, public discussion of the options turned less on empirical data than on notions of what kind of system was most consistent with "American" values. For Barry Jacobs, laissez-faire market exchange was the American way of allocating goods. In a *USA Today* guest column, Jacobs wrote, "Compensating the donor for blood or a kidney is the American way. . . . When it comes to deciding what to do with our bodies, Congress is not a better judge than the individual. . . . Only in the Soviet Union do human organs belong to the State."[56] Others relied on notions of equality or merit: "Any millionaire with cirrhosis of the liver will gladly pay half a million dollars," stated one opponent of organ sales. "That's not considered to be the American way."[57] Anyone seeking to substitute a new mode of organ procurement for organized voluntarism, however, would have faced an uphill battle.

What impact might market mechanisms play in shaping public confidence? Clearly, some Americans were donating organs altruistically, and at the NOTA hearings, speaker after speaker emphasized that introducing payment could undermine the existing system before its full potential was realized. "The realization of profit from the retrieval and sharing of donated organs and tissues," Keith Johnson of the Association of Independent Organ Procurement Agencies testified, "could very rapidly turn off public acceptance of the concept of organ donation."[58] In contrast, although for-profit firms were volunteering corporate jets and beepers in service of transplantation,[59] there was little precedent for commercialized organ procurement. References to Richard Titmuss's research on paid blood donation, with its attendant health risks, were words of caution. Ironically, one aspect of Jacobs's congressional testimony that provoked intense opposition was his insistence that all living kidney donors, whether paid or not, should be required to pass a psychiatric examination. "Do I have to make what I consider a humanitarian decision, then defend that before a psychiatrist or psychologist?" asked one congressman.[60]

When President Ronald Reagan signed NOTA into law in 1984, with no psychiatric exam statutorily required, Reagan expressed his confidence that it "str[uck] the proper balance between private and public sector efforts to promote organ transplantation."[61] Gore's original proposal had called for a National Center for Human Organ Acquisition, housed inside the cabinet Department of Health and Human Services (HHS).[62] In the legislative process, NOTA quickly evolved into a bill that would, in Reagan's words, "support" and "enhance" the "ongoing work" of the "private sector."[63] Even after signing the bill, however, the Reagan administration drew fire from politicians and patients' advocates for failing to follow through with the envisioned budgetary support.[64] In 1986, HHS finally awarded UNOS a $379,200 grant to organize a unitary, "national" organ matching network.[65]

In a statement to the House Committee considering NOTA, David Ogden of the Kidney Foundation expressed his desire to discuss briefly an issue not addressed in the bill—the relationship of foreign nationals to the U.S. transplant system. "The National Kidney Foundation," Ogden asserted, "believes that . . . organs donated by deceased American citizens or their next of kin are inherently intended by the donor to benefit a fellow American citizen, if a suitable recipient can be identified by the matching program in effect at the time." If a "suitable American recipient cannot be identified," Ogden reasoned, donors would not want usable organs to go to waste, so "transplantation to a foreign national" would be "entirely appropriate."[66] Later that year, Georgetown professor of bioethics Warren Reich submitted testimony on the moral implications of allocating organs as "citizens of a global community." In his accompanying oral remarks, Reich distinguished between the ethical issues posed by "the financially capable alien, whom I will call the wealthy alien," and those posed by "the poor alien" or "the destitute alien."[67] Representative Gore, recognizing the sensitivity of donation to allocation policies, responded to Reich's discussion of "egalitarian principle[s]" and "responsibilities to . . . patients" by suggesting that "medical professionals" also had a "responsibility . . . to sustain the rate of voluntary donation in our country."[68] Soon, publicity surrounding foreign nationals' access to donated organs at American transplant centers would galvanize the movement toward a publicly accountable organ allocation system.

In May 1985, the *Pittsburgh Press* revealed that "during a three month investigation," Pittsburgh "doctors bypassed hospital policy that sets transplant priority" to expedite foreign patients' waits. "In at least 27 cases, blood samples from Americans and foreigners were examined, and while suitable cross-matches for the organs were confirmed among the Americans, the kidneys went to foreigners."[69] The chief of surgery at Presbyterian University Hospital, Dr. Henry Bahnson, explained that the usual policy could be waived "for 'compassionate' reasons," such as when a patient was "running short on money to stay in Pittsburgh, or a doctor or the children of doctors or members of the Saudi royal family."[70]

In a series of related articles, the *Press* combined detailed records of blood type and cross-match results with detailed human interest stories juxtaposing foreign and American transplant family's experiences. A relative of a North Carolina car accident victim traced the victim's kidneys, which were "transplanted into" a Saudi national and an Egyptian doctor's son, "both of whom were told to report to the hospital before the lab work on . . . three Americans had been completed." As the news article noted, the latter recipient had been waiting twenty-four days "and had not been on dialysis," whereas a suitable American recipient who had been "passed over" had been on the waiting list for three years and "was running out of . . . sites on her body where doctors [could] connect the dialysis machine."[71] Evidence quickly accumulated that many of the foreign patients obtaining organs at Pittsburgh were wealthy, powerful, or well-connected, and included a "princess" and the wife of "a royal financial advisor to Saudi Arabia's King Fahd."[72] Although the series was copyrighted, the basic contentions were picked up beyond Pittsburgh, and the *Washington Post* similarly found that a high percentage of D.C.-area transplants benefited foreign nationals.[73] At about the same time, "news. . . that some kidneys were being shipped to Japan for transplants there" prompted some California donors to write the words "resident only" on their organ donor's driver's licenses.[74]

The Pittsburgh controversy was the direct outgrowth of an allocation system revolving around local enterprises with global geopolitical orientations. A Cold War belief that providing compassionate care to foreign nationals would build international confidence in America was simply inverted in the inclusion of "diplomatic" considerations among the grounds for "compassionate" exceptions to protocol.[75] The *Press* eventually discovered that the hospital and Pittsburgh surgeons materially benefited from accepting foreign transplant patients, whose surgical fees were four times the average rate charged to American patients. Additionally, the Saudi royal family had donated $650,000 to the university for transplant research. Perks, however, are not necessarily motivations, and reputational considerations almost certainly influenced the Pittsburgh program's stance regarding international patients more than the "four-foot, gold-plated ceremonial sword" that Starzl acknowledged receiving from "Saudis."[76] According to Dr. Bahnson, the *Press* reported, "Presby's position as an international center creat[ed] pressure to accept foreign transplant candidates," not only because transplant expertise was highly concentrated in the United States, but also "because the presence of foreigners enhance[d] the university's prestige."[77] Prestige, in turn, could "draw additional patients, research funding and top-flight medical talent."[78]

Exactly which word in the phrase "Saudi royal" generated more pique was unclear, but the backlash was swift. Whereas before, majoritarian nationalism and free enterprise conspired against egalitarianism, now egalitarianism and majoritarian nationalism militated against transplant institutions' internationally oriented free enterprise. Some egalitarian critics emphasized that their objection was not to the presence of foreign patients on American waiting lists but to an allocation system that favored the wealthy and the well-connected. "If people from other countries need a transplant to live, they should have a chance to get it, but their chance shouldn't be any greater than those of us also waiting," stated one U.S. kidney patient.[79] "It's not American organs going to foreign recipients that is unfair," someone else wrote the *Pittsburgh Press*. "It's donated organs going to the best paying customers, be they foreign or American, that is grossly unjust and scandalous."[80] Other reports, however, suggested that the allegations of preferential treatment for international patients inflamed stridently nationalistic and xenophobic sentiments: " 'Donors,' [Acting Director of the Department of Health and Human Services] Dr. [Edward] Martin said, 'are writing that I didn't sign my donor card to give to a foreign kid. I'm going to tear up my card.' 'There are countless stories of people saying count me out, if you count foreigners in,' added Ronald L. Dreffer, the transplant coordinator at the University of Cincinnati Medical Center. '. . . It's that national spirit.' "[81] In these types of comments, clannish nationalism and egalitarian rhetoric could go hand in hand in a country that constitutionally forbade the granting of titles of nobility. In an oft-quoted comment, an immunologist on a federal transplantation task force remarked, "It's not like we're getting a cross section of foreign nationals. . . . [The economic skew in the foreign patient pool is] not especially fair, so I don't see why we have to be. When they start sending over their shepherds with their bankers, come back and we'll talk."[82] As Howard University transplant surgeon Clive Callendar pointed out, however, such rhetoric about foreign inequalities conveniently overlooked substantial disparities closer to home.

Egalitarian principles could cut in another direction, too: restricting foreigners' access to American transplant institutions would give American citizens privileged access to transplant surgery. But the revelations about foreign patients leaving the United States with Americans' organs tapped into larger patterns of suspicion, indignation, and resentment. Between the early Cold War and the Pittsburgh controversy, a series of global events fostered a sense that American society was under siege by foreigners who would take advantage of Americans' goodwill: Japan's juggernaut economic recovery, America's growing trade deficit, American casualties in Vietnam, an oil embargo by the Organization of Arab Petroleum Exporting Countries, American deaths in airline hijackings, terrorist bombings of U.S. embassies in Lebanon and Kuwait, and the hostage crisis in Iran. As such, in 1984, Sherry Clifton, whose fifty-year-old gospel singer husband, Hardie Clifton, received a Medicaid-financed heart transplant after she called the White House, could explain her frustration with the reimbursement bureaucracy in sweeping terms: "I'm an American citizen. I see what's going on in America, how the United States takes it upon itself to help everybody—all the postwar things we did for Japan, and the Vietnamese refugees—and I'm calling agency after agency, and everybody's saying, 'We don't do this,' and I'm saying, 'Where am I? Am I still in America or off in the twilight zone?' "[83]

Much as ongoing public financial support for dialysis (begun in the early 1970s) had given taxpayers a stake in the 1984 NOTA hearings, taxpayer support for organ transplants and transplant institutions now heightened the public's concern about how organs were allocated. The *Pittsburgh Press* argued, "[P]atients suffering from severe kidney disease are included in federal payment programs. Virtually all costs of treatment and replacement surgery are covered. So the public has a direct financial involvement in transplant decisions and policies."[84]

By August 1985, numerous medical centers had reportedly instituted "quotas" limiting the availability of organs to "foreigners"—under the specter that, if they did not set limits, members of the public would reduce the overall supply by refusing to donate.[85] Today, nonresident aliens' access to cadaver transplants at U.S. hospitals is effectively governed by UNOS policies, including the "5 percent policy" (discussed in Hoffman's essay in this volume). Although Reagan had signed NOTA before the Pittsburgh controversy erupted, the "privileged foreigner" scandal became a foundational event in the transplant community's understanding of UNOS. Thus, a prominent bioethicist would write retrospectively, "In the early '80s it was not uncommon for wealthy foreigners to pay big bucks to push their way to the head of the line for a transplant. This trade got so out of hand that Congress insisted a national system be created to ensure that Americans got first crack at the organs that became available and that organs be distributed in an equitable manner. . . . [UNOS] . . . has had Congress' mandate to keep an eye on the distribution of organs ever since."[86] In this vision, transplant institutions were not just trustees acting on behalf of individual organ donors (as the UAGA implied) but also entrusted by a broad, voting and taxpaying public to impose uniform, accountable rules on all organ transfers (under NOTA).

PUBLIC CONFIDENCE AND A DIVIDED PUBLIC

The "privileged foreigner" scandal, in contrast to the public foreigner figured by Jesica Santillan in 2003, had a direct, if complex, relationship to the problem of how organs should be allocated among U.S. citizens and permanent residents. At least initially, antipathy toward this form of "transplant tourism" provided a basis for crosscutting solidarity among American patients, organ donors, and potential donors. Insofar as the controversy defined equality of access as a core commitment of American society, it had the potential to translate into improved access for patients who were disadvantaged within the pool of U.S. transplant candidates. The media implicitly juxtaposed the transplants to foreign nationals with the high representation of African Americans on the transplant waiting list, appealing to a recognition that the burdens of social inequalities in America often fell heavily on blacks. A *Washington Post* article titled "Foreigners Got High Percentage of Kidney Transplants" noted that "[a]bout 150 D.C. residents, mostly blacks, are waiting for kidneys."[87]

What lasting imprint would the "privileged foreigner" crisis leave on transplant politics? The image of a patient population with privileged access did figure into discussions of racial disparities, but the logic of ABO antigen matching (as discussed in the essay by Cook in this volume) would also become an increasingly important part of debates over privilege, race, and the public confidence in the system. An academic article by legal scholar Ian Ayres et al. critiqued the existing system as one in which "whites dominated the class of recipients having four or more antigens matching," while other patients were left in a lurch (like the American patients in Pittsburgh). Responding to one of the more radical proposals—giving hard-to-match patients bonus points to improve their chances of obtaining a justifiable, if imperfect, transplant—a group of clinical immunologists (inaccurately) echoed the Pittsburgh controversy's "line-jumping"[88] rhetoric: "Anyone claiming black ancestry would be pushed ahead in the line from the first day he or she entered the pool."[89]

Discussion of racial disparities and antigen matching reflected the zero-sum nature of organ allocation in every given case, but the discussion also revealed the perplexing challenge of expanding public confidence over time when levels of confidence differed across demographic groups. Black people were said to donate fewer organs, to face discrimination getting listed for transplant, and to be penalized by an antigen matching system that tilted organ allocation against them. A 1991 *Washington Post* article mentioned "a fear that there would be a backlash to the fact that there are fewer black donors in proportion to the number of blacks awaiting kidney transplants and on dialysis" (as the Pittsburgh revelations had provoked a backlash).[90] Yet, paradoxically, whereas improving black patients' access to organs under these circumstances was a potential source of suspicion or resentment, one reason why more blacks were not becoming organ donors was reportedly "distrust about the donor process."[91] In the years that followed, UNOS gradually but substantially reduced its emphasis on antigen matching. After a recent adjustment to its kidney points system, the network issued a press release quoting Winifred Williams, the physician who chaired the organization's Minority Affairs Committee. Williams noted optimistically, "We hope that our emphasis on ensuring equity will boost the public's confidence in the transplant system. Greater public confidence can also raise people's willingness to become organ donors to help meet the needs of patients."[92]

The antigen-matching debate did not merely threaten to pit minority donors' confidence in organ transfer against the confidence of a majority. Rather, it highlighted the multiplicity of meanings scholars, journalists, and policymakers attached to concepts like "egalitarian" (equality of what?), "minority" (a minority of the whole population or the transplant waiting list?), "equitable," and "trustworthy." The Jesica Santillan story, too, converged with and diverged from the issues animating the Pittsburgh controversy, giving rise to multiple interpretations. An article in *USA Today*, suggesting that Santillan was included on Duke's waiting list in contravention of a UNOS rule "requir[ing] that non-resident organ recipients be in the country legally," revealed the episode's multivalence, as well as its powerful resonance and dissonance with the "privileged foreigner" scandal. "[UNOS] officials have no plans to reprimand Duke for treating Jesica, 17," reporter Tim Friend noted. "The network says limits on transplants to non-resident aliens are designed mainly to ensure that the USA doesn't become a transplant mecca for rich foreigners."[93]

The Santillan episode must be seen as part of a history in which public confidence has been a paramount priority for transplant policymakers, even as competing constructions of public confidence have been difficult to sustain. The persistent scarcity of organs, the increasing diversity of the American public, and patients' extraordinary mobility across national borders all intensify the pressures on maintaining a unified allocation system built on particular forms of public and private confidence. These challenges sometimes give rise to new modalities of organ transfer—either within the UNOS framework or alongside of it—rooted in competing theories of donor and patient confidence.

As Richard Cook has shown, the technical demands of transplantation operate powerfully within the contemporary U.S. organ transfer system, but, as I have shown in this essay, therapeutic efficacy was not the sole, defining principle in the system's creation. The Jesica Santillan case demonstrated that the manifold cultural and political meanings of transplantation could flare into open debate at any point. Reconciling transplantation with some widely shared American values has always required political, economic, and ideological "work."[94] By occasioning a reexamination of the issues of equity and trust in the organ allocation system, the Santillan case reminds us that this work continues unfinished.

NOTES

1. William L. Holmes, "A Year After Botched Transplant, Mother Works for Better Organ Donor System," Associated Press, February 21, 1994.

2. Press Release, United Network for Organ Sharing, "OPTN/UNOS Continues to Improve Accuracy in Donor/Recipient Matching," <http://www.unos.org/news/newsDetail.asp?id=308> (accessed February 6, 2004).

3. See David M. Potter, *People of Plenty* (Chicago: University of Chicago Press, 1954), 92–93.

4. See Amy L. Chua, "The Paradox of Free Market Democracy: Rethinking Development Policy," *Harvard International Law Journal* 41:303 ("the self-reliant individual is less inclined to envy the rich").

5. See, for example, Margaret M. Lock, *Twice Dead: Organ Transplants and the Reinvention of Death* (Berkeley: University of California Press, 2002).

6. For a few intellectuals' assessments of tensions among Enlightenment values that resonate in contemporary America, see, for example, Daniel Bell, *The Cultural Contradictions of Capitalism* (New York: Basic Books, 1976); Robert A. Burt, "Constitutional Law and the Teaching of the Parables," *Yale Law Journal* 93 (1984): 455 ("majority rule is intrinsically at odds with the egalitarian principle"); Chua, "Paradox of Free Market Democracy"; Richard A. Epstein, "Liberty Versus Property? Cracks in the Foundations of Copyright Law," *San Diego Law Review* 42 (2005): 3 (examining a "tension between liberty and property within the natural law tradition of Locke"); James Fitzjames Stephen, *Liberty, Equality, Fraternity*, ed. R. J. White (1873; London: Cambridge University Press, 1967).

7. See Frederick Jackson Turner, *The Frontier in American History* (New York: Holt, 1958), chap. 11, "The West and American Ideals," and chap. 13, "Middle Western Pioneer Democracy" (Address at State Historical Society of Minnesota building dedication, May 11, 1918), at <http://xroads.virginia.edu/7EHYPER/TURNER/> (developed by Michael W. Kidd, 1996).

8. Chua, "Paradox of Free Market Democracy," 292.

9. See Guido Calabresi and Philip Bobbitt, *Tragic Choices* (New York: Norton, 1978).

10. Experimentation with animals suggested that transplants between fraternal twins would also be acceptable in the rare event that they shared a single placenta, exposing the twins' nascent immune systems to each other's tissue. See Tony Stark, *Knife to the Heart: The Story of Transplant Surgery* (London: Macmillan, 1996), 33–34.

11. "Twins Under the Skin," *Time*, October 17, 1955, 84 (emphasis added).

12. Francis D. Moore, *Give and Take: The Development of Tissue Transplantation* (Garden City, New York: Doubleday 1964), 75.

13. See Lock, *Twice Dead.*

14. See Folkert O. Belzer, "Organ Preservation: A Personal Perspective," <http://www.stanford.edu/dept/HPS/transplant/html/belzer.html>.

15. "The Gallup Poll: Majority Would Donate Organs," *Los Angeles Times*, January 17, 1968, A5.

16. Christopher Heredia, "The Ultimate Offering: An Example for the Many Minorities Reluctant to Donate Organs," *San Francisco Chronicle*, January 11, 1999, A13.

17. Arthur J. Snider, "Are Organ Donors Weirdoes?" *Science Digest*, May 1974, 54.

18. Ibid., 191–92.

19. Jesse Dukeminier Jr., "Supplying Organs for Transplantation," *Michigan Law Review* 68 (1970): 817.

20. See, for example, *Kelo v. New London* (2005) (Thomas J., dissenting), approvingly quoting William Blackstone, *Commentaries on the Laws of England* (Oxford: Clarendon Press, 1765), 1:134–35 (" 'the law of the land . . . postpone[s] even public necessity to the sacred and inviolable rights of private property.' ").

21. See "Panel Discussion: Ethical Problems in Medical Procedures," CIBA Foundation symposium, published in G. E. W. Wolstenholme and M. O'Connor, eds., *Ethics in Medical Progress: With Special Reference to Transplantation* (Boston: Little, Brown, 1966), 160.

22. Dukeminier, "Supplying Organs," 836.

23. See Maureen Dowd, "A Lyrical Gift," Editorial, *New York Times*, November 16, 2003, 13.

24. Jeff Stryker, "H.I.V. Patients Get Fresh Hopes for Donor Organs," *New York Times*, December 11, 2001, F6.

25. See Wendy Doniger, "Transplanting Myths of Organ Transplants," in *Organ Transplantations: Meanings and Realities*, ed. Stuart J. Youngner, Rene C. Fox, and Laurence J. O'Connell (Madison: University of Wisconsin Press, 1996), 212–13.

26. Judy Siegel-Itzkovich, "Transplants: The Ultimate Act of Generosity," *Jerusalem Post*, July 28, 1996, Heath, 5.

27. See Lock, *Twice Dead*, for a discussion of the association of organ donation with Christianity and Western philosophy in Japan.

28. Harry Nelson, "For Organ Transplants: 7 Hospitals Here Plan Pool," *Los Angeles Times*, January 9, 1968.

29. "Timeline of Key events in U.S. Transplantation and UNOS History," <http://www.unos.org/whoWeAre/history.asp>; South-Eastern Organ Procurement Foundation, "Brief History," <http://www.seopf.org/intro.htm>.

30. Joey Ledford, "Washington News," United Press International, October 20, 1983.

31. See Paul I. Terasaki, *History of Transplantation: Thirty-five Recollections* (1991),

520–24; and *National Organ Transplant Act: Hearing on H.R. 4080 Before the House Subcommittee on Health and the Environment, Committee on Energy and Commerce,* 98th Cong. (1983), 16–26 (hereafter *Energy and Commerce Hearing*).

32. See Lindsey Gruson, "Center for Transplants and Pittsburgh Ascent," *New York Times*, September 16, 1985, A10.

33. Andrew Schneider and Mary Pat Flaherty, "Donor Organs a Fragile Link between Grief and Hope," *Pittsburgh Press*, May 26, 1985, B9.

34. See Lindsey Gruson, "Center for Transplants and Pittsburgh Ascent," *New York Times*, September 16, 1985, A10.

35. Steve Twedt and Gayle McCracken, "U.S. Panel to Study Transplant Rules," *Pittsburgh Press*, May 13, 1985, A1, A4.

36. See, for example, *H.R. Rep. No. 98–575*, pt. 1, 1983, 19 ("While the Committee believes that the decision to extend Medicaid coverage for one or more organ transplant procedures is appropriately that of each individual State, the Committee does not believe that this decision can equitably be made on a case-by-case basis. . . . Access to organ transplant coverage should not, in the Committee's view, be dependent upon a family's ability to draw sympathetic media coverage and favorable dispensation from elected officials.").

37. See, for example, *Energy and Commerce Hearing*, 3 (statement of Ohio representative Thomas A. Luken, member, House Subcommittee on Health and the Environment) ("Air Force I isn't a national policy"); and Howard Kurtz and James Schwartz, "Organ Transplants Turn into Form of Patronage," *Washington Post*, April 23, 1984, A1.

38. Charles Fiske quoted in Kurtz and Schwartz, "Organ Transplants Turn into Form of Patronage."

39. Ibid., quotation from A1, A6.

40. Raymond G. Shultze quoted in ibid.

41. Quoted in Howard Kurtz, "Organ Transplants Turn Into a Form of Patronage," *Washington Post*, April 23, 1984, A6.

42. Congressman Al Gore quoted in Margaret Engel, "Va. Doctor Plans Company to Arrange Sale of Human Kidneys," *Washington Post*, September 19, 1983, B9 ("Putting organs on a market basis . . . seems to be something inconsistent with our view of humanity. . . . Prostitution is illegal for reasons that are similar. So is slavery.").

43. Dr. Harold Meryman, quoted in ibid.

44. *Energy and Commerce Hearing*, 281 (statement of Samuel Gorovitz). See also Nicholas Wade, Editorial Notebook, "The Crisis in Human Spare Parts," *New York Times*, October 4, 1983, A26 (noting that some critics claimed the plan incorporated "the worst features of . . . colonialism").

45. *Energy and Commerce Hearing*, 56 (testimony of Roger W. Evans, Research Scientist, Health and Population Study Center, Battelle Human Affairs Research Centers).

46. See *National Organ Transplant Act: Hearing on H.R. 4080 Before the House Subcomm. on Health, Comm. on Ways and Means*, 98th Cong. (1984), 33 (hereafter *Ways and Means Hearing*).

47. *Energy and Commerce Hearing*, 74 (statement of Texas representative Charles W. Stenholm).

48. Ibid., 74–75 (statement of Kansas representative Dan Glickman).

49. See *Ways and Means Hearing*, 84 (remarks of Carolyn K. Davis, administrator, Health Care Financing Administration, Department of Health and Human Services; and New York Representative Charles B. Rangel).

50. *Energy and Commerce Hearing*, 60 (testimony of Roger W. Evans); 74–75 ("A kidney transplant is estimated to cost between $25,000 and $35,000").

51. Ibid., 28 (statement of Oscar K. Salvatierra).

52. Ibid., 66 (testimony of Roger W. Evans).

53. *Ways and Means Hearing*, 119 (statement of Gail Rempell).

54. *Energy and Commerce Hearing*, 360 (statement of David A. Ogden, president, National Kidney Foundation).

55. *Ways and Means Hearing*, 25 (prepared statement of Tennessee representative Al Gore Jr.).

56. H. Barry Jacobs, "Let Consenting Adults Sell Their Kidneys," *USA Today*, September 27, 1983.

57. Margaret Engel, "Va. Doctor Plans Company to Arrange Sale of Human Kidneys," *Washington Post*, September 19, 1983, B9.

58. *Energy and Commerce Hearing*, 224 (testimony of Keith Johnson, president, Association of Independent Organ Procurement Agencies).

59. See *Ways and Means Hearing*, 39.

60. *Energy and Commerce Hearing*, 244 (asked by Utah representative Howard C. Nielson).

61. Ronald Reagan, "Statement on Signing the National Organ Transplant Act," October 19, 1984, <http://www.reagan.utexas.edu/archives/speeches/1984/101984f.htm>.

62. *Energy and Commerce Hearing*, 9 (statement of Rep. Al Gore).

63. Reagan, "Statement."

64. See, for example, "Backers of Organ Gifts Criticize Reagan Cuts," *New York Times*, January 13, 1987, C9.

65. "U.S. Establishes National Organ Donor Network in Virginia," *New York Times*, October 1, 1986, A24.

66. Ogden statement, *Energy and Commerce Hearing*, 361.

67. *Procurement and Allocation of Human Organs for Transplantation: Hearings Before the House Subcomm. on Investigations and Oversight, Comm. on Sci. and Tech.*, 98th Cong., 1983, 26, 29, 53 (testimony and submitted statement of Warren Reich).

68. Ibid., 29, 64–65 (statements of Warren Reich and Al Gore).

69. Andrew Schneider and Mary Pat Flaherty, "Favoritism Shrouds Presby Transplants," *Pittsburgh Press*, May 12, 1985, A1.

70. Ibid.

71. Andrew Schneider and Mary Pat Flaherty, "Woman Passed over after 3-Year Wait," *Pittsburgh Press*, May 12, 1985, A10.

72. "Saudi Received 2 Kidney Operations after Presby Set Its Transplant Ban," *Pittsburgh Press*, June 30, 1985, A15.

73. See Margaret Engel, "Foreigners Got High Percentage of Kidney Transplants," *Washington Post*, June 10, 1985, C1.

74. Ibid.

75. Starzl quoted in Schneider and Flaherty, "Favoritism," A10.

76. Andrew Schneider and Mary Pat Flaherty, "Foreigners Paid Extra for Kidney Transplants," *Pittsburgh Press* June 30, 1985, A1.

77. Schneider and Flaherty, "Favoritism," A10.

78. Schneider and Flaherty, "Foreigners Paid Extra," A1.

79. Andrew Schneider, "Presbyterian to Revise Kidney Transplant Rule," *Pittsburgh Press*, May 20, 1985, A3.

80. Linda Berry, "Capitalism Blamed," *Pittsburgh Press*, May 19, 1985, B4 (letter).

81. Lindsey Gruson, "Some Doctors Move to Bar Transplants to Foreign Patients," *New York Times*, August 10, 1985, 1.

82. "Transplant priorities," *Pittsburgh Press*, May 24, 1985, C8 (Opinion); Mary Pat Flaherty, "Organ Network Gives Foreigners Lowest Priority," *Pittsburgh Press*, May 23, 1985, A6.

83. Eugene L. Meyer, "Tax Money for Transplant Operations: Who Pays?" *Washington Post*, September 12, 1984, C8.

84. "Transplant Line-Jumping," *Pittsburgh Press*, May 19, 1985, B2 (Opinion).

85. Gruson, "Some Doctors."

86. Arthur Caplan, "Governor Transplant Case Shows Real Issues of System Fairness," in *Moral Matters: Ethical Issues in Medicine and the Life Sciences*, by Arthur Caplan (New York: John Wiley & Sons, 1995), 141.

87. Engel, "Foreigners," C1.

88. "Transplant Line-Jumping," B2.

89. Takemoto et al., "HLA Matching in Renal Transplantation," *New England Journal of Medicine* 332 (March 16, 1995): 752–53 (correspondence).

90. Paul Delaney, "Fighting Myths in a Bid to Get Blacks to Consider Transplants," *New York Times*, November 6, 1991, C17.

91. Kevin Chapell, "Life Goes On: Be an Organ/Tissue Donor," *Ebony*, July 2004.

92. Quoted in Press Release, United Network for Organ Sharing, "OPTN/UNOS Continues to Improve Accuracy in Donor/Recipient Matching."

93. Tim Friend, "Duke Didn't Follow the Rules in Jesica's Transplant," *USA Today*, March 4, 2003, 1D.

94. See Kieran Healy, "Sacred Markets and Secular Ritual in the Organ Transplant Industry," in *The Sociology of the Economy*, ed. Frank Dobbin (New York: Russell Sage Foundation, 2004), 308, 316, 326–27.

CONSUMING DIFFERENCES

POST-HUMAN ETHICS, GLOBAL (IN)JUSTICE, AND THE TRANSPLANT TRADE IN ORGANS

NANCY SCHEPER-HUGHES

Even as Jesica Santillan's story played itself out in the American media, a powerful global crisis was unfolding—an international commerce in human organs. The globalization of organ and tissue markets turns the Santillan story on its head, and provides crucial insight into the ways in which other kinds of people—wealthy, first world, well-insured, and invoking their "right" to transplant were traveling great distances to procure organ transplants illegally in second and third world contexts. Indeed, the deeply entrenched notions of "organs scarcity" and "waste" that so clearly circumscribed the Santillan story were crucial factors shaping these new global trends. Jesica's move from her small town in Mexico to Durham, North Carolina, was only one part of a broader, and far more troubling, movement of desperate people, and organs. And as we shift from the parochial features of the Santillan story to the global arena, it becomes clear that profound questions of ethics, justice, and allocation (not to mention the modernist conceptions of the body, the person, and the meanings of life and death) are being engaged and challenged.

THE GLOBALIZATION OF TRANSPLANT

The neoliberal readjustments societies worldwide have made to meet the demands of economic globalization have been accompanied by a depletion of traditional modernist, humanist, and pastoral ideologies, values, and practices. New relations between capital and labor, bodies and the state, inclusion and exclusion, belonging and extraterritoriality have taken shape. Some of these realignments have resulted in surprising new outcomes (for example, the emergence and applications of democratic ideas and ideals of "medical" and "sexual" citizenship[1] in countries such as Brazil and India, which have challenged international patent laws and trade restrictions to expand the production and distribution of generic, lifesaving drugs), while others (for example, the spread of paid surrogacy in assisted reproduction[2]) have re-produced all-too-familiar inequalities.

Nowhere are these trends more stark than in the global markets in bodies, organs, and tissues that supply the needs of transplant patients who are now willing to travel great distances to procure them. But rather than lament the decline of humanistic social values and social relations, we recognize that the material grounds on which once-cherished values were based have shifted today almost beyond recognition.

The entry of markets (black and gray) and market incentives[3] into organs procurement has thrown into question the tired transplant rhetoric on "organs scarcity." There is obviously no shortage of desperate individuals willing to sell a kidney, a portion of their liver, a lung, an eye, or even a testicle for a pittance. But while erasing one vexing scarcity, the organs trade has produced a new one—a scarcity of transplant patients of sufficient means and independence and who are willing to break, bend, or bypass laws and long-standing codes of medical ethical conduct.

THE GIFT OF LIFE AND TRANSPLANT ETHICS

Jesica Santillan, in becoming a candidate for transplant surgery in North Carolina, entered a moral and ethical "gray zone." From its origins, transplant surgery presented itself as a complicated problem in gift relations. Organ transplantation is the most intensely social of all medical practice. Its existence presupposes a unique trust between society and its physicians, and it is dependent upon the willingness of ordinary people to share their organs and tissues either with a mortally sick loved one or with an unknown "stranger" who was, nonetheless, a member of a larger community network, a social body if you will, of organ trading partners within a system of open-ended reciprocity. Originally, the circulation of organs was restricted to *internal* networks— either among families (as in living, related donation of kidneys among siblings, parents, and children) or among citizens under national programs of cadaveric organs procurement and distribution, like UNOS (United States) or INCUCAI (Argentina) that designate human organs as a scarce and precious "national resource" to be allocated equitably. Organ sharing, an intimate practice, was not intended to meet the needs of foreign guests and visitors, who would not be in a position to reciprocate at some later date.

From the outset, the language of organ sharing—saturated with references to altruism, sharing, gift-giving—has been excessively idealistic, ethical, and, in a subliminal sense, Christian.[4] In traditional transplantation, the "gift of life" is, like "life insurance," a euphemism and a misnomer. In fact, cadaveric donation is really a "gift of death." And the new "moral imperative" to list oneself as an altruistic organ donor represents a modern form of invisible sacrifice. All transplant patients recognize, of course, that their good fortune comes out of the tragedy of another, and they are often vaguely uncomfortable with the excitement they experience on stormy nights when traffic accidents are more likely to occur and produce the organs they need. But they are rarely privy to the secret negotiations and not-infrequent psychological manipulations of the donor's family members while they are in deep grief. Even when living donation is transacted within families, the recipients may be unaware of the conflicts produced by the simple demand for a "spare" organ. Thus, living, related kidney donors, for example, are counseled to avoid bringing up the subject with the recipient. Their gift must be completely "forgotten," a mandate that burdens living donors to guard what is a classic "family secret"—a secret known to all but never discussed.

With the spread of transplant technologies to virtually all parts of the world, closed, internal circulation/consumption of organs has now become open and extraterritorial. The second recent transformation is from living, *related* (familial) organ sharing to living *unrelated* sharing of organs among strangers. Living donation among strangers became feasible following advances in new generations of extremely powerful antirejection medications. Thus, a new demand for unrelated, living donation—both "Good Samaritan" and paid donors—has appeared on the scene.

Altruistic living donation, modeled after the earlier "gifting" of organs from dead donors, has been embraced by fundamentalist Christian churches, especially in the U.S. South. On any given Sunday in small rural towns, one can find evangelical ministers exhorting members of their congregation to come forward and commit themselves to Christ as anonymous organs donors, exemplifying the perfect, the most pure, gift of self. Good Samaritan donors are motivated by faith, to be sure, but also by the search for celebrity, and the desire to compensate for failures in other domains. For "Gabriella Dove," a Good Samaritan donor from northern California, donating her kidney to a stranger in South Carolina represented a solution of sorts to her repeated failures at in vitro fertilization (IVF) therapy. Her voluntary and altruistic nephrectomy (kidney removal) was described by her as "like giving birth," even though she was distressed and disappointed afterward. After all, she didn't get to keep her baby, the seemingly ungrateful sixty-seven-year-old recipient.

For Zell Kravinsky, a hyperactive philanthropist, the distribution of his self-made fortunes in real estate was not sufficient. In 2003, he answered a plea published in a newspaper and "gifted" one of his kidneys to a sick woman he did not know. Encouraged by the result, he considered donating his second kidney to another stranger, and then he began to consider becoming the first total (living) body donor, so he could save even more lives.[5] Kavinsky calculated the number of lives he could rescue by dismantling himself piece by piece. His "perfect gift" of non-reciprocal "selfless love" was rejected, of course, by doctors as pathological, a kind of altruistic suicide. Even on his own social utilitarian terms, however, Karvinsky's math was off. If he factored in the continued risk of organ rejection and the wear and tear of diseases on his immune-suppressed recipients, he would come up with a quite different equation of years of human life saved, minus his own, of course.

Even in the context of the frank buying and selling of kidneys via the global trade in body parts, selling an organ is often redefined so as to retain elements of the gift relationship. Thus, the British moral philosopher Janet Ratcliffe-Richards has argued in the *Lancet* that since many kidney sales are motivated by altruistic goals—feeding a family or procuring expensive medical treatment for a sick child—donations can partake of both sale *and* gift simultaneously. Similarly, Leonardo de Castro, a bioethicist at Manila's Jesuit University, explained kidney selling in Manila's watery slums as providing an opportunity for individual penance and restitution. In his comments to me he made reference to the cultural practice of self-flagellation during Holy Week rituals among the poor in the Philippines: "Self-flagellation [is] a culturally prescribed way of making up for past mistakes by [showing that] one is willing to go to the extreme to manifest one's sincerity. Organ donation (even with selling) fits this penitential mode of Catholicism. We should reserve the individual's freedom to make decisions regarding his body or parts, while recognizing that even radical acts of self-mortification are safely anchored in religious and cultural traditions."

From its inception, transplant medicine put severe demands on modernist conceptions of the body, the person, and the meanings of life and death. Transplantation demanded a radical redefinition of death, to allow the immediate "harvesting" of organs from bodies neither completely dead nor yet still living, which to this day still troubles many of the world's religious leaders and a surprising number of medical specialists[6]—not to mention the relatives of the nearly dead, who so often refuse to allow the term "brain death" to be applied to their loved ones and prevent harvesting from taking place.

Diametrically opposed to the "softer" medical ethic of the clinic and the emergency room, which is based on a commitment to save the sickest, transplant ethics originally operated on the less "civil" ethic of the lifeboat and of the battlefield, which is based on a commitment to save the salvageable and to allow the sickest to die. But as transplant capabilities developed and the desires for transplant have "democratized," medical consumers have begun to challenge the old battlefield triage and are demanding an end to "wartime" rationing based on scarcities that could be addressed by applying neoliberal market principles to organ harvesting and thereby legally tapping into the bodies of the *living*.

This move to organs markets has required a radical breach with, or a highly selective use of, classical medical ethics, based worldwide on a blend of Aristotelian theories of virtue (wisdom, courage, temperance, and justice), and the Hippocratic ethic of purity, loyalty, compassion, and respect for the dignity of the individual. In the Hippocratic tradition of medical ethics, with its markedly individualist conception of physician responsibility and virtue, the physician may be seen as owing his loyalties to the patient alone, as if society—let alone the rest of the world—did not exist. In recent years, and in response to the privatization and commercialization of medicine (transplant in particular), many surgeons now espouse a frankly posthumanist utilitarian ethic based on the moral philosophy of John Stuart Mill[7] and Jeremy Bentham[8] but stripped of its original social content and concerns. Thus, in a much cited essay in the *Lancet*,[9] Dr. Michael Friedlaender, of Hadassah Hospital in Jerusalem, explained his about-face with respect to accepting the "greater good" that can result from adopting a utilitarian ethic toward the individual's right to buy (or sell) a kidney: "Recently I was told that I am a utilitarian. I had always considered myself a humanitarian, but I have since developed some doubts about my beliefs." He cites, approvingly, the large number of his kidney patients, both Jews and Arabs, who have traveled abroad for a transplant (Jews to Eastern Europe and Arabs to Iran and Iraq) with a purchased kidney from a living "donor." I would do the same, he said.

The kidney trade evokes a timeless moral and ethical "gray zone"[10]—the lengths to which it is permissible to go in the interests of saving or prolonging one's own life at the expense of diminishing another person's life or sacrificing cherished cultural and political values (such as social solidarity, justice, or equity).

THE ORGANS WATCH PROJECT

Although at first blush the Jesica Santillian story might seem disconnected from the global story of organs traffic, the case shares many of the same structures and sentiments, including urgent demands to expand possibilities and options for transplant; the refusal by those seeking organs of older systems of rationing on which UNOS and other national systems of organs sharing are based; and the emergence of a new class of nonspecialized intermediaries and organs brokers (in the Santillan case the prominent role played by Mack Mahoney, a Durham, North Carolina, building contractor who tirelessly advocated on behalf of Jesica's transplant). While Mahoney's interventions were not part of the extensive organs trade, they were nevertheless similar to the role of organs transplant advocates, for example, in Israel who initiate campaigns to raise the funds needed for illicit internationally based transplant operations.

The Organ Watch documentation and medical human rights project was formed, in the absence of any other organization of its kind, to respond to the need for independent surveillance of new organs markets and brokers. At the Heart of this project are a few basic questions: How does the human organs market function? Who are the key players? How are the relations between organized crime and illicit transplant medicine structured? Whose needs are privileged? What invisible sacrifices are demanded? What "noble lies" are concealed in the tired transplant rhetoric of gifting, scarcities, and human needs? Although our investigation of the global trade offered answers strikingly different than those in the Santillan story, the worldwide organs trade and its key features (illicit practice, crime, need, privilege, exploitation, and sacrifice) certainly intersect in crucial ways with the themes surrounding Santillan.

In the course of our research we have interviewed kidney patients in their homes, clinics, and hospital beds to try to understand the specific conditions of their suffering. My associates and I[11] have followed a much smaller number of them from their dialysis clinics to meetings with brokers and intermediaries in suburban shopping malls and hotel lobbies, and from there to illicit surgeries in rented operating rooms of public and private hospitals, some resembling the clandestine back-alley abortion clinics of the 1940s and 1950s. We have tracked down some notorious organs brokers, only to discover that many began as desperate kidney sellers themselves, who were later hired by their surgeons as local kidney hunters. We have met with local kidney sellers in township *shabeens* in Soweto, in squatter camps in Manila, in shantytowns in Brazil, in jails in Israel, in smoke-filled bars in Chisenau, and in the wine cellars of Mingir in Moldova.[12]

In short, we have gone to many of the places where the economically and politically dispossessed—including refugees, the homeless, street children, undocumented workers, prisoners, AWOL soldiers, aging prostitutes, cigarette smugglers, petty thieves, and other marginalized people—are lured into selling their organs. At the same time, we have followed, observed, and interviewed at length and at their sites of "operation" over 100 international surgeons and transplant specialists who are knowledgeable about or implicated in illicit surgeries, and we have interviewed their lawyers and their often far-flung medical and financial intermediaries (that is, brokers) who make these surgeries possible.

In the following discussion I contrast the *variable* meanings and medical and social consequences of selling (or buying) a body part (in Israel, Moldova, and the Philippines) with a growing consensus in the international transplant community that supports a patient-centered ethic that includes the right to purchase advanced, expensive, and experimental biomedical/surgical procedures, as well as to buy and sell body parts from the living and the dead. Both are compatible with neoliberal economics.

Indeed, commercialized transplant exemplifies better than any other biomedical technology the reach of economic liberalism. Transplant technology trades comfortably in the domain of postmodern biopolitics, with its values of disposability and free and transparent circulation. The uninhibited circulation of bought and sold kidneys exemplifies a neoliberal political discourse based on juridical concepts of the autonomous individual subject, equality (at least, equality of opportunity), radical freedom, accumulation, and universalism, expressed in the expansion of medical rights and medical citizenship.

Despite this neoliberal rhetoric, in fact, it is far-flung networks of organized crime that are responsible for putting into circulation and bringing together ambulatory organ buyers, outlaw surgeons, illicit and sometimes makeshift transplant units, and clandestine laboratories in an example of what economist Jagdish Bhagwati refers to as "rotten trade."[13] Rotten trade refers to any trade in "bads"—arms, drugs, stolen goods, and hazardous and toxic products, as well as traffic in humans, babies, bodies, and slave labor. The organs trade is fueled by a dual "waiting list," one formed by sickness, the other by misery.

We have found almost everywhere a new form of globalized "apartheid medicine" that privileges one class of patients, organ recipients, over another class of invisible and unrecognized "nonpatients," about whom almost nothing is known.

In the context of this globalized system, Jesica Santillan appears to have crossed the divide—moving in a direction unlike those traversed by so many transplant tourists of her time. Millennial, or "second coming," capitalism[14] has facilitated the spread of advanced medical procedures and biotechnologies to all corners of the world, producing strange markets and "occult econo- mies." Together, these have incited new tastes and desires for the skin, bone, blood, organs, tissue, and reproductive and genetic material of others. No- where are these processes more transparent than in the field of organ trans- plants that now takes place in a transnational space, with both donors and re- cipients following new paths of capital and technology in the global economy.

The spread of transplant technologies initially created a global scarcity of transplantable organs at the same time that economic globalization released an exodus of displaced and "surplus" persons to do the shadow work of production and to provide bodies for sexual and medical consumption. The "open" global market economy provided the ideal conditions for an unprece- dented movement of people, including mortally sick bodies traveling in one direction and "healthy" organs (encased in their human packages) in another direction, creating a bizarre "kula ring" of international body trade. Like any other business, the organs trade is driven by a simple market calculus of supply and demand. Its brokers organize and bring together affluent kidney buyers from Japan, Italy, Israel, and Saudi Arabia with the stranded Moldovan and Romanian peasants, Turkish junk dealers, Palestinian refugees, AWOL soldiers from Iraq and Afghanistan, and the unemployed stevedores of Ma- nila's slums from whom they will buy a lifesaving commodity.

Transplant tourism is vital to the medical economies of rapidly privatizing clinical and hospital services in poorer countries that are struggling to stay afloat. The "global cities"[15] in this nether economy are not London, New York, Tokyo, and Frankfurt, but Istanbul, Lima, Lvov, Tel Aviv, Chisenau, Bombay, Johannesburg, and Manila. However, the United States has not been isolated from this global market that pits desperate transplant patients against equally desperate poor people, each trying to find a solution to basic problems of human survival. Transplant tourism packages, arranged in the Middle East, have brought hundreds of affluent kidney patients to U.S. transplant centers for surgeries conducted with paid donors or with cadaver organs that are otherwise described as painfully scarce.[16]

Until Organs Watch protested it, the University of Maryland Medical Cen- ter advertised its kidney transplant program in Arabic, Chinese, Hebrew, and

Japanese on its Web site.[17] Mt. Sinai Hospital in New York City published promotional advertisements on its transplant capabilities in the *Wall Street Journal* and in the *International Herald Tribune*. The United States is very democratic in at least one sense—anyone with enough cash, regardless of where they come from, can become a "medical citizen" of the United States and be transplanted, even with a scarce, "made in the U.S.A." transplant organ.

On the one hand, the spread of transplant technologies, even in the murky context of illicit surgeries, has given the possibility of new, extended, or greatly improved life to a select population of mobile kidney patients from the deserts of Oman to the rain forests of Central Brazil.[18] On the other hand, the spread of "transplant tourism" has exacerbated older divisions between North and South, core and periphery haves and have-nots, spawning a new form of commodity fetishism in demands by medical consumers for a quality product—"fresh" and "healthy" kidneys purchased from living bodies. In general, the circulation of kidneys follows the established routes of capital from South to North, from poorer to more affluent bodies, from black and brown bodies to white ones, and from females to males, or from poor males to more affluent males. Women are rarely the recipients of purchased or purloined organs anywhere in the world. We can even speak of organ donor versus organ recipient nations.

The commodified kidney is, to date, the primary currency in transplant tourism; it represents the gold standard of organ sales worldwide. In recent months, however, markets in part-livers from living vendors are beginning to emerge in Southeast Asia.

TRANSFORMING DIFFERENCE—BIO-SOCIALITY: "KIDNEY KIN"

New forms of social kinship and "bio-sociality" must be invented to link strangers, even at times political "enemies," from distant locations who are described by the operating surgeons as "a perfect match—like brothers," while they are prevented from seeing, let alone speaking to, each other. If and when these "kidney kin" meet at all, it will be by accident and like ships passing in the night, as they are wheeled, heavily sedated, on hospital gurneys into their respective operating rooms, where one surgeon *removes* the seller's kidney of last resort and the other *inserts* the buyer's kidney of opportunity.

Because "sharing organs" among the living is an ultimate act of bodily commitment, even if it occurs among strangers from far-flung places and for money, kidney buyers and sellers often try to seek each other out and make claims on each other. Kidney buyers fear they may "reject" a kidney purchased from an angry or resentful seller who, after the fact, may harbor ill will toward the buyer. Meanwhile, kidney sellers often feel that they are "family" to the buyer, their underprivileged and barefoot country cousin, their "kidney kin," and feel they have the right to demand help. "A life for a life," Alberty da Silva, thirty-eight, from a slum in Recife, Brazil, said of his plea for continued financial help from Luanne "Hinks," the woman from New York City who bought his kidney. The transplant transfer brought both of them across the Atlantic to South Africa, where the kidney removal and transplant took place at a private, formerly Catholic hospital, St. Augustine's. Alberty defended his honor, saying that although he was paid something ($3,000) for his kidney, his kidney was still a priceless "gift": "Isn't a life worth much more than that?" And Luanne sent a Christmas card to Alberty offering to send a gift to the man who saved her life:

> "Dear Alberty: How are you feeling? I hope and pray that all is well with you and your family. My husband and myself are doing well and putting our faith in God to keep us well. I hope you haven't forgotten me, because I'll never forget you for giving me my life back. I was close to death and you gave me your kidney. I'd like to send you a gift for Christmas but I am not sure this is your correct address . . . God Bless you, Luanne."

In all, the strange markets, excess capital, occult medical economies, renegade surgeons,[19] and local rings of "kidney hunters" with links to an international Mafia[20] exist side by side with desperate sellers, panic-stricken kidney buyers, and international organ "brokers with hearts of gold," all trying to redefine the illicit traffic as a meritorious humanitarian act and the bartered kidney as a "paid gift." The emergence of new zones of abandonment generating the formation of so-called kidney belts and itinerant kidney sellers is a troubling subtext in the story of late-twentieth- and early-twenty-first-century globalization.

MEDICAL MIGRATIONS: SCENES FROM THE FIELD

The trajectory of Jesica Santillan, from the small town of Arrondo Hoyo through Guadalajara, across the U.S. border into Texas and finally to Louisburg, North Carolina, was the consequence of Jesica's mother's quest for the life of her mortally sick child and was but one variant of medical migrations. In recent decades, ever increasing numbers of people are crossing borders in search of advanced medical procedures they cannot get at home, in pursuit of experimental procedures such as genetic therapies, reproductive technologies, AIDS therapies, etc. These new medical migrants include the poor and the affluent, the desperate and the dissatisfied. Among the ranks of these brave new medical travelers are European tourists in Southeast Asia and Latin America for cosmetic surgeries, North African migrants who enter France on medical visas, Americans traveling to Montreal for generic drugs, alcohol- and drug-addicted Argentineans and Brazilians visiting upscale medicalized health spas in Cuba, and Israelis traveling to Turkey and South Africa for kidney transplants alongside ruined Moldovan peasants and debt-plagued Brazilian slum dwellers hiding out in depressing "safe" houses (in the shadow of five-star private hospitals) to which they were trafficked as half willing/half coerced kidney providers. Medical migrations like these reveal the intersections and disjunctions in the contemporary global politics of health. The specificities, differences, connections, and tensions among these diverse forms of medical travel reveal the shape of desires and needs, the biopolitical imperative for health, self-enhancement, consumer-driven health care, and the possibilities and the damages released through globalization.

Jesica Santillan's story (as one variant of cross-border medical migration) offers a critical vantage point for exploring globalization and transnationality. It also brings into relief what is at stake for the desperate pursuit of life, health, and medical technologies in the world today. Jesica's story and other scenes of transplant tourism described in this essay raise important questions: How are innovations in medicine, and biotechnology brought together in emergent biomedical global-scapes? What benefits, risks, and dangers are associated with these travels and their social, political, and medical outcomes? In what ways do the regulatory apparatuses of transnational organizations, nation-states, and private industries shape the contours of new medical migrations?

Avraham R., a retired lawyer of seventy, stepped gingerly out of his sedan at the curb of the Beit Belgia Faculty Club at the University of Jerusalem in July 2000. The dapper gent, a grandfather of five, had been playing a game of "chicken" with me over the past two weeks, ducking my persistent phone calls. Each time I asked the genial grandfather for a face-to-face interview, he demurred: "It's not to protect me," he said, "but my family." Then, one afternoon, Avraham surprised me, not only agreeing to meet me, but insisting that he come over to my comfortable quarters, where, over a few bottles of mineral water, he explained why and how he had come to the decision to risk traveling to an undisclosed location in Eastern Europe to purchase a kidney from an anonymous "peasant" and to face transplant in a spartan operating room ("I have more medicines in my own medicine chest than they had in that hospital," he said.) rather than remain on dialysis at Hadassah Hospital, as his nephrologist had suggested.

Avraham was still eligible for a transplant, but at his age, his doctors warned, such a long operation was risky. Dialysis, they told him, was really his best option. But Avraham protested that he was not yet ready for the "medical trash-heap," which is the way he and many other Israeli kidney patients now view hemodialysis. And, like a growing number of kidney patients, he rejected the idea of a cadaver organ (the "dead man's organ") as "disgusting" and unacceptable:

> Why should I have to wait years for a kidney from somebody who was in a traffic accident, pinned under a car for many hours, then in miserable condition in the I.C.U. [intensive care unit] for days and only then, after all that trauma, have that same organ put inside me? That organ isn't going to be any good! Or worse, I could get the organ of an old person, or an alcoholic, or someone who died of a stroke. That kidney has already done its work! No, obviously, it's much better to get a kidney from a healthy person who can also benefit from the money I can afford to pay. Believe me, where I went the people were so poor they didn't even have bread to eat. Do you have any idea of what one, let alone five thousand dollars, means to a peasant? The money I paid him was "a gift of life" equal to what I received.

In December 2001, during an early snowstorm, I ducked into a small, dark, subterranean wine cave in the rustic little village of Mingir, Moldova. There, once out of earshot of his elderly father and beyond the prying eyes of disapproving neighbors, twenty-two-year-old Vladimir, a skinny lad with a rakish metal stud in his lip, explained how he had been approached a few years earlier by Nina, a local kidney hunter, who arranged his passport, visa, and bus ticket to Istanbul, a bumpy eighteen-hour overnight ride, for what he thought would be a job. With the demise of the Soviet Union, the agricultural economy of rural Moldova collapsed in the mid-1990s. Here, in the heart of central Europe, economic globalization has meant one thing only for agricultural villagers—that 40 percent of the adult population has had to leave home to find work abroad. Today, Moldova is the poorest country in Europe: an indigenous "third world" within European borders.

Once in Istanbul, Vladimir was housed in the basement of a run-down hotel facing a notorious Russian "suitcase market" in the tough immigrant neighborhood of Askary. He shared the space with several other Moldovan villagers, including a few frightened village girls barely out of high school. First, Nina arrived to break the news to one of the girls that her "waitressing" job would be in a bar where "exotic" dancing was required. Then Vladimir was told that he was wanted for more than pressing pants. He would start by selling a few pints of his blood, and once a "match" was found, he would be taken to a private hospital where he would give up his "best" kidney for $3,000, less the cost of his travel, room, and board and the fees for his "handlers." And a few days later Vlad was told that an elderly transplant patient from Israel, who had traveled to Istanbul with his private surgeon, was matched and ready to go. When Vlad demurred, Nina arrived with her pockmarked, pistol-carrying Turkish boyfriend, who told Vladimir that he was quickly losing patience. "Actually," Vlad says ruefully, "If I had refused to go along with them, my body minus *both* kidneys, and who knows what else, could be floating somewhere in the Bosporous Strait."

Safely home again—or so they think—hapless kidney sellers such as Vladimir face ridicule and ostracism. Both kidney sellers and female sex workers are held in contempt in rural Moldova as shameless prostitutes. Months and even years later, these young men suffer from feelings of shame and regret—like Nicolae, a twenty-six-year-old former welder from Mingir, who broke down during an interview in December 2000, calling himself "a disgrace to my family, my Church, and my country."

While kidney selling is deeply stigmatized in Moldova, where it is symbolically linked to prostitution, it is a routine event in the slums and shantytowns of Manila in the Philippines, even though the operation has put a great many young men out of work there. "No one wants a kidney seller on his work team," an unemployed kidney seller and father of three told us, while his wife fumed at him from across the room.

Bangon Lupa is a garbage-strewn slum built on stilt shacks over a polluted and feces-infested stretch of the Pasig River that runs through the shantytown on its way to Manila Bay. In Bangon Lupa, "coming of age" now means that one is legally old enough to sell a kidney. But, as with other coming-of-age rituals, many young men lie about their age and boast of having sold a kidney when they were as young as sixteen years old: "No one at the hospital asks us for any documents," they assured me. The kidney donors lied about other things as well—their names, addresses, and medical histories, including their daily exposure to the general plagues of the third world—TB, AIDS, dengue, and hepatitis, not to mention chronic skin infections and malnutrition.

In this *barangay* of largely unemployed stevedores, I encountered an unanticipated "waiting list" comprised of angry and "disrespected" would-be kidney sellers who had been "neglected" and "overlooked" by the medical doctors at Manila's most prestigious private hospital, St. Luke's Episcopal Medical Center. When word spread that I was looking to speak to kidney sellers, several scowling and angry young men approached me to complain: "We are strong and virile men, and yet none of us has been called up to sell." Perhaps they had been rejected, the men surmised, because of their age (too young or too old), their blood type (difficult to match), or their general medical condition. But whatever the reason, they had been judged as less valuable kidney vendors than some of their lucky neighbors, who now owned new VCRs, karaoke machines, and expensive tricycles. "What's wrong with me?" a forty-two-year-old man asked, thinking I must be an American kidney hunter. "I registered six months ago, and no one from St. Luke's has called me. . . . But I am healthy. I can lift heavy weights. And my urine is clean." Moreover, he was willing, he said, to sell below the going rate of $1,300 for a fresh kidney.

When one donor is rejected, another, younger and more healthy looking family member is often substituted. And kidney selling becomes an economic niche in some families that specialize in it. Indeed, one large extended family in Bangong Lupa supplied St. Luke's Hospital with a reliable source of kidneys, borrowing strength from across the generations as first father, then son, and then daughter-in-law each stepped forward to contribute to the family income.

THE CONSUMERS—THE EXPANSION OF
MEDICAL CITIZENSHIP AND COMMODITY FETISHISM

In recent years, the frustrations of Americans (for example) with the UNOS system, the long waiting times for transplants, and the national rules of the transplant system have not only stimulated medical tourism but raised new questions about the nature of medical citizenship. Who has a right to scarce resources donated as part of a national trust? Should undocumented immigrants, like Jesica Santillan, have the right to participate in dialysis and transplant—the only and exceptional form of nationalized health care in the United States? The question is belied, of course, by the special provisions (the 5 percent rule) made by UNOS to allow mostly wealthy foreign patients to be transplanted with bonafide U.S. donor organs "for humanitarian reasons." Here, the recent controversy at St. Vincent's hospital in Los Angeles in which the transplant staff bypassed nine of its own patients to transplant a liver into a Saudi national and the outrage that this occasioned is instructive, all the more so when it was revealed that the Royal Embassy of Saudi Arabia had paid the hospital $339,000 for the Saudi patient's transplant and hospital care, plus undisclosed fees to the doctors, an amount that was about 30 percent higher than the hospital would have been paid by insurance companies and government programs.[21] On the other hand, transnational organizations and organ sharing compacts, such as Eurotransplant, have eroded the nationalism of earlier systems that defined donated organs as a kind of community-based property, and these organizations have advanced late modern notions of universal medical citizenship based on human rights to basic health care and lifesaving procedures. To be sure, similar issues about the nature and limits of medical citizenship also emerged in the Santillan story in 2003 (see the essay by Meslin et al. in this volume), but these questions take on different meanings in the context of the expanding "free markets" in organs.

Finding an available supply of organ vendors was only a partial solution to the new scarcities produced by transplant technologies. The tempting "bioavailability" of poor bodies has been a primary stimulus to the "fresh organs" trade. Today, a great many eager and willing kidney sellers wait outside transplant units; others check themselves into special wards of surgical units that resemble "kidney motels," where they lie on mats or in hospital beds for days, even weeks, watching color television, eating chips, and waiting for the "lucky number" that will turn them into the day's winner of the kidney transplant lottery. Entire neighborhoods, cities, and regions are known in transplant circles as "kidney belts" because so many people there have entered the kidney trade.

More difficult is locating patients of sufficient economic means to pay for these expensive operations, as well as sufficiently courageous to travel to the largely third world locations where people are willing to self-mutilate in the interests of short-term survival. Here is a classic problem in microeconomics —one of supply- and demand-side sources separated by vast geographies, different cultures, and even fierce religious and political hostilities.

Who, for example, would imagine that, in the midst of the long-standing religious and ethnic hostilities and an almost genocidal war in the Middle East, one of the first "sources" of living donors for Israeli kidney transplant patients would be Palestinian guest workers; or that, as recently as March 2002, Israeli patients would be willing to travel to Istanbul to be transplanted in a private clinic by a Muslim surgeon who decorates his waiting room with photos of Ataturk and a plastic glass eye to ward off evil? Or that transplanted kidneys would be taken from impoverished Eastern Orthodox peasants from

Moldova and Romania who came to Turkey to sell smuggled cigarettes until they ran into the famous kidney brokers of Askary flea market?

New transplant-patient advocacy groups have sprung up in many parts of the world, from Brazil to Israel to Iran to the United States, demanding unobstructed access to transplant and to the lifesaving "spare" organs of "the other," for which they are willing to pay a negotiable, market-determined price. They justify the means by recourse to the mantra that the organ will "save a life." However, many kidney patients in the first world with access to hemodialysis reject it as an option, weakening the "lifesaving" argument. The problem is that dialysis, even as a bridge while waiting for transplant, is increasingly viewed by sophisticated kidney activists today as unacceptable suffering. In September 2000, a twenty-three-year-old university student from Jerusalem flew to New York City for a kidney transplant with an organ purchased from a local "donor," arranged through a broker in Brooklyn. The cost of the surgery ($200,000) was paid for by his Israeli "sick funds" (medical insurance that is guaranteed to all Israeli citizens). Noteworthy in his narrative is an almost seamless "naturalization" of living donation accompanied by a rejection of the artificiality of the dialysis machine:

> Kidney transplant from a living person is the most natural solution because you are free of the [dialysis] machine. With transplant you don't have to go to the hospital three times a week to waste your time, for three or four hours. And after each dialysis you don't feel very well, and you sleep a lot, and on weekends you feel too tired to go out with your friends. There are still a lot of poisons in the body and when you can't remove them, you feel tired. Look, it isn't a normal life. And also you are limited to certain foods. You are not allowed to eat a lot of meat, salt, fruits, vegetables. Every month you do tests to see that the calcium level is OK, and even so your skin becomes yellow. Esthetically, it isn't very nice. So, a kidney transplant from a living donor is the best, and the most natural solution.

Similarly, many kidney activists reject conventional "waiting lists" for organs as archaic vestiges of wartime triage and rationing, or reminiscent of hated socialist bread lines and petrol "queues." In the present climate of biotechnological optimism and biomedical triumphalism, any shortage, even of body parts, is viewed as a basic management, marketing, or policy failure. The ideology of the global economy is one of unlimited and freely circulating goods. And these new commodities are evaluated, like any other, in terms of their quality, durability, and market value. In today's organs market, a kidney purchased from a Filipino costs as little as $1,200, one from a Moldovan peasant, $2,700, and one from a Turkish worker, up to $8,000, while a kidney purchased from a housewife in Lima, Peru, can command up to $15,000 in a private clinic.

BIOETHICS—THE HANDMAIDEN OF FREE MARKET MEDICINE

Questions of illegality and the corruption of waiting lists in the United States (where donor organs allocated by UNOS to designated individuals on the waiting list are sometimes treated by transplant surgeons as their prize rather than belonging to the designated patient) shadowed the Santillan case and the bungled transplant that could and should have been avoided. But the problems of outlaw surgeons, corruption, and malfeasance are far more pronounced in the world of international transplant tourism, where national laws and international regulations are simply disregarded.

Whether in the United States or in the larger global context, transplant operations are imbued with magical beliefs about "resurrection" and "new life" that endow transplant surgeons with a power (and charisma) so absolute that it can easily lend itself to abuse. Surgeons described as operating with "golden hands"—when the only "gold" in sight is ill-gotten gains through transplant tourism packages brokered by thieves—bioethicists serving as handmaidens rather than as much-needed critics and skeptics, and economic contradictions produced in the illogical blend of public and private systems of payment have threatened the integrity of this distinguished field of medical surgery. For example, both UNOS in the United States and South African law both define all donated organs as precious "national resources" and as public property. Meanwhile, relatively open (though still illicit) organs and tissues markets coexist in both nations undermining the goodwill and public trust required by the national system.

What goes by the wayside in these new medical transactions are the modernist conceptions of bodily holism, integrity, and human dignity, not to mention traditional Islamic and Judeo-Christian beliefs in the "sacredness" of the body. Free market medicine requires a divisible body with detachable and demystified organs to be seen as ordinary and "plain things," simple material for medical consumption. But these same "plain" objects have a way of reappearing and returning like the repressed, when least expected, almost like medieval messengers and gargoyles from the past, in the form of highly spiritualized and fetishized objects of desire. As Veena Das once wryly observed, "An organ is *never* just an organ."[22]

Indeed, the highly fetishized kidney is invested with all the magical energy and potency that the transplant patient is looking for in the name of "new" life. As Avraham, the Israeli kidney buyer put it: "I was able to see my donor [from a village in Eastern Europe]. He was young, strong, healthy, and virile— *everything* I was hoping for."

It might be fair to ask if the life that is teased out of the body of the living donor bears any resemblance to the ethical life of the free citizen (*bios*) or whether it is closer to what Giorgio Agamben, drawing on Aristotle's *Politics*, referred to as *zoe*—brute, bestial, or bare life, the unconscious, unreflective mere life of the species?[23] Thomas Aquinas would later translate these ancient Greek concepts into medieval Christian terms that distinguished the natural life from the good life.[24]

But neither Aristotle nor Aquinas is with us. Instead, medical practitioners consult and take counsel from the new specialists in bioethics, a field finely calibrated to meet the needs of advanced biomedical biotechnologies. Even as conservative a scholar as Francis Fukuyama refers to the "community of bio-ethicists" as having "grown up in tandem with the biotech industry . . ." and are at times nothing more than sophisticated (and sophistic) justifiers of whatever it is the scientific community wants to do."[25]

The field of bioethics has to date offered little resistance to the growth of markets in humans and body parts. Many bioethicists now argue that the real problems are outdated laws, irrelevant regulatory agencies (such as UNOS), and archaic norms that are out of touch with social and economic realities. They point to the "quiet revolution" of those who have refused to face premature death with equanimity and "dignity" while waiting for a cadaver organ.[26] Some argue for a free trade in human organs; others, like the philosopher Janet Radcliffe-Richards, argue for a regulated market. In the meantime, the rupture between practice and the law can be summarized as follows: while commerce in human organs is illegal according to the official legal codes of virtually all nations where transplant is practiced, nowhere are the renegade surgeons (who are well known to their professional colleagues), organs brokers, and kidney buyers (or sellers) pursued by the law, let alone prosecuted. It is easy to understand why kidney buyers and sellers would not be the focus of prosecution under the law. Compassion rather than outrage is the more appropriate response to their acts. But the failure on the part of governments, ministries of health, and law enforcement agencies to interrupt the activities of international transplant outlaws and their holding companies, money-laundering operations, and Mafia connections can only be explained as an *intentional* oversight.

Indeed, some of the most notorious outlaw transplant surgeons are the medical directors of major transplant units who serve on prestigious international medical committees and on ethics panels. None have been censured by their own profession, though a few have been investigated, and some live in self-imposed social isolation. But all practice their illicit surgeries freely, though some move their bases of international operations frequently so as to avoid medical or police surveillance. One of transplant medicine's most notorious outlaws, Dr. Zaki Shapira, who recently retired from Bellinson Medical Center near Tel Aviv, served on the prestigious international "Bellagio Task Force" investigating the global traffic in organs, of which I was also a member.[27] In one of his subsequent trips to Italy, he was the recipient of a prestigious human service award. Meanwhile, one of Dr. Shapira's "transplant tour" patients from Jerusalem provided me with copies of his medical and financial records that led to a fraudulent medical society in Bergamo, Italy, to whom the patient had sent the $180,000 that his illicit transplant (in Turkey) had cost.

The impunity of these transplant outlaws concerns more than government lassitude and obvious professional corruption. Outlaw surgeons are also protected by the charisma that accompanies their seemingly miraculous powers over life, death, and adverse circumstances. As much as his younger colleagues worry about Dr. Shapira's questionable ethics, they praise his surgical technique and his "golden hands." The head of the Turkish medical ethics committee lamented that Dr. Yusef Somnez, the "Doctor Vulture" of Istanbul fame, was one of Turkey's most celebrated transplant surgeons. "Somnez is the man who put transplant on the map in Turkey," he said.[28]

Some transplant surgeons moreover see themselves as "above the law," a tradition they inherited from the early days of transplant, when the "founding fathers," such as Christiaan Barnard in South Africa and Thomas Starzl in the United States, battled against prevailing social norms and those who resisted transplant's redefinition of death to allow the removal of "fresh" organs to transplant from neo-morts or quasi-morts. That same sense of embattlement continues today among transplant surgeons who may publicly support international regulations against buying and selling organs but who privately say that this is the *only solution* to organ scarcities. In the face of illicit transplants involving paid donors, many surgeons simply look the other way. Others actively facilitate sales, while others counsel kidney patients for transplant trips overseas and care for them on their return from a trip to South America, South Africa, or China, where organs are purchased from the living or (as in the case of China) taken from an executed prisoner.

In the rational choice language of contemporary medical ethics, the conflict between nonmalfeasance ("do no harm") and beneficence (the moral duty to perform good acts) is resolved in favor of the market and consumer-oriented principle that those able to broker or buy a human organ should be allowed to do so. Paying for a kidney "donation" is viewed as a potential "win-win" situation that can benefit both parties.[29] Individual decision-making and patient autonomy have become the final arbiters of medical and bioethical values. Social justice and notions of the "good society" hardly figure at all in these discussions. In the post-humanist context, the idea of virtue in suffering and grace in dying can only appear as patently absurd. But the transformation of a person into a "life" that must be prolonged or saved at any cost has made life into the ultimate commodity fetish. A belief in the absolute value of a single human life saved or prolonged at any cost ends all ethical inquiry and erases any possibility of a global social ethic. And the traffic in kidneys reduces the human content of all the lives it touches.

MEDICINE AND THE MAFIA

Illicit transplant transactions are obviously complex and require expert teamwork among technicians in blood and tissue laboratories, dual surgical teams working in tandem, nephrologists, and postoperative nurses. Travel, passports, and visas must be arranged. These awesome organizational requirements are arranged in many parts of the world by a new class of organs brokers, ranging from sophisticated businessmen, medical insurance agents, and travel agents to criminal networks of armed and dangerous Mafia to the local "kidney hunters" of Istanbul, Bangong Lupa, and Mingir. In Israel and the United States, religious organizations, charitable trusts, and patient advocacy organizations sometimes harbor organs brokers. I have identified a large network operating between Israel and several cities in the United States on both coasts. Some have recruited organ donors locally, while others have recruited Russian and Moldovan immigrants, ex-prisoners, and other marginalized people who have been smuggled into the United States as tourists.

The outlaw surgeons who practice their illicit operations in rented, makeshift clinics or, just as often, in operating rooms of some of the best public or private medical centers in the city do so under the frank gaze of local and national governments, ministries of health, regulatory agencies, and professional medical associations. In short, the illegal practice of transplant tourism, which relies on an extensive network of body brokers and human traffickers, is a public secret, one that involves some of the world's most prestigious hospitals and medical centers. Transplant crimes—even when they explode into gunfire and leave a trail of blood—go officially undetected and unpunished. Even the most aggressive surgeons can find themselves trapped and more deeply involved in "the business" than they had ever anticipated.

But in addition to organized crime, the organs business is also not infrequently protected by military and state interests, particularly during periods of political conflict and war. A footnote to the story of military terrorism during (and following) the "Dirty War" in Argentina and the dictatorship years in Brazil is that doctors there provided—in the case of Argentina—not only children for military families but also blood, bones, heart valves, organs, and tissues for transplant. These parts are taken from the bodies of the politically "disappeared" and from the socially disappeared, including the captive populations such as the mentally retarded in state institutions, such as the infamous Montes de Oca and Open Door asylums in Lujan, Bsás province. There are indications that the organs trafficking business in Eastern Europe began amid the chaos and dehumanization of the death camps during the genocides in the former Yugoslavia.

Israel is a major player in the global market for organs, a market that began in the West Bank and moved to nearby Arab countries. Israeli citizens purchase, proportionally, the largest number of organs per capita in the world. Caught between a highly educated and medically conscious public and a very low rate of organ donation, the Israeli Ministry of Health has expedited the expansion of transplant tourism by allowing Israeli patients to use their national insurance to pay for transplants conducted elsewhere, even if illegally. The cost of the transplant "package" increased from $120,000 in 1998 to $200,000 in 2001. The cost includes the air travel, the bribes to airport and customs officials, the "double operation" (kidney extraction and kidney transplant), the rental of operating and recovery rooms, and the hotel accommodation for accompanying family members. The donor fee of between $3,000 and $15,000 (depending on the status of the donor) is also included.

Shady business men and their medical associates have formed "corporations" with ties to illicit medical centers and rogue transplant units (public and private) in Turkey, Russia, Moldova, Estonia, Georgia, Romania, Brazil, South Africa, and the United States. The specific sites of the illicit surgeries are normally kept secret from transplant patients until the day of travel. And the locations are continually rotated to maintain a low profile. The surgeries are performed at night in rented operating rooms. In one organized plan, Israeli patients and doctors (a surgeon and a nephrologist) flew to a hospital in a town on the Turkish-Iraqi border for illegal transplants with kidneys procured from Iraqi soldiers and guest workers. In another plan, Israeli and Turkish doctors and their patients traveled to Estonia for transplants using unemployed workers from elsewhere in Eastern Europe.

In a third scenario, kidney sellers were recruited from the slums and favelas of Recife, Northeast Brazil (by brokers including a military police officer), and sent by plane to Durban and Johannesburg in South Africa, where they were met by South African brokers who "matched" up these unfortunates with Israeli patients arriving from Tel Aviv. In this instance, South African surgeons operated independently, without Israeli surgeon accomplices.

The participation of South Africa's largest health maintenance organization (HMO), Netcare, and Israel's national insurance programs in the illegal multimillion-dollar transplant tourism business, which has made Israel into something of a pariah in the international transplant world, and also sullied South Africa's "grand" tradition of transplant medicine, requires some explanation. In Israel, the absence of a strong culture of organ donation, an inadequate national system of cadaver organs "capture," and the pressure exerted by angry transplant candidates have contributed to a belief (in Ministry of Health circles) that each patient transplanted abroad is one less angry and demanding client at home. More troubling, however, is the involvement of Ministry of Defense personnel who sometimes "accompany" transplant tourists abroad. To date, roughly half of all kidney transplant patients in Israel were transplanted abroad via illicitly arranged transplant tours. The corruption of South Africa's private hospitals, surgeons, and HMOs is the result of the collapse of public support for transplant surgery, previously provided under the apartheid regime for white South Africans. The channeling of public funds for primary health care has inadvertently resulted in a rampant privatization and commercialization of tertiary medical care, including transplant surgery. Indeed, if transplants are to happen at all in South Africa today, they must be paid for by private insurance. This paved the way for the flowering of illicit transplant tourism. Do we need to explain why Northeast Brazil was an ideal location for the recruitment of desperate and hungry kidney sellers? Despite President Lula's "Zero Hunger" program, hunger and other raw needs are commonplace there, making young, strong, Afro-Brazilian men, in particular, appealing candidates for kidney forfeit.

BEYOND BIOETHICS—REGULATING THE
BLACK MARKET IN ORGANS

If a living donor can do without an organ, why shouldn't the donor profit and medical science benefit?—Janet Ratcliffe-Richards, The Lancet, 1998

The Santillan case provoked a powerful chauvinistic anti-immigration reaction. Rather than grieve the unfortunate and "accidental" death of Jesica, the public response was dominated by a perverse national sentiment that cast Jesica as a "winner" of an ill-fated organ that was denied to an American who thereby "lost" their shot at a new life. In the wake of Jesica's second bungled transplant, calls for reexamining the rules and for better enforcement emerged. Some political leaders like Senate Majority Leader and transplant surgeon Bill Frist (R-Tenn.) have proposed legislation aimed at increasing organ donation rates by invoking market-oriented strategies including travel and subsistence reimbursements for living donors. This legislation opens the door for paying people to travel and donate their organs to strangers.

From the exclusively market-oriented "supply and demand" perspective that is gaining ground among transplant specialists and bioethicists today, the buying and selling of kidneys is viewed as a potential solution to the global scarcity in organs and as a "win-win" situation that benefits both parties. In viewing the solution this way, however, the human and ethical dilemmas are reduced to a simple problem in management. The problems with this rational solution are many. The arguments for "regulation" are out of touch with the social and medical realities operating in many parts of the world, but especially in second and third world nations. The medical institutions created to "monitor" organs procurement and distribution are often dysfunctional, corrupt, or compromised by the power of organs markets and the impunity of the organs brokers, and of outlaw surgeons willing to violate the first premise of classical medical bioethics: above all, do no harm.

Philippine secretary of health Manuel Dayrit had two proposals on his desk at the time of my interview with him in February 2002. The first would create a government-regulated kidney bank (to be called KIDNET) that would allow poor people to sell and deposit a kidney into a virtual "organs bank" that would presumably make kidneys available to all Philippine citizens who needed them. Dr. Dayrit was, however, reluctant to discuss just how the Ministry of Health might set a "fair price" for a poor person's kidney, preferring to leave this task to the free market. Dr. C., the director of a large private hospital in Manila, agreed: "Some of our 'donors' are so poor that a sack of rice is sufficient. Others want medical care for their children, and we are quite prepared to provide that for them." The second proposal is a government-sponsored program to grant death row prisoners (most of them killers) a reprieve in exchange for donating a kidney. Their death sentence would then be replaced by life imprisonment. Supporters of this program believe that the donor incentives program could end up convincing society that the death penalty is a terrible waste of a healthy body. "Organ donation is a medical equivalent of Catholic Lenten rites of self-flagellation," Professor Leonardo Castro, of the University of the Philippines, said in defense of the prisoner organ donation incentives program.

For most bioethicists, the "slippery slope" in transplant medicine begins with the emergence of an unregulated market in organs and tissue sales. But for the critical medical anthropologist, the ethical slippery slope occurs the first time one ailing human looks at another living human and realizes that inside that other body is something capable of prolonging or enhancing his or her life. Dialysis and transplant patients are highly visible, and their stories are frequently reported by the media. Their pain and suffering are palpable. But while there is empathy—even a kind of surplus empathy—for transplant patients, there is little empathy for the donors, living and brain dead. Their suffering is hidden from the general public. Few organ recipients know anything about the impact of the transplant procedure on the donor's body. If the medical and psychological risks, pressures, and constraints on organ donors and their families were more generally known, transplant patients might want to consider opting out of procedures that demand so much of the other.

In the absence of any national or international registries of living donors or mandatory reporting laws concerning complications following living donation for the donor/seller, there is really no reliable data on the medical/psychological risks and complications suffered by living organ donors anywhere in the world. In the United States, two kidney donors have died during the past eighteen months and another is in a persistent vegetative state as a result of donation.[30] The fact that many living donors have either died immediately following the surgical procedure or are themselves in dire need of a kidney transplant at a later date sounds a cautionary note about living donation and serves as a reminder that nephrectomy (kidney removal) is not a risk-free procedure.[31]

Bioethical arguments supporting the right to sell an organ are based on Euro-American notions of contract and individual "choice." But the social and economic contexts make the "choice" to sell a kidney in an urban slum of Calcutta or in a Brazilian *favela* or Philippine shantytown anything but a "free" and "autonomous" one. Consent is problematic with "the executioner" —whether on death row or at the door of the slum resident—looking over one's shoulder. Asking the law to negotiate a fair price for a live human kidney goes against everything that contract theory stands for. When concepts such as individual agency and autonomy are invoked in defending the "right" to sell an organ, anthropologists might suggest that certain "living" things are not alienable or proper candidates for commodification.

The problems multiply when the buyers and sellers are unrelated, because the sellers are likely to be extremely poor and trapped in life-threatening environments where the everyday risks to their survival are legion, including exposure to urban violence, transportation- and work-related accidents, and infectious disease that can compromise their kidney of last resort. And when that spare part fails, kidney sellers often have no access to dialysis, let alone to organ transplant. While poor people in particular cannot "do without" their "extra" organs, even affluent people need that "extra" organ as they age, and when one healthier kidney can compensate for a failing or weaker kidney.

Transplant surgeons have disseminated an untested hypothesis of "risk-free" live donation in the absence of *any* published, longitudinal studies of the effects of nephrectomy among the urban poor living anywhere in the world. The few available studies of the effects of neprectomy on kidney sellers in India and Iran are unambiguous.[32] Even under attempts (as in Iran) to regulate and control systems of "compensated gifting" by the Ministry of Health, the outcomes are devastating. Kidney sellers suffer from chronic pain, unemployment, social isolation and stigma, and severe psychological problems. The evidence of strongly negative sentiments—disappointment, anger, resentment, and even seething hatred for the doctors and the recipients of their organs—reported by 100 paid kidney donors in Iran strongly suggests that kidney selling there represents a serious social pathology.

Our research and fieldwork among kidney sellers in Moldova, Brazil, and he Philippines, which included diagnostic exams and sonograms, determined that kidney sellers face many postoperative complications and medical problems, including hypertension and kidney insufficiency, without their having access to adequate medical care or medications. Kidney sellers find themselves weakened, sick, and unemployable because they are unable to sustain the demands of heavy agricultural or construction work, the only labor available to men of their skills. Kidney sellers are often alienated from their families and coworkers, excommunicated from their churches, and excluded from marriage. The children of kidney sellers are ridiculed as "one-kidneys."

Kidney sellers we examined in Moldova had no access to postoperative medical care following their illicit "nephrectomies" (kidney removal) in Turkey, the United States, and Russia. We had to coax young kidney sellers to accept a sonogram at the expense of Organs Watch. Some said they were ashamed to appear in a public clinic, as they had tried to keep the sale a secret. Others said they were afraid of learning negative results from the tests. If medical problems were discovered, they would be unable to pay for necessary treatments or medications. Above all, they feared being labeled as "weak" or "disabled" by their employers and coworkers, or as "inadequate" males by girlfriends and wives. "No young woman in the village will marry a man with the tell-tale scar of a kidney seller," a village elder in Mingir told us. Sergei said that his mother was the only person who knew the reason for the large, saberlike scar on his abdomen. His young wife believed that he had been injured in a construction accident while he was away in Turkey.

IS REGULATION THE ANSWER?

How can a national government set a price on a healthy human being's body part without compromising essential democratic and ethical principles that guarantee the equal value of all human lives? Any national regulatory system would have to compete with global black markets that establish the value of human organs based on consumer-oriented prejudices, such that in today's kidney market Asian kidneys are worth less than Middle Eastern kidneys and American kidneys are worth more than European ones. The circulation of kidneys transcends national borders, and international markets will coexist and compete aggressively with any national, regulated systems. Putting a market price on body parts—even a fair one—exploits the desperation of the poor, turning suffering into an opportunity. And the surgical removal of nonrenewable organs is an act in which medical practitioners, given their ethical standards, should not be asked to participate. Surgeons whose primary responsibility is to provide care should not be advocates of paid self-mutilation, even in the interest of saving lives.

Market-oriented medical ethics creates the semblance of ethical choice (for example, the right to buy a kidney) in an intrinsically unethical context. Bioethical arguments about the right to sell an organ or other body part are based on cherished notions of contract and individual "choice." But consent is problematic when a desperate seller has no other option left but to sell an organ.

The demand side of the organs scarcity problem also needs to be confronted, especially the expansion of waiting lists to include patients who would previously have been rejected. Liver and kidney failure often originate in public health problems that could be treated more aggressively preventively. Ethical solutions to the chronic scarcity of human organs are not always palatable to the public, but they also need to be considered. Foremost among these are systems of educated, informed "presumed consent," in which *all* citizens are assumed to be organs donors at brain death unless they have officially stipulated their refusal beforehand. This practice, which is widespread in parts of Europe, preserves the value of organ transplant as a social good in which no one is included or excluded on the basis of their ability to pay.

DUAL CITIZENSHIP IN THE KINGDOM OF THE SICK

The material needs of my neighbor are my spiritual needs.—Emmanuel Levinas, Nine Talmudic Readings

Situated in the larger global context of transplant tourism, Jesica's family's migration from Mexico to the United States in the quest of what should have been a lifesaving procedure was subject to the same pressures that motivate Americans and Europeans to travel to China, the Philippines, Peru, and South Africa for illicit transplants they cannot easily get at home. Sickness and death are the great social levelers. As Susan Sontag opened her famous broadsheet, "Illness as Metaphor," "Illness is the dark side of life, a more onerous citizenship. Everyone holds dual citizenship in the kingdom of the well and in the kingdom of the sick. Although we all prefer to use only the good passport, sooner or later each of us is obliged, at least for a spell, to identify ourselves as citizens of that other place."[33]

I conclude with a reminder of the radical premise entailed in organs sharing that envisioned a "commons" of the body, with the body as a gift, meaning also a gift to one's self. In the most simple Kantian or Wittgensteinian formulation, the body and its parts are not proper candidates for commodification and sale because they are inalienable from the body-self. The body provides the grounds of certainty for saying that one has a "self" and an existence at all. Humans both *are* and *have* a body. For those who view the body in more collectivist terms as a gift (whether following Judeo-Christian, Buddhist, or animistic religious traditions or following a socialist ethic) the body cannot be sold, while it may be re-gifted and re-circulated in humanist acts of generosity and caritas.

From its origins, transplant surgery presented itself as a complicated problem in gift relations and gift theory, a domain to which sociologists and anthropologists from Marcel Mauss to Levi-Strauss to Pierre Bourdieu have contributed mightily. The spread of new medical technologies and the artificial needs, scarcities, and commodities that they demand have produced new forms of social exchange that breach the conventional dichotomy between gifts and commodities and between kin and strangers. While many individuals have benefited enormously from the ability to get the organs they need, the violence associated with many of these new transactions gives reason to pause. Are we witnessing the development of bio-sociality or the growth of a widespread bio-sociopathy?

The division of the world into organ buyers and organ sellers is a medical, social, and moral tragedy of immense and not yet fully recognized proportions.

NOTES

This essay is drawn from sections of my forthcoming book, *The Ends of the Body: The Global Traffic in Human Organs* (New York: Farrar, Straus & Giroux).

1. On biological citizenship, see Adriana Petryna, *Life Exposed: Biological Citizens after Chernobyl* (Princeton: Princeton University Press, 2002); on sexual citizenship, see Nancy Scheper-Hughes, "AIDS and the Social Body," *Social Science & Medicine* 39 (7) (1994): 991–1003.

2. See Elizabeth Roberts, "Examining Surrogacy Discourses: Between Feminine Power and Exploitation," in *Small Wars: The Cultural Politics of Childhood*, ed. Nancy Scheper-Hughes and Caroline Sargent (Berkeley: University of California Press, 1998), 93–110.

3. See Francis Delmonico, Robert Arnold, Nancy Scheper-Hughes et al., "Ethical Incentives—Not Payment—For Organ Donation," *New England Journal of Medicine* 346 (25) (2002): 2002–5; James Stacey Taylor, *Stakes and Kidneys: Why Markets in Human Body Parts are Morally Imperative* (Burlington, Vt.: Ashgate, 2005); and Mark J. Cherry, *Kidney for Sale by Owner: Human Organs, Transplantation, and the Market* (Washington, D.C.: Georgetown University Press, 2005).

4. While exhortations to altruism and heroic acts are found in all world religions, the emphasis in organ donation on bodily self-sacrifice and charity toward strangers strongly resonates with a Christian ethic. The passion and death of Christ offers a ready divine model of "suffering-for-the-other" and of bodily commitment, explicit in the Last Supper's culminating moment: "This is my Body, Take this and eat. Go and do likewise," which to this day motivates altruistic organ donation among many people. The resonances between transplant ethics and a "sacramental" approach to life fostered an early acceptance of organ transplantation by the Vatican and the Catholic Church, even though it necessitated a redefinition of death—that is, brain death—for purely practical, utilitarian reasons: to facilitate the removal of still lively and animate body parts from dying individuals. This transplant slight- of-hand was accepted with-

out debate within the Vatican, creating an interesting paradox. While the definition of when life begins remains a vexed, even hexed, theological subject, the definition of death was left up to the transplant doctors alone.

5. See Ian Parker, "The Gift," *New Yorker*, August 2, 2004, 54–63.

6. For example, Alan Shewmon, a respected pediatric nephrologist at UCLA, has argued persuasively that on neurological grounds alone, while the brain dead are incontestably and probably irreversibly dying, they are quite simply not yet dead. Margaret Lock, who has exhaustively explored the topic of brain death, refers to the brain dead as "*as good as* dead." Alternatively, I call them the "good enough" dead. But the point is that the brain dead are not dead in the more usual "deader than a door nail" sense of the term.

7. See John Stuart Mill, "Utilitarianism," in *Ethical Theories: A Book of Readings*, ed. A. I. Melden (Englewood Cliffs, N.J.: Prentice-Hall, 1967), 391–434.

8. Jeremy Bentham, "An Introduction to the Principles of Morals and Legislation," in Melden, ed., *Ethical Theories*, 367–90.

9. Michael Friedlaender, "The Right to Sell or Buy a Kidney: Are We Failing Our Patients?" *The Lancet* 359 (March 16, 2002): 971–73.

10. This is a reference to Primo Levi's description, in his book *The Drowned and the Saved*, of the extent to which inmates of the concentration camps would collaborate with the enemy in order to survive.

11. In each of the nine countries where I have conducted field research for Organs Watch, I have been assisted by local researchers, human rights activists, journalists, and younger colleagues and graduate students in medical anthropology, public health, medicine, and the law. Professor Lawrence Cohen, my primary Organs Watch associate, has worked primarily in India and also with local colleagues and medical and graduate students.

12. This project has been a thoroughly collaborative one. Lawrence Cohen and I cofounded Organs Watch in November 1999 as a research, documentation, and medical human rights project. In each of the nine countries in which I have worked, I have collaborated with younger anthropologists, medical students, and law students, as well as with human rights workers, political journalists, and documentary filmmakers.

13. Jagdish Bhagwati, "Deconstructing Rotten Trade," *SAIS Review* 22 (1) (2002): 39–44.

14. Jean Comaroff and John Comaroff, eds., *Millennial Capitalism and the Culture of Neoliberalism* (Durham, N.C.: Duke University Press, 2001).

15. See Saskia Sassen, *The Global City: New York, London, Tokyo* (Princeton: Princeton University Press, 1991).

16. The United Network for Organ Sharing (UNOS) allows 5 percent of organ transplants in U.S. transplant centers to be allotted to foreign patients. However, only those centers reporting more than 15 percent foreign transplant surgery patients are audited.

17. See, for example, the Arabic (as well as Hebrew and Japanese) version of the university's advertisement at <http://www.umm.edu/transplant/arabic.html>.

18. In São Paulo Hospital, Mariana Ferreira and I encountered Dombe, a Suyá Indian from the forest of Mato Grosso who, to our amazement, faced kidney transplant (including two rejection crises) with remarkable equanimity and calm. See Nancy Scheper-Hughes and Mariana Leal Ferreira, "Domba's Spirit Kidney—Transplant Medicine and Suyá Indian Cosmology," in *Disability in Local and Global Worlds*, ed. B. Ingstad and S. Reynolds (Berkeley: University of California Press, in press).

19. See Marina Jimenez and Nancy Scheper-Hughes, "Doctor Vulture—The Unholy Business of Kidney Commerce," part one of a three-part series in *The National Post* (Toronto), March 30, 2002, B1, B4–B5.

20. See Flavio Lobo and Walter Fangaaniello Maierovitch, "*O Mercado dos Desperados*," *CartaCapital*, January 16, 2002, 30–34.

21. Charles Ornstein, "Transplant Unit Said to Have Ignored Priority List," *Boston Globe*, September 28, 2005, <http://www.boston.com/news/nation/articles/2005/09/28/transplant—unit—said—to—have—ignored—priority—list/>.

22. Quoted in Nancy Scheper-Hughes, "Rotten Trade: Millennial Capitalism, Human Values, and Global Justice in Organ Trafficking," *Journal of Human Rights* 2 (June 2003): 197–226.

23. See note 10.

24. Both Giorgio Agamben, *Homo Sacer: Sovereign Power and Bare Life*, trans. Daniel Heller-Roazen (Stanford: Stanford University Press, 1998), 2–3, and Hannah Arendt, *The Human Condition* (Chicago: University of Chicago, 1958), 12–49, treat the translation from ancient Greek to Church Latin in slightly different ways.

25. Francis Fukuyama, *Our Postmodern Future* (New York: Farrar, Straus & Giroux, 2002), 204.

26. "Offering Money for Organ Donation Ethical, HHS Committee Says," AP/ Nando Times, December 3, 2001.

27. See David Rothman et al. "The Bellagio Task Force Report on Global Traffic in Human Organs," *Transplantation Proceedings* 29 (1997): 2739–45.

28. Related to the author during an interview in Istanbul in 2001.

29. See Janet Radcliffe-Richards et al., "The Case for Allowing Kidney Sales," *The Lancet* 352 (1998): 1951.

30. "Man Keeps Vigil for Comatose Wife Who Gave Him Kidney, Life," *The Holland Sentinel*, February 15, 2001.

31. "The Live Donor Consensus Conference," *Journal of the American Medical Association* 2001 (284) (2000): 2919–26.

32. See Madhav Goyal, R. Mehta, L. Schneiderman, and A. Sehgal, "The Economic Consequences of Selling a Kidney in India," *Journal of the American Medical Association* 288 (13) (October 2, 2002): 1589–93; Javaad Zargooshi, "Iranian Kidney Donors: Motivations and Relations with Recipients," *Journal of Urology* 165 (2001): 386–92; and Javaad Zargooshi, "Quality of Life of Iranian Kidney 'Donors,'" *Journal of Urology* 166 (5) (November 2001): 1790–99.

33. Susan Sontag, *Illness as Metaphor* (New York: Farrar, Straus, and Giroux, 1978), 3.

3

CITIZENS AND FOREIGNERS/ ELIGIBILITY AND EXCLUSION

SYMPATHY AND EXCLUSION

ACCESS TO HEALTH CARE FOR

UNDOCUMENTED IMMIGRANTS

IN THE UNITED STATES

BEATRIX HOFFMAN

When the editors approached me about writing this essay, I had already been researching immigrants' access to medical services for my book on the history of the right to health care in the United States. Initially, I expected to show how the Jesica Santillan case fits into that history. It turned out, however, that Jesica's story does not actually fit very neatly. First of all, the Santillan family came to the United States to seek medical care for Jesica; most undocumented immigrants avoid the health care system as much as possible, and very few migrate solely for medical reasons. Second, Jesica's family had the financial means to purchase her transplant because her mother had health insurance through her job, and because a private organization raised thousands of dollars on her behalf. Even though the undocumented are eligible for transplants under United Network for Organ Sharing (UNOS) rules, the only public insurance program that covers indigent immigrants (Emergency Medicaid) specifically excludes organ transplants, and most undocumented workers lack private health insurance.[1] Jesica's case, therefore, was far from typical.

But there was one crucial way in which the Santillan case did typify the history of immigration and health care in America, and this was in its ongoing tension between the impulses of exclusion and generosity. Strict immigration laws prevented Jesica from entering the country legally or receiving a humanitarian parole and forced her family to make the dangerous, expensive, and unlawful journey across the border. National organ transplant rules then made Jesica eligible for a transplant despite her immigration status, but Medicaid rules forbid the government from paying for the transplant. The INS tried to deport the Santillans, but local citizens and even a conservative senator intervened on the family's behalf. Duke University, businessman Mark Mahoney, and the employer of Jesica's mother were praised for their generosity when they helped Jesica get her first transplant but were later castigated by immigration opponents for "wasting" precious medical and financial resources on a noncitizen.

These seemingly contradictory impulses of sympathy and exclusion have historically been embodied in the nation's immigration policy, which has veered between exclusion, quotas, amnesties, guest worker programs, deportations, raids, employer sanctions, and border crackdowns, and sometimes several of these at once.[2] It is perhaps not surprising that attitudes toward health access for the undocumented have reflected the nation's erratic immigration policies. As I outline below, U.S. policies on immigrant health care have been fragmentary, contradictory, or nonexistent. Although the general trend has been to officially exclude undocumented immigrants from every type of health care except emergency care, this history is punctuated with examples of great generosity toward individuals. In this way, the Santillan case *is* reflective of the history of immigrants and health care in America, and indeed of the paradoxes of the American health care system itself.

Access to health care in the United States rests on a basis of categorization and exclusion, of defining who is deserving of and able to receive what services based on income, insurance coverage, past health conditions, and myriad other factors, and the nation is notorious for its growing number of uninsured. At the same time, Americans are proud of the generosity of their health care system, with its long history of charity and voluntarism. Private medical philanthropies, individual giving, the coin box on the convenience store counter raising money for a local child's leukemia treatment, are just as integral a part of the American health system as hospitals, the American Medical Association, and insurance companies. While seemingly paradoxical, these impulses of exclusion and charity together drive the engine of American health care, allowing Americans the comforting notion that "we don't let people die in the streets" even as universal access to care grows increasingly elusive. Similarly, the clashing notions of welcome and exclusion in U.S. immigration policies serve to maintain our economic system, with its cyclical increases and decreases in requirements for immigrant labor and concurrent demands that this labor be bought as cheaply as possible. The apparently baffling contradictions of the Santillan case, then, make it not a historical curiosity but a window onto the complex workings of American immigration and health care policy.

ACCESS AND RIGHTS TO HEALTH CARE BEFORE 1986

The history of undocumented immigrants' access to health care is particularly elusive for several reasons. By definition, the undocumented leave few written records. The term "undocumented" itself is a recent one, and throughout the twentieth century it was often difficult to distinguish "legal" from "illegal" immigrants and migrants to the United States. In the Southwest, for example, all residents of Mexican descent were referred to as "Mexican," including those who had been in the United States for generations.[3] This led to great fluidity in border areas; longtime residents might be treated like foreigners in their own land, but Mexican migrants could also be treated like locals. Mutual aid societies, founded throughout the Southwest in the 1870s, intended to serve both immigrants and longtime residents of Mexican descent, and membership in the societies usually included some health care provision. In the mining community of Bisbee, Arizona, the company-owned Copper Queen Hospital treated numerous workers with Spanish surnames; its records from the 1910s did not distinguish between citizens and non-citizens.[4] At the same time, when access was restricted, the restrictions applied to longtime "legal" residents and recent arrivals alike. While some county and private hospitals in the Southwest and California seem to have treated both Mexican and Anglo patients, other health facilities were strictly segregated by national origin. In Los Angeles in the 1920s, for example, separate public health clinics were established for "Americans" and "Mexicans," the latter ones intended to serve both U.S. citizens and Mexican nationals.[5]

Migrant farmworkers, undocumented or not, historically have endured the poorest health conditions and the least access to health care of all socioeconomic groups in the United States. However, because of their importance to the agricultural economy and the fact that they by definition crossed state boundaries, their health problems have received the attention of the federal government. The Migrant Health Act of 1962 originated in concerns about migrants' supposed propensity to contagious disease. Mexican workers entering the country to work in the bracero and other contract labor programs were required to pass through Public Health Service stations at the border, where they were "dusted with an insecticide, vaccinated, examined for evidence of venereal disease, given a . . . chest X-ray, and examined for any other condition which would make the laborer inadmissible or unfit for agricultural work."[6] Once workers had passed through the stations, the government turned over responsibility for their health to employers. Reliance on employer voluntarism predictably proved ineffective, and by the early 1960s health conditions among migrant laborers had become a national scandal.

Congressional sponsors of the Migrant Health Act of 1962, which provided federal grants to local health providers willing to care for migrant workers, argued that the legislation was intended to protect American citizens from contagious disease, sustain the agricultural labor force, and even to fight the Cold War. "[Q]uite apart from humanitarian considerations," the act would "help assure in the national interest the continued availability of an essential labor supply." One New York congressman told a committee hearing that "the plight of the migrant worker is foreign to our American institutions. This long-festering sore in our society and our economy provides a propaganda weapon for those who oppose our traditions and ideals." Arguments about national interest and labor demands, rather than the health needs or rights of the migrants themselves, helped the Migrant Health Act pass in 1962.[7] Currently, over 100 migrant health centers receive federal funding, but advocates estimate that only 10 to 15 percent of migrants ever use the services. Undocumented workers fearing deportation are reluctant to attend these clinics, and, due to low literacy levels, many are not even aware of the clinics' existence, which are advertised primarily through pamphlet literature.[8]

Sometimes, undocumented workers in need of medical help turned to local indigent care services. Medical care for the poor in the United States was traditionally a county responsibility that in the twentieth century became guaranteed by state statutes. County and municipal health systems were required to provide care to local indigent residents; the statutes made no reference to citizenship requirements, and most public hospitals and county welfare programs did not inquire into immigration status. In general, communities with public hospitals (such as Los Angeles and Chicago) seemed to offer greater access than those who relied on private practitioners and institutions to provide indigent care (such as in most rural areas). Local taxpayers occasionally objected to the use of county funds to pay for immigrants' health care. In 1940, an anti-immigrant Mexican American newspaper complained about "county charities" that "provide aliens and their families food, clothing, shelter, and medical care without work." In 1980, a taxpayers' group sued L.A. County to "stop the expenditure of public funds to pay for non-emergency health care for undocumented persons," but lawyers argued successfully that the state of California required counties to "provide health services to *all* indigent residents," including the undocumented.[9]

But basing access on local residency was a double-edged sword for migrants and immigrants. Local indigent care facilities had strict requirements for proving residency, usually demanding not only a local address but also utility bills, employment verification, and other documents. Such requirements likely prevented many undocumented immigrants from ever approaching the local hospital or health center. In some communities, residential requirements were "durational," meaning a patient was required to have resided in the county for at least six months before becoming eligible for indigent medical care. In the absence of a citizenship requirement for indigent care, residency requirements provided a legal basis for hospitals and other county and public health facilities to deny care to recent immigrants, or to deny reimbursement to providers willing to treat them.

In 1971, a Mexican-born migrant worker launched the first successful constitutional challenge to residency requirements for medical care. Henry Evaro, a legal resident of Arizona, traveled to Phoenix to find work as a welder. He had been there less than a month when he had a severe asthma attack and went to the emergency room of the private Memorial Hospital. Evaro was so sick that he needed admission as an inpatient; Memorial called Maricopa County Hospital and asked them to take him, since he was indigent. The county hospital refused because Evaro had not resided in the county for at least a year, as required by Arizona State statute. The welder remained at Memorial for eleven days, and the hospital sued the county to pay for Evaro's care. On February 26, 1974, the U.S. Supreme Court ruled in *Memorial Hospital v. Maricopa* that durational residency requirements for medical care were an unconstitutional violation of the equal protection clause of the Fourteenth Amendment since they "impinged on the right of interstate travel by denying newcomers basic necessities of life."[10]

It was not *Memorial*, however, but another Arizona case the following year that would firmly establish a legal right to emergency care for the undocumented. On February 10, 1972, two young children at home in the border town of Naco, Sonora, Mexico, were severely burned when a stove exploded in their kitchen. Relatives rushed the children across the border to the nearest hospital, Phelps Dodge Company's Copper Queen Hospital in Bisbee, Arizona, but a nurse refused to even allow them into the emergency room. Instead, she glanced at the burned children crying in the back seat of the car and told the driver to take them to the county hospital in Douglas, Arizona, eighteen miles away. The boy and girl both survived, but their parents sued Copper Queen, alleging that the hospital's refusal of care had aggravated the children's injuries and prolonged their convalescence. When the case reached the Arizona Supreme Court, the resulting decision, *Guerrero v. Copper Queen*, stated that "nonresident aliens" could not be excluded from hospitals' duty to provide emergency care. The justices based their decision rather narrowly on the existing Arizona State statute regarding private hospitals' requirements to provide emergency care, which did not exclude noncitizens. Until state legislators chose to make an exception in the case of immigrants, the *Guerrero* decision concluded, hospitals would be required to treat all emergency cases.[11] The *Guerrero* decision is still cited today as a major precedent for the federal, universal right to emergency care in the United States.

The *Memorial* and *Guerrero* decisions laid the groundwork for a legal basis for immigrants' right to health care. However, they also coincided with a growing backlash against immigration. In the severe economic downturn of the 1970s, politicians and some of the public blamed immigrants for taking American jobs and burdening the welfare state. The 1965 amendments to the Immigration and Nationality Act drastically reduced the number of Mexicans eligible for legal residency, forcing many more immigrants to enter illegally; between 1968 and 1976, the number of annual deportations of undocumented Mexicans increased from 151,000 to 781,000.[12] When Congress added the Supplemental Security Income program to Social Security in 1972, it explicitly denied coverage to undocumented immigrants. Then, in 1973, the U.S. secretary of health, education, and welfare issued a regulation denying Medicaid eligibility to any alien who was not a permanent resident or "otherwise permanently residing in the United States under color of law."[13] For the first time, undocumented immigrants were specifically excluded from Medicaid.

THE BACKLASH: IRCA AND WELFARE REFORM

The Immigration Reform and Control Act of 1986 (IRCA) further restricted immigrants' access to health care. The law excluded some categories of *legal* immigrants from Medicaid during their first five years in the country, and new sanctions against employers undoubtedly made it harder for the undocumented to get jobs that might provide health insurance. That same year Congress amended the federal Medicaid statute to bar aid to undocumented immigrants for "any condition short of a medical emergency," thereby creating the program known as Emergency Medicaid. Emergency Medicaid continued the nation's trajectory of setting apart emergency care for special coverage.[14] The program is extremely restrictive, excluding single adults over eighteen and childless couples under sixty-five, and covers nothing outside of acute care in the hospital for sudden-onset conditions.[15] As mentioned before, Emergency Medicaid does not cover organ transplants.

In the early 1990s, some states continued to provide undocumented immigrants with nonemergency services such as prenatal care and immunizations. Politicians sought to remove the supposed "immigration incentive" of such care through measures like California's Proposition 187, which attempted to bar undocumented immigrants from using nonemergency health services. The Personal Responsibility and Work Opportunity Reconciliation Act (PRWORA), the 1996 "Welfare Reform" passed by a Republican Congress and signed into law by President Clinton, dramatically cut back on immigrants' (including legal immigrants) access to health care and welfare programs. PRWORA declared all state aid to the undocumented illegal unless states chose to pass new enabling legislation. Some states attempted to continue offering care, but others took the opportunity provided by PRWORA to eliminate most health services to the undocumented. In 1996, for example, California governor Pete Wilson ordered state employees to stop giving prenatal care to undocumented women, and in 2003 a Texas district attorney began a criminal investigation of local hospitals that offered such care.[16] Both of these actions were successfully challenged by health care providers and advocates for immigrants, as was Proposition 187.

State attempts to either end or provide nonemergency care continue to be mired in legal challenges and confusion, and Emergency Medicaid remains the only federal health program officially available to undocumented immigrants. Unofficially, many locally funded health clinics offer some nonemergency care for immigrants. At Alivio Medical Center in Chicago, for example, which provides $1 million a year in uncompensated care, more than half of the patients are undocumented.[17] School-based clinics are an important source of care for children of undocumented parents. This contradictory and patchwork system of care—official policies of exclusion and cutbacks coupled with tolerance of provision at the local level—reflects the nation's inability to come to terms with the realities of immigration and the health needs of undocumented workers.

IMMIGRATION AND HEALTH CARE IN NORTH CAROLINA

Until Jesica Santillan's case, most of the debate and legislative activity around immigrants' access to health care took place in areas of the country with traditionally large Spanish-speaking immigrant and migrant populations: the Southwest, California, and New York State. Jesica's story highlights one of the major shifts in immigration patterns in the last decade. Fewer Mexican nationals are heading for the heavily immigrant neighborhoods of the urban West and Southwest; their destinations increasingly are small, rural towns in the Midwest and Southeast. In North Carolina, the immigrant population increased by 72 percent between 2000 and 2004.[18] According to a federal estimate, the state currently has 206,000 undocumented residents.[19] As a heavily agricultural state, North Carolina has long been dependent on migrant labor, but the composition of the migrant workforce has shifted dramatically in the past twenty years, from primarily African American to primarily Mexican.[20]

Immigrants to North Carolina face extreme difficulty in obtaining health care. In 2003, 69 percent of Hispanics in North Carolina whose primary language was Spanish had no health insurance. In comparison, 32 percent of English-speaking Hispanics, 19 percent of African Americans, and 13 percent of whites in North Carolina lacked health coverage.[21] Immigrants lack health insurance primarily because they are concentrated in job sectors that do not provide health coverage, such as agriculture, and in jobs with wages insufficient to purchase health insurance or health services.

Although the private Duke Endowment was renowned for its health care philanthropy in the state, at the time of the Santillans' arrival the Duke University Medical Center was not actually the top provider of charity care in central North Carolina. That distinction went to WakeMed, a community hospital in Raleigh, and the University of North Carolina hospitals.[22] While Duke was not known primarily for its indigent care or its care for immigrants or migrants, its transplant capabilities were world famous. It was also one of the few hospitals in the country providing heart-lung transplants for children. This is what Jesica and her family had heard about Duke in Mexico.

A RIGHT TO ORGAN TRANSPLANTS?

At the time of Jesica's arrival, the UNOS policy of allowing (or limiting) 5 percent of organs to go to noncitizens had been in place for over a decade. The 5 percent policy originated in the mid-1980s, when public outrage was sparked by media coverage of wealthy foreigners, including members of the Saudi royal family, traveling to the United States to receive transplants. At one Pittsburgh transplant center, for example, 28 percent of donated kidneys went to wealthy foreigners between 1984 and 1985.[23] UNOS was urged by some to ban transplants to noncitizens altogether, but experts argued that immigrants were an important source of organ donations (see Eric Meslin's essay in this volume for more discussion of this argument, and see Jed Adam Gross's essay for more on the Pittsburgh case). The UNOS guidelines refer only to non-citizens and do not explicitly mention undocumented immigrants.

Following the Santillan case, letters to newspaper editors nationwide railed at the unfairness of scarce organs going to someone who had deliberately violated U.S. laws by entering illegally, but others pointed out that undocumented immigrants actually donate *more* than the 5 percent of organs they are entitled to receive.[24] "In North Carolina, Latino families are among the most likely groups to say yes to donating a family member's organs," reported the Raleigh *News and Observer*. "Latino consent rates ran about 78 percent during the first six months of [2002], compared with 62 percent for other groups."[25]

Not only do immigrants donate more organs than they are entitled to receive, they actually end up receiving far fewer than the 5 percent designated by UNOS. Only slightly over 1 percent of organs actually to go undocumented immigrants annually.[26] Transplant centers are not required to provide organs to noncitizens and many refuse to do so. A Raleigh newspaper found at least two cases of undocumented immigrants who died after being refused transplants at U.S. hospitals.[27] Children's Memorial Hospital in Chicago underwent a storm of negative publicity when it refused a liver transplant to eleven-year-old Ana Esparza in 2001. Ana, who was near death, finally underwent the transplant at a Florida hospital, and Children's agreed to pay for her follow-up care and also offered transplants to two other undocumented children.[28] As for Duke, it was far from being a center of transplantation for the undocumented. According to UNOS data, "Of 2,541 people who received transplants at Duke from Jan. 1, 1988, to Nov. 30, 2002, there were no 'nonresident aliens' recorded, although eight people did not specify their citizenship status."[29] The UNOS 5 percent marker, then, clearly has not established a guaranteed right to organ transplants for noncitizens. And Emergency Medicaid's denial of reimbursement to hospitals performing such transplants made immigrants' access to organs even more elusive (this was the reason given by Children's Memorial for refusing Ana Esparza's transplant).

When Jesica Santillan arrived in North Carolina, then, she was ostensibly eligible for an organ transplant, and Duke did indeed put her on the waiting list for a heart and lungs. However, Duke wanted to be paid, and as an undocumented immigrant Jesica had no right to government assistance and Duke had no right to government reimbursement for her care. But because of her unique situation as a young female with a devastating illness, Jesica was able to tap into two other funding mechanisms for her care: employer health insurance and private charity. Jesica's plight led to widespread sympathy for her family among locals in their town of Louisburg, sympathy that helped Jesica's mother find a job with health insurance and led businessman Mack Mahoney to begin aggressive fund-raising on her behalf. Had Jesica relied only on official governmental and organ network policies, she would likely not have received a transplant. Instead, like many Americans (especially children) who cannot afford catastrophic medical expenses, she ended up relying on the charitable impulses of private citizens.

THE POLITICS OF CHARITY AND SYMPATHY

Jesica's second transplant and her subsequent death led to extensive discussions in the media about immigrants' "deservingness" of organ transplants and of U.S. health care in general. As Leo Chavez shows in his essay in this book, immigration opponents capitalized on Jesica's tragedy to demand further restrictions on immigration and on health services for the undocumented. The Santillan case and its aftermath, however, also elicited extensive public and media sympathy for Jesica and her family. The Santillan tragedy led to powerful outpourings of both compassion and anti-immigrant invective, highlighting Americans' continuing confusion, unease, and ambivalence about the country's immigration policies and its health care system.

As Eric Meslin points out, there is widespread acceptance of the "idea that charity and humanitarianism are necessary features of the U.S. health care system that result from inequities generally." The Santillans themselves were aware of this. Jesica's family came to the United States not to seek Medicaid but because they had heard about the Children's Miracle Network, a private charity that helped pay for children's organ transplants at major hospitals, including Duke.[30]

It was not this national charitable network, however, that enabled Jesica to receive a transplant. Rather, the Santillans ended up relying on a particularly southern tradition of local benevolence. The family settled in Louisburg, North Carolina, and Jesica was accepted onto the transplant waiting list at Duke, with the knowledge that a heart-lung transplant would cost around $500,000, not including follow-up care. When Louisburg home developer Mack Mahoney read Jesica's story in the local paper, he decided he had to help. Mahoney created a private charity, "Jesica's Hope Chest," solely to raise money for the transplant. When traditional fund-raising efforts fell short, Mahoney enlisted building suppliers and contractors to donate materials and labor to build houses that then would be sold and the proceeds donated to Jesica's cause. According to Mahoney, "Soon, the whole community was involved in the effort. Individuals, local business groups, churches and many civic organizations were working to raise money for the first 'Jesica's House.' "[31] Mahoney also helped Jesica's mother find a job at the local college—a janitorial position that, amazingly, included health insurance coverage.

Jesica's case appealed not only to Mahoney and other local supporters but even to North Carolina senator Jesse Helms, no supporter of immigration, who "reportedly interceded on [Jesica's] family's behalf when INS officials considered deporting them."[32] Such a remarkable outpouring of support seemed to be the polar opposite of the anti-immigrant reactions to Jesica's case that later emerged. This might be understood, then, as a story of American acceptance of immigrants and of Jesica's right to medical citizenship. But the public support for Jesica was based not on her immigration status but on other factors that made it possible for her supporters to ignore or downplay that status. These factors were Jesica's youth, her gender, and the severity of her medical condition (and probably her beauty as well). Mahoney repeatedly referred to Jesica as a "little girl," a "baby girl," and "my baby." Mahoney himself had lost a baby years earlier, making these pronouncements about a seventeen-year-old a bit more understandable.[33] Mahoney also seemed to play the role of the southern patriarch whose benevolence was rooted in paternalism (a paternalism that emerged quite harshly as a desire to control Jesica in the Mahoney interview cited by Carolyn Rouse in her essay in this volume).[34]

Sympathy for children plays an important role in America's welfare state and private charity systems. Government programs are more popular when they are aimed at children rather than able-bodied adults; such programs as Head Start and, more recently, the State Children's Health Insurance Programs expansion of Medicaid, and children's charities (particularly medical charities) are extremely well funded and generate much publicity. And not only was Jesica a young female whose teenage dreams could be embodied by a "Hope Chest"; she was placed in an even more vulnerable condition by the nature of her illness, which would shortly kill her if she did not receive the transplant. As an increasingly familiar member of the local community, Jesica was an "identified life" of the type discussed in Nancy King's essay in this book, a known individual who elicited public sympathy even as the broader social problems she embodied (immigration, the high cost of health care, organ shortages) went unaddressed.

Jesica's age, gender, and medical condition added up to a state of "innocence" that trumped her illegal status. It is difficult to imagine such an outpouring of public support on behalf of, for example, a forty-five-year-old undocumented Mexican male farm laborer in need of a liver transplant (especially if the liver disease were due to excessive drinking). The confluence of factors in Jesica's favor made her unusually well positioned to attract charitable support—support that was significant enough (alongside her mother's insurance) to convince Duke to go ahead with the transplant.

AFTERMATH: BACKLASH RHETORIC VERSUS POLICY REALITY

Although her local supporters never wavered, much of the broader public sympathy for Jesica seemed to evaporate after she received the second transplant, and media coverage became increasingly critical. As Leo Chavez's essay details, the Santillan case quickly became a flashpoint for anti-immigrant sentiment. John A. Mulhall of upstate New York wrote in a newspaper editorial, "Why were Jesica Santillan and her mother, illegal aliens from Mexico who knowingly broke our laws, even at Duke University and not in an INS holding cell?"[35] Feelings against Jesica and her family reflected anxiety not only about unchecked immigration but also about the scarcity of organs and high medical costs. Sixty-five-year-old Jackie Mills of Raleigh, North Carolina, told a reporter, "I definitely would not want [my organs] to go to an illegal alien. I don't think they should be able to come in here and take our hospital and take our medicine and turn around and sue us."[36]

The image of illegal immigrants using up precious health care resources came to a head in the aftermath of the Santillan case, but such arguments were not new. Since the 1970s, hospitals in U.S.-Mexico border areas had claimed that immigrants were "swamping" emergency rooms and "flooding" local health facilities, and they used these images to argue for increased federal funding to hospitals.[37] In 2003, shortly after Jesica's death, the Bush administration finally agreed to include $1 billion for uncompensated emergency care for undocumented immigrants in its Medicare Modernization Act.[38]

The new legislation infuriated immigration opponents who saw it as a subsidy for illegal immigrants. California congressman Dana Rohrabacher introduced a bill requiring hospitals accepting the funds to report undocumented patients to the Department of Homeland Security, which would then begin deportation proceedings. Rohrabacher used the Santillan case to argue that immigrants were depleting crucial health care resources that should be reserved for U.S. citizens. "We all remember Jesica Santillan, said Rohrabacher. "She was an illegal alien who died after receiving not one, but two, heart and lung transplants in North Carolina. . . . There are American citizens who desperately need organs, and they are being knocked out of line by a family who broke the law to come here. . . . If we cannot provide medical care for our senior citizens, we cannot provide them medicines, how is it that we can provide $1 billion to treat illegal immigrants. . . ? My bill . . . is meant to deal with this travesty. If passed, it will signal to the leadership that the American people no longer will stand for this type of providing services for illegal immigrants."[39]

Despite strong anti-immigrant sentiment in his home state, Rohrabacher's in the measure in the U.S. House of Representatives was defeated in May 2004 by a vote of 331 to 88. One year later, on May 9, 2005, the Centers for Medicare and Medicaid Services announced that hospitals would not be required to ask patients about their immigration status in order to be eligible for the new federal funds. Instead, reimbursements to hospitals would be based on statistical estimates of state and local undocumented populations. For each of the next four years $4.9 million from this fund has been allocated to North Carolina.[40]

In this case, at least, anti-immigration rhetoric failed in the face of other forces: the power of the hospital lobby, which used immigrants' medical needs to tap into a new source of funding; pressure from medical practitioners and immigrants' rights groups, who argued that demanding to know patients' immigration status would discourage seriously ill people from seeking care; and finally, acknowledgment of the reality that the population of undocumented immigrants is large and growing and that ignoring their health needs is not in the nation's best interest.

Jesica Santillan's tragedy both highlighted and obscured central themes in U.S. immigration and health care. Most significantly, her case reflected the historical ambivalence and contradictions of U.S. attitudes and policy toward immigrants. Jesica and her family experienced the clash between generosity (employer benefits, private charity, a policy allowing immigrants to receive organ transplants) and exclusion (a dangerous border crossing, threats of deportation, Medicaid limitations). In the media and in public opinion, Jesica was portrayed as both a deserving innocent and a callous lawbreaker—the "angel" versus "thieving immigrant" dichotomy analyzed by Susan Morgan et al. in this volume's opening essay. Her case represented the continuing irrationality of the U.S. health care system, in which spectacular technology and expensive medical miracles flourish alongside the denial of basic health coverage and services to millions. It is notable that while health care "rationing" is supposedly anathema to Americans, during the Santillan case rationing was discussed explicitly and openly. The case lay at the intersection of two areas—organ transplantation and immigrant health access—where shortages and scarcity are endemic and are explicitly acknowledged. In discussions of Jesica Santillan, Americans were able to express—sometimes openly, sometimes in more coded terms—their own anxieties about scarcity and rationing in health care.

In other, significant ways, Jesica's story was highly untypical and thus obscures as much as it reveals. It is extremely rare, for example, for undocumented immigrants to get employer health insurance, to have local Anglos create a charity on their behalf, or to receive an organ transplant. It is also very rare for Mexicans to enter the United States solely to seek medical care. Perhaps the most important way that the Santillan case obscures the typical immigrant experience is that it focused the debate around a highly unrepresentative case of medical immigration (see the cartoon in Leo Chavez's essay showing immigrants coming for "free health care"). In doing so, it distracted from the major reasons people come to the United States: poverty in their home country and unceasing demand for their labor in this country.

These realities were vividly depicted in a news article that appeared shortly after Jesica's death. Alfredo Corchado, a reporter for the *Dallas Morning News*, traveled to the Santillan's home village of Arroyo Hondo in Jalisco, Mexico. Corchado found that Jesica's was only one of many desperate journeys that the villagers of Arroyo Hondo had taken over the northern border. Jesica's great-uncle, Bernardo Torres, had been a farmworker in the United States in the 1940s, when the U.S. government created the bracero guest worker program to meet a severe shortage of labor in the Southwest. After Torres returned to Mexico, over the next decades he saw more than one of his fellow villagers depart for the United States, only to come back in coffins—"people who died at the hands of smugglers, fell victim to the heat and brutality of the deserts or drowned in the Rio Grande." Jesica Santillan was in many ways an untypical immigrant, but her determination, her desperation, and her sad end made her not so different from many others who seek work and dignity in the United States. " 'Sometimes we search for a better life, only to find death,' said Torres, 70, as he quietly sobbed. 'That's life.' "[41]

NOTES

1. Undocumented immigrants actually use less health care (apart from labor and delivery care) than nearly every other group in the population. They fear that using the health care system will require them to disclose their immigration status, that it will

open them up to accusations of being a "public charge" if and when they apply for legal status, and that it will be unaffordable. Undocumented immigrants tend to live in agricultural areas and inner cities, the parts of the country that are most likely to be strapped for health services. Workers' dependence on employers is another factor limiting access to health care; some employers may take workers to a doctor, but many workers are also afraid to tell employers about illness or injury for fear of losing their jobs (or even, as Leo R. Chavez describes in *Shadowed Lives*, of being dumped at the border by the employer.) And undocumented immigrants are, of course, overwhelmingly concentrated in low-wage jobs that do not provide health insurance. See Marc L. Berk, Claudia L. Schur, Leo R. Chavez, and Martin Frankel, "Health Care Use Among Undocumented Latino Immigrants," *Health Affairs*, July/August 2000, 51–64; Leo R. Chavez, "Undocumented Immigrants and Access to Health Services: A Game of Pass the Buck," *Migration Today* 11 (1) (1983): 15–19; Leo R. Chavez, Estevan T. Flores, Marta Lopez-Garza, "Undocumented Latin American Immigrants and U.S. Health Services: An Approach to a Political Economy of Utilization," *Medical Anthropology Quarterly* 6 (1) (March 1992): 6–26; Leo R. Chavez, *Shadowed Lives: Undocumented Immigrants in American Society* (Fort Worth, Tex.: Harcourt Brace Jovanovich College Publishers, 1992), 74–75; and "Increasing Share of U.S. Uninsured are Immigrants," *Wall Street Journal*, June 14, 2005, D6.

2. Mae M. Ngai, *Impossible Subjects: Illegal Aliens and the Making of Modern America* (Princeton, N.J.: Princeton University Press, 2004).

3. David G. Gutierrez, *Walls and Mirrors: Mexican Americans, Mexican Immigrants, and the Politics of Ethnicity* (Berkeley: University of California Press, 1995), 91; Ngai, *Impossible Subjects*, 8.

4. Gutierrez, *Walls and Mirrors*, 75, 96; Admissions Log, Copper Queen Hospital, Cochise County Historical Society, Bisbee, Arizona. On mutual aid societies, see also Jose Amaro Hernandez, *Mutual Aid for Survival: The Case of the Mexican American* (Malabar, Fla.: Robert E. Krieger Publishing Company, 1983).

5. Emily K. Abel, " 'Only the Best Class of Immigration': Public Health Policy toward Mexicans and Filipinos in Los Angeles, 1910–1940," *American Journal of Public Health* 94 (6) (June 2004): 932–39. On the bracero program, see Ngai, *Impossible Subjects*.

6. Norma J. Robinson, "The Public Health Program for Mexican Migrant Workers," *Public Health Reports* 73 (9) (September 1958): 851–60.

7. "Health Clinics for Migratory Farmworkers: Hearing before a Subcommittee of the Committee on Interstate and Foreign Commerce, House of Representatives," February 13, 1962 (U.S. Government Printing Office, 1962), 13.

8. Tina Castañares, M.D., "Outreach Services," *Migrant Health Issues Monograph Series*, No. 5, April 2002, National Center for Farmworker Health, Inc., Texas.

9. Mexican American Movement newspaper quoted in Gutierrez, *Walls and Mirrors*, 137; "Access Upheld for California Undocumented," *Health Advocate: Newsletter of the National Health Law Program*, No. 124, September 1981.

10. *Memorial Hospital v. Maricopa County*, Supreme Court of the United States, 415 U.S. 250; 94 S. Ct. 1076; 39 L. Ed. 2d 306; 1974 U.S.; *Memorial Hospital and Henry Evaro v. Board of Supervisors and Maricopa County*, Case No. 251236, Maricopa County Superior Court, Clerk's Office; Interview Transcript, Augusto Ortiz, M.D., May 26, 1994, 5, *Medicine and Health Care Delivery in Southern Arizona*, Arizona Historical Society Oral History Project, Arizona Historical Society. Since the 1996 welfare reform legislation, discussed below, states are again allowed to impose residency requirements for welfare services; see David A. Donohue, "Penalizing the Poor: Durational Residency Requirements for Welfare Benefits," 72 *St. John's Law Review* 451, Spring 1998.

On the residency debate in California, see Chavez, "Undocumented Immigrants," 18.

11. Deposition of Katie Perazzo (nurse), Bisbee, Arizona, May 18, 1982, Superior Court of Cochise County; *Guerrero v. Copper Queen Hospital*, Supreme Court of Arizona, 112 Ariz. 104; 537 P.2d 1329; 1975 Ariz. (July 18, 1975).

12. Ngai, *Impossible Subjects*, 261.

13. 38 Fed. Reg. 30, 259 (1973), reprinted in *Lewis v. Grinker*, 965 F.2d at 1212.

14. See Beatrix Hoffman, "Emergency Rooms: The Reluctant Safety Net," in *Bringing the Past Back In: History and Health Policy in the United States*, ed. Rosemary Stevens, Charles Rosenberg, and Lawton R. Burns (New Brunswick, N.J.: Rutgers University Press, forthcoming 2006).

15. The Omnibus Budget Reconciliation Act of 1986, Pub. L. No. 99–509, 100 Stat. 1874, 2057 (1986). The program was preserved by Congress in the 1996 welfare reform; Lucette Lagnado, "Emergency Medicaid Policy Binds Sick Immigrants Without an Exit," *The Wall Street Journal*, October 18, 2000, A1.

16. Katherine Eban Finkelstein, "Medical Rebels: When Caring for Patients Means Breaking the Rules," *The Nation*, February 21, 2000, 11–17; Jeffrey T. Kullgren, "Restrictions on Undocumented Immigrants' Access to Health Services: The Public Health Implications of Welfare Reform," *American Journal of Public Health* 93 (10) (October 2003): 1630–33.

17. Ana Mendieta, "Hospitals Pay Medical Costs of Undocumented," *Chicago Sun-Times*, December 11, 2001, 8.

18. Joel Millman, "Low-Wage U.S. Jobs Get 'Mexicanized,' But There's a Price," *Wall Street Journal*, May 2, 2005, A2.

19. Sarah Avery, "Hospitals Face Care Quandary," *News and Observer* (Raleigh, N.C.), September 25, 2004, A1.

20. For an illuminating study of immigrant labor in rural North Carolina, see Leon Fink, *The Maya of Morganton: Work and Community in the Nuevo New South* (Chapel Hill: University of North Carolina Press, 2003).

21. Harry Herrick and Ziya Gizlice, "Spanish-Speaking Hispanics in North Carolina: Health Status, Access to Health Care, and Quality of Life Results from the 2002 and 2003 NC BRFSS Surveys," State Center for Health Statistics (Raleigh, N.C.) Study No. 143, *SCHS Studies*, July 2004. This study also found that only 12 percent of Hispanics in North Carolina received Medicaid.

22. In fiscal year 2004, WakeMed claimed to spend $68.2 million for charity care; UNC, $48 million; Duke, $28.8. See Avery, "Hospitals Face Care Quandary."

23. Lindsey Gruson, "Some Doctors Move to Bar Transplants to Foreign Patients," *New York Times*, August 10, 1985, 1.

24. Diana Washington Valdez, "Mexican Teen's Death Stirs Debate," *El Paso Times*, March 2, 2003.

25. Christina Headrick and Vicki Cheng, "Some Link Citizenship, Transplants," *News and Observer* (Raleigh, N.C.), March 4, 2003, A1.

26. "Undocumented Immigrants in U.S. Donate More Organs Than They Receive," *Transplant Week*, March 9, 2003, <www.transplantweek.org/members/Vol14?News/041001.htm>.

27. Headrick and Cheng, "Some Link Citizenship, Transplants," A1.

28. Mendieta, "Hospitals Pay Medical Costs," 8. The other children were Samira Ocampo, age thirteen, and Jesus Ramirez, age twelve, who both received stem cell transplants. Ocampo died of complications from the transplant.

29. Headrick and Cheng, "Some Link Citizenship, Transplants," A1.

30. Apparently the Santillans heard about the Children's Miracle Network from Jesica's aunt, an undocumented worker in the North Carolina tobacco fields. See Avery Comarow, "Jesica's Story," *U.S. News and World Report*, July 28, 2003, 51. According to the organization's Web site (<www.cmn.org>), "Children's Miracle Network Hospitals . . . provide $2.5 billion in charity (uncompensated) care each year; Treat 98% of all children needing heart or lung transplants."

31. "What Is the History of Jesica's Hope Chest?" <www.4jhc.org/index.html>.

32. Allen Johnson, "Who Lives, Who Dies, Who Pays? Jesica's Sweet Sad Song Plays On," *News and Record* (Greensboro, N.C.), March 9, 2003, H2.

33. It is also notable that most of the media, and some of the authors in this volume (including me), refer to "Jesica" rather than "Santillan" or "Ms. Santillan." This familiar usage of her first name emphasizes her youth, even though she was nearly eighteen.

34. The literature on the history of southern benevolence and paternalism is large; a few examples include James C. Cobb, *The Most Southern Place on Earth: The Mississippi Delta and the Roots of Regional Identity* (New York: Oxford University Press, 1994); Bertram Wyatt-Brown, *Southern Honor: Ethics and Behavior in the Old South* (New York: Oxford University Press, 1983); and Eugene D. Genovese, *Roll, Jordan, Roll: The World the Slaves Made* (New York: Vintage, 1976).

35. John A. Mulhall, "How Many Died While Illegal Alien Got Two Heart-Lung Transplants?" *The Post-Standard* (Syracuse, N.Y.), February 27, 2003, A13.

36. Headrick and Cheng, "Some Link Citizenship, Transplants," A1.

37. A 2002 Border Counties Coalition study, funded by the U.S. Department of Health and Human Services after pressure from influential Arizona senator John Kyl, determined that 25 percent of uncompensated care costs ($190 million) to border hospitals were attributed to undocumented immigrants; See MGT of America, Inc., and U.S. Border Counties Coalition, "Medical Emergency: Who Pays the Price for

Uncompensated Emergency Medical Care Along the Southwest Border?" 2002, available at <www.bordercounties.org>. Since all such statistics must be estimates due to the fact that hospitals do not ask patients about immigration status, it is impossible to determine their accuracy; see Lisa Richardson, "Immigrant Health Tab Disputed," *Los Angeles Times*, May 18, 2003. Other studies have found that undocumented immigrants' use of emergency rooms is minimal; Chavez, Flores, Lopez-Garza, "Undocumented Latin American Immigrants"; Veronica Bucio, "Misperceptions Won't Cure Our ER Crisis" (op-ed), *Houston Chronicle*, January 7, 2002, A24.

38. I have found no evidence that the Santillan case played a role in the passage of this legislation.

39. Speech by Dana Rohrabacher, "Stemming Uncontrolled Illegal Immigration," House of Representatives, May 12, 2004, available at <www.votesmart.org/speech—detail.php?speech—id=40989>.

40. Centers for Medicare and Medicaid Services, <www.cms.hhs.gov/providers/section1011/state—alloc.asp>.

41. Alfredo Corchado, "Village Shocked Over Transplant Death," *Salt Lake Tribune*, February 24, 2003. The article by the reporter for the *Dallas Morning News* was picked up by the Salt Lake City paper.

ELIGIBILITY FOR ORGAN TRANSPLANTATION TO FOREIGN NATIONALS

THE RELATIONSHIP BETWEEN CITIZENSHIP, JUSTICE, AND PHILANTHROPY AS POLICY CRITERIA

ERIC M. MESLIN, KAREN R. SALMON, & JASON T. EBERL

The events and commentary surrounding Jesica Santillan's access to multiple organ transplants raise profound questions about the criteria used to justify her receiving these organs, and whether her status as a citizen of another country should have had any bearing on whether she was eligible to receive the organs and the related care. In the wake of September 11, with public and governmental scrutiny about one's country of origin having intensified, these questions about citizenship, justice, and the role of the state take on new meaning.

This essay examines the salient issues from the perspectives of moral and political philosophy, philanthropy, public policy, and bioethics. These disciplinary approaches provide a perspective on the Santillan case that is intended to complement other approaches in this book. We approach the problem of eligibility to transplantation using two different but interrelated lenses. The first lens considers the extent to which citizenship (or its virtual equivalent in the United States: resident alien status) is a morally relevant criterion for distinguishing between those who are eligible to access high-end technologies, like transplantation, and those who are not eligible. This is both a matter of political philosophy, since citizenship is fundamentally a political construction, and of moral philosophy, since the scarcity of organs forces society to make ethical distinctions about who should receive organs when not all who need them can.

The argument that organs are justly distributed first and foremost, or even exclusively, to citizens presupposes that what is at stake is an issue of fairness in the distribution of scarce resources; from this perspective, the problem of access to organ transplantation by foreign nationals is understood as one of fair entitlement to the resource.[1] If citizenship is not a morally relevant criterion for limiting access, then access by foreign nationals will have to be assessed using other criteria. The public policy question asks whether any policy using citizenship status alone can be implemented fairly. We argue that it cannot. But we also claim that citizenship status is a relevant criterion for determining who is eligible for transplantation—that is, some moral weight may be attached to the status of being legally permitted to live and work in the United States and thereby able to access certain health care benefits—yet it is not so compelling that it cannot be trumped. For example, the weight of this claim diminishes if the individual's citizenship status more closely resembles that of an undocumented foreign national,[2] illegal immigrant, or casual tourist. Ultimately, we conclude that even if citizenship has minimal moral weight, it should not be used as a basis for national policy for limiting access to transplantation. It is, in the language of philosophical argumentation, neither necessary nor sufficient.

The second lens considers whether, and to what extent, philanthropy can be used as a basis to determine if foreign nationals may be eligible for organ transplants in the United States. Not unlike the citizenship argument, the philanthropy argument has a set of presuppositions, including but not limited to the idea that charity and humanitarianism are necessary and foundational features of the U.S. health care system—necessary, of course, but not sufficient. Health care philanthropy is a key component of what is generally seen as a flawed U.S. health care system—flawed in that it permits gross inequities in access to even basic care by tens of millions of people. Since some gaps in health care coverage are currently filled by social philanthropy— specifically through unreimbursed "charity care"—it is reasonable to extend this model to the organ transplantation problem. According to this approach, the problem of access to organ transplantation by foreign nationals may be understood as one of "equivalent philanthropy": that is, if citizens may be the recipients of charity care, then so too may noncitizens. It follows that any limitations on access will be determined by other factors, such as need or urgency (the current criteria), as well as the extent to which a hospital system (or, as in the case of Jesica, a benevolent private citizen) can afford to be charitable.

We argue that, while there is a difference between the social philanthropy that is built into the system and the individual philanthropy of wealthy sponsors, this approach also suffers from certain limitations. There are different consequences of philanthropy for hospitals, communities, care providers, and society in general, not all of which may be desirable.

THE FIRST LENS: THE MORAL RELEVANCE OF
CITIZENSHIP AND JUSTICE

It is difficult to dismiss lightly the idea that citizenship is a morally relevant category of political and ethical concern in matters of public policy. Since Socrates debated with Crito about the merits of following the law as a prerequisite of being a citizen of Athens, most democratic states have come to appreciate the value society places on the rights, privileges, and responsibilities associated with citizenship. Recall Socrates' argument for staying in prison, accepting his sentence, and not trying to escape and save his own life: "And suppose the laws were to reply, 'Was that our agreement? Or was it that you should abide by whatever judgment the state should pronounce?' And if we were surprised by their words, perhaps they would say, 'Socrates, don't be surprised by our words, but answer us; you yourself are accustomed to ask questions and to answer them. What complaint have you against us and the state, that you are trying to destroy us? Are we not, first of all, your parents?' "[3] Socrates' argument—that by remaining in society one has a civic duty to adhere to its laws *as if the state were one's parents*—is a dramatic piece of political philosophy. At once, it provides the basis for the social contract that would inform the eighteenth- and nineteenth-century political philosophies of Hobbes, Locke, and Hume and hints at some of the more worrisome forms of totalitarianism—particularly those that grant the state powers to enforce certain laws, even when such laws may violate individual liberty. This particular view of citizenship is at odds with a more pragmatic political philosophy that would suggest that citizens have a civic duty, *qua citizen*, to speak, to challenge, to argue, and even to debate the very laws themselves.[4]

A less extreme notion of citizenship is one in which specific rights can be claimed exclusively by those who are either born a citizen or choose to become naturalized as a citizen.[5] This notion sees citizenship as a status that entitles one to certain benefits (for example, obtaining a passport, voting, or running for president) with a modest set of obligations, one of which is to comply with the law. But clearly there is more to such claims than mere materialist entitlements.[6] As Leo Chavez notes in his essay in this book, "The Santillan case forces us to . . . observe the biopolitics surrounding citizenship that are so essential to the representations of Jesica Santillan." We think Chavez is right, especially in light of the ongoing public conversation about the multiple ways in which citizenship—far from being merely a legal category of status acquired by an individual at birth or through naturalization—is also a heavily political category of status that can be used by the state to provide benefits to some and not others; other categories include tax-paying status, whether one has a criminal record, or (historically) one's race or ethnicity. One of the challenges in thinking through the way in which citizenship functions as a moral category in the Santillan case is determining which category, legal or political, is operative at any given moment. Any understanding of this case using this first lens, must, in our view, necessarily recognize the inherent tension that exists between these two ideas. Indeed, a cynic might suggest that questions of citizenship, tax-paying status, etc., are just stalking horses for the notion of "who deserves the organ"?[7]

One version of the citizenship argument has been offered (though not fully defended) by James Dwyer, who characterizes the debate about undocumented foreign nationals' eligibility for health care as one pitting nationalists against humanists.[8] Nationalists argue that illegal immigrants are not entitled to, and therefore should be denied, public benefits because they are in the country illegally: they have failed to comply with relevant immigration policy. This argument is based on the single and tenuous claim that compliance with the law is a condition of eligibility to all public goods. But few examples are needed to demonstrate the weakness of the argument since many natural-born citizens fail to follow laws and are not in any jeopardy of losing their eligibility. Of course, when specific laws are broken, particularly criminal laws, then individuals forfeit certain liberty rights during the period of their incarceration. Interestingly, access to medical treatment is not one of these forfeited rights. Nor, as the country learned in a recent Indiana case of a death row inmate who wanted to donate his liver to his sister either prior to or after his execution, do prisoners forfeit their right to donate organs or to receive them.[9] In contrast with nationalists who would bar the door to noncitizens, humanists would "employ a discourse of human rights . . . [and] emphasize the right of all human beings to medical treatment, as well as the common humanity of aliens and citizens, pointing to the arbitrary nature of national borders."[10] Humanists defend the view that citizenship status is not a relevant criterion for discriminating between those eligible for care and those who are not eligible. The clear conclusions from each of the positions are that nationalists would prohibit undocumented foreign nationals from receiving U.S.-based organ transplant services while humanists would not.

Dwyer finds both positions untenable and proposes a third perspective: that there is a social responsibility to care for undocumented foreign nationals, not because they have a right to care (as the committed humanist might argue), but rather because in many respects illegal immigrants are social members (of society).[11] This argument works well in the case of existing undocumented foreign workers—perhaps the same people eligible for President Bush's proposed guest worker program. It even works for Jesica, an individual whose family came into the country illegally in hopes of a transplant that she was unlikely to receive in her host country. But let's examine this argument further. It is known that a member of the Santillan family was already established in Louisburg, North Carolina, where the family would come to illegally reside.[12] Jesica attended a local Louisburg school, while her mother, Magdalena, took a job as a housekeeper for Louisburg College, and her father, Melecio, obtained employment as a construction worker. The family's efforts to raise money for Jesica's transplant and the community's philanthropic response by creating Jesica's Hope Chest, where nearly $500,000 was raised toward her transplantation, suggest that they had become a valued part of the community.

Given these initial observations, how should we assess whether citizenship ought to count in this type of case? And perhaps more directly: Can citizenship ever function only as an impartial criterion for determining whether Jesica should have received these organs? One answer may be found in the recommendations of the former Task Force on Organ Transplantation, which tackled the issue head on in 1996. The task force recommended that a ceiling be placed on the number of nonresident aliens that could be on the national waiting list for kidneys, and that nonresident aliens could be placed on a waiting list for hearts or livers but would receive an organ only if no U.S. citizen could benefit from it.[13] This position is not as restrictive as the one proposed several years earlier by Jeffrey Prottas, who argued that residency status is a necessary rationing strategy to protect against reduction of the supply of available organs.[14] Admittedly, if citizenship is irrelevant to establishing eligibility for receiving an organ, residence may raise similar challenges. In other words, must the recipient live in the same community, state, nation, hemisphere in which the organ is available?[15] Drawing such a line may be difficult but not impossible, since established law and practice recognizes the difference between temporary visitors, including casual tourists with no intention of working, and temporary workers.

Other examples of the general argument for limiting access to organs by foreign nationals include:

- Any payment for transplant services that cannot be recovered (either directly or through general taxation) places an additional tax and financial burden on citizens.
- Making organs available to anyone will decrease the supply generally to

U.S. citizens either directly (organs going to foreign nationals are removed from circulation and hence are no longer available to U.S. citizens) or indirectly (disappointment with the apparent unfairness of this system will discourage people from donating).

- It is unfair as a matter of distributive justice to allow people to receive the benefit of an organ if they are not a member of the community that provides it.
- It is ethically and economically unsound to permit "free riders" in a system.

Many of these arguments have been skillfully dispensed with by others so we will do no more than provide reminders of some of the more successful counterarguments. Dena Davis showed more than a decade ago why the political category of citizenship should not be used to discriminate against individuals who need care.[16] The argument that permitting access to organs by undocumented foreign nationals places an unfair tax burden on the tax-paying public is less about citizenship and more about the facts surrounding taxation. Little is needed to show why this argument fails. Most Americans pay many types of taxes: value-added tax, sales tax, gasoline tax, cigarette tax, etc. Some Americans do not pay all of these taxes. The same applies to undocumented foreign nationals. The major differences are with state and federal *income* taxes and *property* taxes, which one would expect that foreign nationals without proper documentation to live or work would avoid paying for fear of being discovered and deported. But some Americans can be counted among those who do not pay income tax or property tax because they either fall below the income level required to pay income taxes or do not own a home and thus are not subject to property taxes.

The contribution of tax-paying undocumented foreign nationals helps support Dwyer's argument that illegal immigrants are members of our society. But declaring people to be members of society with the implication that they may be eligible for the benefits of that society does not solve the problem entirely, either. It is obvious that "society," like "community," is differently interpreted depending on whether the term is defined by political scientists, demographers, elected officials, cultural/ethnic groups, or social anthropologists. Who would deny that on September 11 or in the immediate aftermath of the Indonesian tsunami or Hurricane Katrina the local orientation of community was (at least temporarily) enlarged to include a regional, national, or more global orientation?

However, there is a larger issue surrounding the taxation of undocumented foreign nationals. Two decades ago, James Nickel argued, "If counties that fund public hospitals have any valid complaint, it is not that undocumented immigrants don't pay taxes, but that the taxes mostly go to the federal government while the costs of providing services to these people fall disproportionately on states and counties."[17] A decade later, Karen Pallarito targeted the costs of health care for undocumented foreign nationals in individual states and hospitals, focusing on Florida and Texas (states with the largest immigrant population). She found that the problem of unpaid taxes among undocumented foreign nationals was, as Nickel described, a problem at the state and local level, where hospitals have provided immigrant care and are left with billions of dollars in unpaid services.[18]

Both reports concur regarding the contribution (via taxation) of undocumented foreign nationals; indeed, that contribution takes place on a federal level. Rather, the dispute lies in the extent or reach of their tax contribution and its effect on their eligibility for the benefits readily available to citizens. Indeed, the same taxes paid by citizens also go primarily to the federal government, and yet many citizens qualify for unreimbursed "charity" care from locally supported hospitals. Although some of these citizens may pay local/state income and property taxes, some (probably many) of them don't pay these taxes if their income level is low enough for them to qualify for charity care. Thus, if citizenship (via taxation) obligates people to support social institutions, then the vagaries of American taxation cannot be the proxy for the determination of who is eligible for organ transplantation and who is not.

The claim that increased public attention to organ transplants for noncitizens would cause a general decline in overall organ donation (based on the perception that organs were not going to citizens first) is similarly flawed. Many versions of the argument for this claim exist, including those based on the empirical premise that there is a causal relationship between an open-door or permissive policy for providing organs and a decrease in the number of organs.[19]

Citizenship, it would seem, ought to play some role in any assessment of access to U.S. organs for transplant by foreign nationals—that is, some moral weight may be attached to the status of being legally permitted to live and work in the United States and thereby eligible to obtain access to certain health care benefits. But this weight is not so compelling that it cannot be trumped by other claims and considerations. There are two reasons why it should not be given significant weight in this assessment. First, as we have argued, the concept of citizenship can be interpreted legally, politically and morally in very different ways. Even when citizenship is used as an impartial rule of access, it runs counter to the idea that responding to a person's urgent medical needs can legitimately be limited by a political criterion, such as the legal status of his or her presence in the country. Second, we are not convinced that citizenship will always be used in this impartial way. There are too many examples (many of which are discussed elsewhere in this volume) of situations in which the underserved, disadvantaged, and disempowered are at increased risk of discrimination. The lens of citizenship, in our view, functions heuristically at best—providing us with a window into areas of political and moral discussion that are not comfortably broached in this country. This does not mean that citizenship should be rejected outright as a category of moral reflection, since it gives us much to think about. In considering Jesica's case, citizenship lets us assess her situation in important ways: How would we feel if she were legally entitled to be in the United States on a JI student visa or an HI-B work visa? What if she were in the United States after having fled a tortuous regime and, while requesting political asylum, learned of her illness? A United Network for Organ Sharing (UNOS) spokesperson has already shed light on such hypothetical cases: "We do not differentiate between whether a transplant patient has legal or illegal immigration status."[20] But this determination only gets us part of the way. Even if Jesica's family had, as we believe, a reasonable expectation that she would be eligible for access to transplantation irrespective of her citizenship status, this expectation in no way ensures that a particular institution has an *obligation* to provide the organs (and related services).

But the lens of citizenship will forever be clouded by other pragmatic political realities. Imagine Jessica's situation, but change her ethnic background, socioeconomic status, race, gender, etc., and one quickly recognizes how heavy the political and moral baggage that accompanies any apparently impartial assessment of whether one deserves or should be allowed to receive a transplant. For example, would we think differently about her (or the case itself) if she were the daughter of a wealthy Saudi industrialist who has both political and economic influence? Or, what if she were from a middle-class Canadian family, as opposed to a poverty-level Mexican family? The arguments about citizenship and legal status do not disappear, however. Instead they provide a context for asking the broader social question, to which we now turn: How ought society respond to cases like Jesica's?

THE SECOND LENS: PHILANTHROPY AS
A MORAL BASIS FOR PROVIDING HEALTH CARE

If society has difficulty requiring that resources be diverted from those legally entitled to be in the United States to others who do not enjoy this status, does the debate end here? How should the United States—a country without a comprehensive and universal health care system—respond to situations like Jesica's? Where might we look for solutions? The usual (albeit unsuccessful) location for many proposed solutions is in the architecture of the failed U.S. health care system, a system that un- or underinsures more than 44 million Americans (another reason why citizenship cannot function effectively as a criterion of access). Years of debate and public policy initiatives have not altered what appears to be a fundamental truth about access to health care in the United States: the country apparently is not prepared to make a commitment to ensure that all who live here can access even basic health care. This is especially shameful given that this lack of commitment is more a reflection of a series of political decisions about the place of health care as part of the government's obligations to citizens than of a reasoned assessment of the costs to be incurred.[21]

We will leave for another time, and for other contributors to this volume, to comment on this issue in any further detail. Instead we turn our attention, and thus the second lens, to another approach: What about relying on the altruistic and philanthropic motivations of physicians, surgeons, nurses, administrators, transplant coordinators, and other members of the society as a response to cases like Jesica's? Prima facie, organ *donation* is an act of social philanthropy involving (usually) a gift to a stranger, and most of the cases capturing public attention of individuals from other countries who obtain transplants in the United States involve the benevolence of an individual, group, or institution.[22] What can a philanthropic approach contribute to this discussion?

HISTORY OF PHILANTHROPY

The history of literature, philosophy, and society records many efforts to codify obligations and expectations related to philanthropic giving, or charity. The Code of Hammurabi (twenty-first century B.C.E.), Jewish, Christian and Muslim scriptures, the Elizabethan Poor Laws of 1601, the founding of "almshouses" in New York City and Baltimore in the eighteenth and nineteenth centuries, and early discussions by the American Medical Association

(AMA) all make reference to social philanthropy.[23] For example, the 1847 AMA *Code of Medical Ethics* included the following expectations:

- A physician should be "ever ready to obey the calls of the sick."
- "There is no profession, by the members of which, eleemosynary [charity] services are more liberally dispensed, than the medical."
- "Poverty . . . should always be recognized as presenting valid claims for gratuitous services."
- "To individuals in indigent circumstances, such professional services should always be cheerfully and freely accorded."[24]

In recent years, the academic study of philanthropy and charitable giving has focused on private action for the public good, often taking as a starting point the idea of one common good or of giving to one particular charity. Included in this broad idea is the study of the public good of improving health. Philanthropic giving is often associated with "charity," the kindly and sympathetic disposition to aid the needy or suffering, and it has a long philosophical tradition. Aquinas, for instance, wrote that charity is "the root of all virtues." Milton said of charity that it is "the soul of all the rest" of the virtues. In terms of social responsibility, Montesquieu observed: "The state is frequently obliged to supply the necessities of the aged, the sick, and the orphan . . . the alms given to a naked man in the street do not fulfill the obligations of the state, which owes to every citizen a certain subsistence, a proper nourishment, convenient clothing, and a kind of life not incompatible with health."[25] In agreement with this sentiment, Kant argued: "The government is justified and entitled to compel those who are able, to furnish the means necessary to preserve those who are not themselves capable of providing for the most necessary wants of nature."[26]

Following the dire days of the Depression, which witnessed a rise in private insurance and government-subsidized care and a decline in private charity/philanthropy, the United States began taking steps to institutionalize portions of a public health care system based on its tendency to rely on *charity* rather than a right to universal health care as matter of social welfare. A prominent example is the Hill-Burton Act (1946), which provided funds for the development and improvement of hospitals. Hill-Burton funded facilities that "agreed to provide a 'reasonable volume of free or reduced cost care' to 'individuals unable to pay' and to make service 'available to all' in the general service area without discrimination."[27]

MODELS OF PHILANTHROPY

To fulfill the moral mandate to provide charity to those in need, several models exist that reflect particular ethical attitudes, motivations, and goals to be achieved.[28] For example, someone may act charitably because of an *egoistic* concern to demonstrate their power or to provide themselves with an "insurance policy" in case they will one day have to rely on others' charity: "Do unto others so that they'll do unto me." Of course, while those who follow this model may give the appearance of philanthropic donation, it is actually just an exercise of enlightened self-interest. At the other end of the spectrum, there is the truly *compassionate* person who feels sympathy for those in need and is emotionally moved to respond to immediate crises. The question arises, though, of whether acting compassionately, by responding to immediate need, is sufficient to avoid those in need becoming perpetually dependent on philanthropic donation and never becoming self-sufficient.

Here, the *utilitarian* philanthropist argues that we must "produce the greatest good for the greatest number of people." To accomplish such a goal we must move beyond the motivation to respond to immediate need and address the underlying root causes of such need. A purely utilitarian approach to philanthropy, however, does not necessarily provide a sufficient motivation to act charitably in a given situation. Although utilitarians are free from the motivation of self-interest, unlike egoists, they will respond charitably in a particular set of circumstances only if it promotes the best outcome for the majority of people involved. Hence, whether undocumented foreign nationals should receive organs in general, or whether Jesica in particular should have been eligible for (not one but two) transplant procedures, depends on the calculation of whether the majority of people involved would be benefited or harmed.

Our colleague Richard Gunderman has referred to another philanthropic model, one he calls "donation to liberate." The goal of this model is not to fulfill ego-centered interests or produce only the greatest good for the majority but to make recipients of charity self-sufficient and actually transform them into givers themselves. This model reflects a definition of "generosity" in which a philanthropist "begets or produces" goodness by being attuned to other people's potential. The goal in such a model is to cultivate the virtuous character of both givers and recipients, who then become givers, by unleashing their philanthropic potential.

Any of these models may support the donation of organs to undocumented foreign nationals, albeit not without certain limitations. The egocentric donor might have the capacity to see themselves in Jesica's situation, a native of one country requiring a transplant that is available only in another country. The compassionate donor might sympathize with Jesica's condition and seek to alleviate her immediate need, as many people in North Carolina apparently did by giving to her cause. It is difficult to see how utilitarians would justify providing organs to undocumented foreign nationals, given the limited amount of available organs and financial resources; utilitarians may even conclude that we should not spend medical resources on transplants at all but instead focus on preventative measures that would reduce the need for transplants. It is worth noting, though, that utilitarianism holds as a fundamental tenet that the ethical calculation of what would maximize overall net welfare must be *impartial*, recognizing that each person involved "counts as one and no more than one" regardless of any other possible discriminatory conditions such as ethnicity or nationality. Therefore, if the practice of organ transplantation is at all justifiable on utilitarian grounds, then we should not deny someone a transplant simply because of their citizenship status. Finally, the idea of "donation to liberate" applies to the present case insofar as those who receive organs, or their families, may become organ donors and thereby increase the pool of available organs for transplant.

HEALTH-RELATED PHILANTHROPY AND THE DONATION OF THE BODY

There are several ways in which both public and private philanthropic giving have taken hold in the development of health care initiatives and policy. We further note that the donation of blood, body parts, organs, and now human tissues and DNA, share a family resemblance: the donors' motivations can be traced to an important sense of self, altruism, and community. A research team at the Indiana University Center for Bioethics recently completed a year-long study of these issues in a project titled "Heath Related Philanthropy: The Donation of the Body (and Parts Thereof)."[29] The finding most relevant to this essay that emerged from this work was that there is no single policy approach that enjoys sufficient public support to ensure access to organs. Factors such as gender, geography, age, income, and religiosity all contribute in different ways to the motivations people have for participating in the organ donation system. As of this writing (October 2005), we continue to analyze data from a national survey of more than 1,000 individuals who were asked about their views concerning the donation of blood, organs for transplant and other therapies, and their bodies to science for education and research—as contrasted with the traditional philanthropic donations of time and money. Initial findings show little or no correlation: that is, the reasons that people offer for their willingness to donate blood are not the same as the reasons they offer for why they may be willing to donate an organ after death, or their body to science. Similarly, the reasons people offer for donating money and time are quite different from those they give for donating blood, organs, tissue, or bodies.

We think these preliminary findings are important to the discussion of Jesica Santillan for two reasons. First, if studies like this involving the public can be carried out in a way that accurately captures their future intentions (and there is much to be done to validate our study), then it would be worth asking the public for their views about whether they would be more or less willing to sign donor cards and donate organs if they knew that their organs might be given to foreign nationals. Second, if one of the values of this kind of study lies in its ability to combine two different types of social philanthropy (traditional giving of money and time, and what we have called "health-related philanthropy," in which one literally donates a part of themselves), then it is likely that we can assess a more nuanced public policy analysis of the relationship between access to organs and access to broader public goods, like indigent health care.

This latter point is especially important for Jesica's case. During the course of Jesica's treatment, Duke University Hospital stated, "The duty of the hospital is to provide health care to all people, regardless of immigration status."[30] Not only did Duke make good on that policy in Jesica's case, it established a $4 million endowment in her memory. The fund provides additional support services for Hispanic pediatric patients and their families receiving treatment at Duke University Medical Center.[31] Duke hospital launched the Jesica Santillan Fund by committing to donate $1 million by 2008. William J. Fulkerson, M.D., CEO of Duke University Hospital, recognized the importance of the charitable giving of available resources, from the perspective of a health care facility, when he stated, "It is important that a broad range of services— temporary housing, food, ministerial services, social services, interpreters, etc., is available for the families, especially those without economic means."[32]

Duke's benevolence may be exceptional, but it did not occur in a complete vacuum. UNOS has a policy that up to 5 percent of transplanted organs may go to non-U.S. residents per year; but overall, it has been left to the individual institutions and providers to set their own policies.[33] Moreover, most would recognize in Duke's actions an obvious public relations motivation that would lead to reciprocal donations to Duke: to be seen as a well-motivated giver puts one in a desirable position of being identified as a worthy recipient of future philanthropy. (Wailoo and Livingston, in their essay in this volume, also highlight this reality—that such institutions exist within a broader moral economy.)

Duke's situation is not unlike that faced by other hospitals in the United States. Clarian Health Partners, Inc., is a state-wide health network in Indiana that includes both not-for-profit and for-profit institutions. In Indianapolis, three Indiana University hospitals—Riley Hospital for Children, Indiana University Hospital and Methodist Hospital—are part of the Clarian Health Partners network. Clarian is also one of the largest transplant centers in the United States. The merger agreement that established Clarian, between the Methodist Church and Indiana University, includes a values statement that explicitly references "charity, equality and justice in health care." Clarian recently adopted an "International Humanitarian Policy" in which they outline the process under which undocumented foreign nationals can receive charity care under exceptional circumstances. Undocumented foreign nationals are grouped with anyone who is not a U.S. citizen or a legal resident of the United States. Foreign tourists, business people away from home, and visiting students also fall within this category. This grouping of undocumented foreign nationals with other foreigners is rare among other health care providers. In addition to defining the groups of people that fall within the International Humanitarian Policy, Clarian gives examples of the type of charity care that it is willing to provide and examples of relevant kinds of procedures. Furthermore, the policy includes the conditions that must be met in order for a person to qualify for charity care. These conditions include

- obtaining both a physician and executive sponsor,
- the willingness of physicians to "waive their professional fees associated with or incidental to proposed procedure," and
- a humanitarian form that must be filled out by the patient, physician, and executive sponsor.

However, Clarian limits its charitable assistance to foreign nationals to emergency, nonelective services, thereby ruling out charitable support for most transplant services.

Given this tendency for the United States to rely on charity to support a portion of its health care services, what would a philanthropic approach look like as applied to organ transplantation for undocumented foreign nationals? At the very least, such an approach would lay to rest citizenship as a criterion of access or support and turn directly to a criterion of medical need and urgency. Such an approach would expect that private individuals and organizations would step forward to fill the gap created by the chronic shortage of organs and the imminent need of patients. Some decisions would be based on pragmatic considerations: Is the case for supporting undocumented foreign nationals a compelling one for the organization? Is it consistent with its mission or values? We also suspect that some decisions would be based on a type of social altruism. But, prima facie, altruism is not a sufficient incentive for individuals to *donate* cadaveric organs: an altruistic attitude does not entail philanthropic activity.[34] There is a chronic and distressing shortage of organs available for transplant in this country with hundreds of people dying every day on waiting lists. If altruism is not working to grow supply, what is the likelihood that a similar motivation will inform the distribution of this scarce resource?

One avenue is to supplement pure philanthropy with a more pragmatic type of philanthropy, known as "justice as reciprocity." In contrast with the argument that justice demands some form of fair distribution of resources, justice as reciprocity means that individuals are entitled to a benefit in return for their contributions to an enterprise or society. Tom Beauchamp and James Childress defend an understanding of obligations of beneficence in health care based on reciprocity: "Many obligations of beneficence are appropriately justified by implicit arrangements underlying the necessary give-and-take of social life."[35] This notion of justice views societies as "enterprises that are run for the mutual benefit of their citizens" and in which the citizens "give meaning to their affiliation by providing for each other, by sharing benefits and burdens. Contributions such as paying taxes, obeying the law, and serving in the military are repaid with benefits such as access to public facilities, safety against crime and foreign invasions, and social assistance in times of need."[36] In this way, the indigent are members of society and contribute in ways that generate an obligation (based on the balance between contributive and distributive justice) to repay them with access to health care. Larry McCullough argues that, because foreign nationals, whether or not they are documented, have made economic contributions to society through their work, they are entitled to some public resources in virtue of the property rights that their labor helped create: "The key feature they possess in common with citizens and legally resident foreign nationals is contribution to the national society; this contribution is independent of citizenship and immigration status. Thus, their property rights in and to transplantation services would be no different from those of any other citizen or legally resident foreign national."[37] This argument owes its origin in part to John Locke, who argued that "mixing" our own individual labor with natural material resources provides us with a *natural right of property* over whatever we thereby produce. The argument that one is entitled in direct proportion to what one has contributed is especially attractive for the present discussion because it recognizes and permits the obvious incommensurability between the type of contribution people may make and the benefit that they would receive.

Undocumented foreign nationals and illegal immigrants make many economic, cultural, religious, social, and political contributions to U.S. society. Their economic contributions alone are significant considering that they often provide a considerable amount of labor for the workforce and pay certain taxes, such as sales tax when they buy goods and services and gas taxes when they purchase gasoline. Permitting them access to the benefits of transplantation is understood as a form of reciprocity, since they are not paying directly for the organs. But, then, no one pays directly for organs, any more than anyone who is taxed pays directly for atomic submarines.

Note that in this sense justice as reciprocity is not identical to justice as contribution. If it were, we could point out that for some groups there is a legitimate expectation of entitlement to organs based on contribution. For example, it has been estimated that in 2001 twice the number of undocumented Hispanics *donated* organs as *received* organs.[38] Is this an outpouring of generosity on their part, or are other exploitative factors (economic, political, social) at work? Despite the possibility that such donations may not be motivated purely by altruism or given with voluntary informed consent, the fact of Hispanics' significant material contribution is undeniably evident. Nevertheless, although organ donation is an enormous contribution, both personally and socially, this does not immediately render the entire Hispanic population (legal or illegal) eligible to receive organs for transplant if their medical conditions require it. And we know that a depressingly small number of people in the United States actually donate organs every year and yet still believe that they are entitled (not merely eligible) to organs. We also know that some organs are retrieved from foreign donors who died in the United States on vacation or during periods of visa-authorized work.

CONCLUDING THOUGHTS:
REASONABLE LIMITS AND THE ROLE OF POLICY

In *The Enforcement of Morals*, Lord Patrick Devlin asked, "To what extent should society use the law to enforce its moral judgments?"[39] Fifty years later, with the availability of technologies to save and extend life, this has emerged as one of the dominant questions for those struggling to develop regulatory policy.[40] Most would agree with the claims that the law often reflects public morality, and that what is ethical ought to be permitted and what is unethical ought to be prohibited.[41] Finding this balance can be a tremendous challenge. Given this, it is reasonable to ask whether *policy* is the appropriate response. Should there be a national policy for providing transplantation services to individuals without recognized documentation? Or would it be better to provide guidance to local officials—health care entities and organ procurement organizations—and allow them to develop policy where needed? Certainly there are advantages to policy, not the least of which is transparency and accountability. But it should also give us pause that the volume of transplants into undocumented foreign nationals is still rather small. Existing UNOS policy limits transplants to foreign nationals (nonresident aliens and resident aliens) to no more than 5 percent per year. Data from UNOS (1988–2005) show that at no time has this upper limit been met. Looking at the last three years, the following information is available. In 2005, of the 28,110 transplants performed, 216 were on nonresident aliens and 874 were on resident aliens, for a total of 1,090 (3.4 percent). For 2004, of the 27,038 transplants performed, 192 were on nonresident aliens and 717 were on resident aliens, for a total of 909 (3.3 percent). And for 2003, the year of the Santillan story, of the 25,468 transplants performed, 203 were on nonresident aliens and 572 were on resident aliens, for a total of 775 (3.04 percent).[42] Given this information, is this a problem that warrants a new policy?

We worry that exceptional cases will be used to set policy that eventually turns out to be neither fair nor practical. Like most instances in which taking different perspectives reveal different features of an argument, our decision to direct two different lenses on the case of Jesica Santillan is an effort to provide a new orientation to some old and some new problems. And yet so many other questions are left out of focus (to push the metaphor a bit harder) —about the history of U.S. immigration policy, trade policy (including NAFTA), national security, homeland security, labor policy, and the like. This suggests, as Beatrix Hoffman discusses in her essay in this book, that there are certain dangers in using immigration issues as a proxy for health care reform, and vice versa. Similarly, examining the case through a "philanthropy" lens provides a brief glimpse into the world of public charity, necessarily missing out on the important discussions about constructing a health care system in the United States that provides a basic level of health care to all who live here, along with those who might emigrate to the United States. It also leaves out discussions of the country's history of public health initiatives and the significant rise of private health care philanthropy (for example, the Rockefeller, Carnegie, Ford, and Gates Foundations). Gaps in perspectives among public beliefs already exist in the examination of Jesica's story. We have countered some of these perspectives, such as the mistaken beliefs about the extent of contributions made by legal and illegal immigrants living in the United States. We worry, though, not that Jesica's story will be retold as different stories depending on the political, medical, or ethical perspective adopted by the storyteller, but quite the opposite: that we will be so overwhelmed by the many layers and complexities that her story reveals that we will adopt a single story that is understandable (to us), simple and wrong.

NOTES

This essay is the product of many hands, including, most relevantly, a year-long study group undertaken at the Indiana University Center for Bioethics, titled "Health Care Philanthropy: The Donation of the Body (and Parts thereof)." For more information on the study group, go to <http://www.bioethics.iu.edu/pubstudy.html>. The study group was supported by a grant from the Indiana University Center on Philanthropy. The Center for Bioethics is supported in part by the Indiana Genomics Initiative (INGEN), which itself is supported by the Lilly Endowment, Inc. We are grateful for comments by Steven Ivy and Richard Gunderman on an earlier draft, to the organizers and participants at the Rutgers Conference, and to the external reviewers for their helpful suggestions for improving the essay.

1. This topic is discussed extensively in Rosamond Rhodes's essay in this book.

2. The phrase "undocumented foreign nationals" is an admittedly cumbersome one, given that it must apply to a variety of ethical, legal, and political categories of persons. For example, it is used to cover what have been termed "illegal aliens," "undocumented aliens," "undocumented workers," and "unauthorized aliens," among others. According to the Internal Revenue Service, an "Illegal Alien" is also an "Undocumented Alien." The definition of an illegal alien is "an alien who has entered the United States illegally and is deportable if apprehended, or an alien who entered the United States legally but who has fallen "out of status" and is deportable." "Undocumented alien" and "illegal alien" are used interchangeably on the IRS Web site. See Internal Revenue Service, Department of the Treasury, <http://www.irs.gov/businesses/small/international/article/0,,id=129236,00.h tml> (accessed March 29, 2006). "Undocumented workers" are non-U.S. citizens who are not authorized to work in America and lack immigration status. (Nick Beermann, "Liability in More Ways Than One: Employing Undocumented Workers," <http://library.findlaw.com/2003/Sep/30/133064.html (accessed March 9, 2005). An "unauthorized alien" has been defined with respect to the employment of an alien at a particular time when the alien is not at that time either an alien lawfully admitted for permanent residence, or

authorized to be so employed by 8 USCS § 1324a (2005) or by the Attorney General. (United States Code Service, 8 USCS § 1324a 2005).

3. F. J. Church, trans., *Euthyphro, Apology, Crito* (Indianapolis: Bobbs-Merrill, 1956).

4. This is not, of course, a complete interpretation, since Plato's *Apology* illustrates quite clearly that Socrates believed he had a duty to challenge, argue with, and debate the status quo.

5. There are certain differences. For example, individuals wishing to become naturalized U.S. citizens are required to swear an oath of allegiance to "protect and defend the Constitution against enemies foreign and domestic" and "to take up arms on behalf of the United States of America"; neither of these pledges is required by persons who are born citizens. On the other hand, male citizens are required to register for Selective Service (the draft) at eighteen years of age. So there are similar expectations, even though no explicit oath is taken.

6. The main question we address in this essay is whether citizenship is a morally relevant criterion for determining *eligibility* for transplantation. Eligibility is, of course, quite a different notion from *entitlement*. No one is actually entitled to organs, even if they are desperately sick. One may be entitled to many things as a result of one's legal status, but organs are not one of them.

7. We are grateful to one of our anonymous reviewers for reminding us that the concept of desert is embedded in any discussion of access to organs.

8. J. Dwyer, "Illegal Immigrants, Health Care and Social Responsibility," *Hastings Center Report* 34 (2004): 34–41.

9. V. Ryckaert, "Set to Die, Inmate Asks to Give Liver to His Sister, *Indianapolis Star*, May 12, 2005. The inmate, Gregory Scott Johnson, was executed on May 25, 2005. The Indiana governor denied the request to donate but on narrow grounds that medical contraindications precluded the donation. For more on this case, see <http://www.bioethics.iu.edu/deathrow.html>. See also U.S. Department of Justice, Federal Bureau of Prisons, Program Statement: Patient Care, HSD/HPB P6031.01, January 15, 2005, Section 38: Organ Donation by Inmates and Section 39: Inmates as Recipients of Organ Transplants, <http://www.bop.gov//policy/progstat/6031–001.pdf>.

10. Dwyer, "Illegal Immigrants," 38.

11. Ibid.

12. David Resnick, "The Jesica Santillan Tragedy: Lessons Learned," *Hastings Center Report* 33 (2003): 15–20.

13. J. F. Childress, "Ethical Criteria for Procuring and Distributing Organs for Transplantation," in *Organ Transplantation Policy: Issues and Prospects*, ed. James F. Blumstein and Frank A. Sloan (Durham, N.C.: Duke University Press, 1996), 87–113.

14. J. Prottas, "Nonresident Aliens and Access to Organ Transplantation," *Transplantation Proceedings* 21 (3) (1989): 3426–29.

15. We thank our colleague Richard Gunderman for posing this challenge.

16. D. Davis, "Organ Transplants, Foreign Nationals, and the Free Rider Problem," *Theoretical Medicine* 13 (1992): 337–47.

17. J. Nickel, "Should Undocumented Aliens Be Entitled to Health Care?" *Hastings Center Report* 16 (1986): 19–23.

18. K. Pallarito, "Bridging the Gap: Health Care Reform and Illegal Aliens," *Modern Health Care* 4 (1994): 24–33.

19. O. Jonasson, "In Organ Transplants, Americans First?" *Hastings Center Report* 19 (1986): 24–25.

20. "Report Claims Duke Violated Transplant Laws: Interpretation Of UNOS Requirements For 'Non-Resident' Patients Under Scrutiny," March 4, 2003, WRAL.com, <http://www.wral.com/news/2018036/detail.html> (accessed March 8, 2005).

21. N. Jecker and E. M. Meslin, "United States and Canadian Approaches to Justice in Health Care: A Comparative Analysis of Health Care Systems and Values," *Theoretical Medicine* 15 (1994): 181–200.

22. D. K. Martin and E. M. Meslin, "The Give and Take of Organ Procurement," *Journal of Medicine and Philosophy* 19 (1994): 61–78.

23. R. G. Newman, *National Study of Charity Care Services in U.S. Hospitals* (Ann Arbor: UMI Dissertation Services, 1994).

24. American Medical Association, *Code of Medical Ethics* (New York: Willow Wood & Company, 1847), 93, 105–6.

25. C. Montesquieu, *The Spirit of Laws*, trans. T. Nugent, rev. J. V. Prichard (Chicago: Encyclopedia Britannica, 1952).

26. I. Kant, *The Science of Right*, trans. W. Hastie (Chicago: Encyclopedia Britannica, 1952).

27. Newman, *National Study of Charity Care Services.*

28. We are grateful to Richard Gunderman for sharing his perspectives on this issue, many of which were discussed in a lecture, "Donation and Human Excellence," delivered to the Health Related Philanthropy Study Group at Indiana University–Purdue University Indianapolis in March 2004.

29. Indiana University Center for Bioethics (IUCB), "Health Related Philanthropy: The Donation of the Body (and Parts Thereof)," vol. 1, Final Report of the Health Related Philanthropy Study Group, December 2004, <http://www.bioethics.iu.edu/pubstudy.html>; IUCB, "Health Related Philanthropy: The Donation of the Body (and Parts Thereof)," vol. 2, Survey on Health-Related Philanthropy in the United States, Summary of Methods and Findings, June 2004, <http://www.bioethics.iu.edu/HRP survey.pdf>.

30. "Report Claims Duke Violated Transplantation Laws."

31. J. Molter, "Duke University Hospital Announces Fund to Honor Jesica Santillan," <http://dukemednews.duke.edu/news/article.php?id=6556> (accessed March 2, 2005).

32. Ibid.

33. United Network of Organ Sharing, Policy 6 § 3: Transplantation of Non-Resident

Aliens," <www.unos.org/policiesandbylaws/policies/docs/policy—18.doc> (accessed March 8, 2005).

34. We characterize "altruism" as a moral *attitude* of concern for the welfare of others or selflessness, whereas "philanthropy" is altruistic *activity* engaged in by individuals or organizations to increase human well-being.

35. T. L. Beauchamp and J. F. Childress, *Principles of Biomedical Ethics*, 5th ed. (New York: Oxford University Press, 2001).

36. Nickel, "Should Undocumented Aliens Be Entitled to Health Care?"

37. L. B. McCullough, "Commentary: Psychosocial and Citizenship Status of Patients Needing Transplant," *Cambridge Quarterly in Health Care Ethics* 4 (1996): 236–38.

38. "Undocumented Immigrants in U.S. Donate More Organs Than They Receive," *Transplant Week*, March 9, 2003, <www.transplantweek.org/members/Vol14?News/041001.htm> (accessed March 8, 2005).

39. P. Devlin, *The Enforcement of Morals* (New York: Oxford University Press, 1957).

40. T. Caulfield, L. Knowles, and E. M. Meslin, "Law and Policy in the Era of Reproductive Genetics," *Journal of Medical Ethics* 30 (2004): 414–17.

41. D. Orentlicher, *Matters of Life and Death: Making Moral Theory Work in Medical Ethics and the Law* (Princeton: Princeton University Press, 2001).

42. Organ Procurement and Transplantation Network (OPTN), data as of March 24, 2006, from <http://www.optn.org/latestData/advanceddata.asp>.

IMAGINING THE NATION,

IMAGINING DONOR RECIPIENTS

JESICA SANTILLAN AND THE

PUBLIC DISCOURSE OF BELONGING

LEO R. CHAVEZ

By what mechanisms, precisely, do social forces ranging from poverty to racism become embodied *as individual experience?*—*Paul Farmer,* Pathologies of Power, 2003

Jesica Santillan's story is simple but tragic: Jesica, seventeen years old, suffered from a birth defect that left her heart and lungs unable to function properly. Her only chance for survival was a transplant to replace the defective organs. She underwent surgery at Duke University Medical Center on February 7, 2003.[1] Tragically, the transplanted organs were of a different blood type from Jesica's.[2] Doctors quickly found new organs and transplanted those into Jesica's body, but it was too late. Jesica's brain had experienced too much damage. Jesica died on February 22, 2003.[3]

By the time of her death, and most surely after, Jesica came to embody more than the tragedy of an untimely death. Jesica's body came to signify a national tragedy, the nature of which has come to be refracted in many ways, as the multifaceted topics in this book indicate. As an allegory of contemporary U.S. immigration and medical history, Jesica's story is now a part of our history, and, as such, I am reminded of Walter Benjamin's apt observation that "History dissolves into images." The image left behind by Jesica's story can be read at various levels. At the denotive level, there are the basic elements in the brief overview of Jesica's story given above.[4] But there is a more complex level, that of connotation, where messages about social and cultural values, narratives, myths, commonsense, and ideologies abound, often in contestation and in competition for primacy.

It is at this more meaningful level of connotation that Jesica's story must be read, for it is here that we find that Jesica's is a story within a story. The larger narrative in which Jesica's tragic tale is embedded is about immigration, about differing perceptions of who is an American, and about the alleged threat posed by some immigrants, particularly Mexicans, to the United States. Only by reading the Santillan saga in relation to this other story can we begin to make sense of what happened, not in biomedical terms but in cultural, social, and political terms.

Jesica and her parents are Mexicans. They were living in Mexico, in 2000, when Jesica's parents decided to bring Jesica to the United States in order to find a way to get Jesica the organ transplants she needed in order to live. Apparently, lacking documents to enter the United States legally, Jesica and her mother crossed into the United States clandestinely with the aid of a coyote, or smuggler. At the time of her transplant, Jesica may have had a humanitarian visa because of her illness,[5] but her immigration status is unclear. It was her original status as an "illegal alien" that carried great currency in the many iterations of her story before and after her death.

Jesica's story is about a Mexican, about an "illegal immigrant," about a sick and dying girl in need of an organ transplant, about medical malfeasance, and about an unnecessary death. But her story is also a window through which we can examine the larger public debate over immigration in general, and Mexican immigration in particular. At the same time, Jesica's experiences, and the public opinion surrounding her case, act as a mirror that reflects the struggles of Americans to reconceptualize what it means to be American in a period of rapid demographic change. In this mirror metaphor, Jesica's story tells us less about Mexican immigrants and more about attitudes among some vocal members of U.S. society. Are organ transplants one of those benefits of citizenship that must be protected? Should persons not in the country legally be allowed to receive organ transplants at all? Should noncitizens only receive an organ transplant after any citizen who needs one? Or as one headline for an article on Jesica put it, "Organ Donation: Should National Origin Matter?"[6]

The Santillan case forces us to reflect on issues of belonging, of legitimacy, and the rewards of membership in the community or nation.[7] For it is here that we observe the biopolitics surrounding citizenship that are so essential to the representations of Jesica Santillan, and that help us to begin to answer Paul Farmer's question at the beginning of this chapter: How did Jesica's individual experiences come to embody debates over citizenship and foreigners, membership in the nation and threats to the nation? By exploring this question, the linking of the biological/body and privileges of citizens take on new meanings, a new biocitizen construction.[8] Benedict Anderson argues that members of modern nations cannot possibly know all their fellow members, and yet "in the minds of each lives the image of their communion. . . . It is imagined as a community, because, regardless of the actual inequality and exploitation that may prevail in each, the nation is always conceived as a deep, horizontal comradeship."[9] However, Jesica, like other "illegal" immigrants, are typically outside the imagined community of the nation, which is underscored by the controversy over organs for immigrants.[10]

Jesica's organ transplants bring into focus the often taken-for-granted assumption that there exists, or should exist, a queue for organ transplants and that citizens should have priority over organs donated by co-nationals. According to the United Network for Organ Sharing (UNOS), transplant centers must provide no more than 5 percent of organ transplants to foreign nationals.[11] In 2002, foreign nationals received 936 of the 22,709 (4.1 percent) organ transplants performed in the United States.[12] In addition, the federal government some time ago discontinued reimbursing hospitals for organ transplants for undocumented immigrants.[13] The queue exists, and at the back of that queue, as much of the public opinion indicates, should be people like Jesica, Mexican undocumented immigrants.

I argue here that the public opinion that surfaced around Jesica's organ transplants must be examined within a national discourse that constructs Mexican immigrants, especially undocumented Mexican immigrants, as a threat to the nation. The construction of "the Mexican illegal immigrant as threat" does not occur in one statement alone but through repetitive statements in various contexts in public discourse. As Judith Butler has observed, the signification attached to bodies, such as Jesica's, "must be understood not as a singular or deliberate 'act,' but, rather as the reiterative and citational practice by which discourse produces the effects that it names."[14] Central to the construction of Jesica and "people like her" are a set of essential binary oppositions that work to establish that she is outside the culturally imagined membership of the nation, that is, she is a "them" rather than a "we," and thus undeserving of benefits, such as organs, reserved as a privilege of membership in the "we." The analysis that follows calls attention to the binary oppositions in the cultural construction of Jesica Santillan.

NATION/THREAT TO THE NATION

The structural oppositions or essential binaries that are so central to the public discourse surrounding the Jesica Santillan case did not just appear suddenly after Jesica's surgeries. They are drawn from a larger national discourse on immigration and, more specifically, on the construction of Mexican immigration as a threat to the nation.[15] For example, a veritable publishing industry has emerged to play to the public's fears of immigration, especially from Mexico. Among the many books on the topic that have appeared since the early 1990s are Peter Brimelow's *Alien Nation*, Arthur Schlesinger's *The Disuniting of America*, Georgie Anne Geyer's *Americans No More*, Patrick J. Buchanan's *The Death of the West*, and Victor Davis Hanson's *Mexifornia*.[16]

Harvard professor Samuel P. Huntington warned about the threat to the nation posed by Mexican-origin people in the United States in an article in the *American Enterprise* magazine in 2000, just three years before Jesica's operation and death: "The invasion of over 1 million Mexican civilians is a comparable threat (as 1 million Mexican soldiers) to American societal security, and Americans should react against it with comparable vigor. Mexican immigration looms as a unique and disturbing challenge to our cultural integrity, our national identity, and potentially to our future as a country."[17]

Jesica's presence was framed not just by the rhetoric of such a well-placed scholar warning about the invasion of Mexicans but by the rapid growth in the immigrant population in North Carolina since the late 1980s.[18] Between 1990 and 2000, the number of foreign-born residents in North Carolina increased from 115,077 to 430,000, representing a 273.7 percent change.[19] North Carolina ranked number one in terms of the percent of change in a state's foreign-born population from 1990 to 2000.[20] About 40 percent of the foreign-born in North Carolina were born in Mexico, and 53 percent were of Latin American origin.[21] The Latino population in North Carolina is less likely than other groups to have medical insurance, and their health issues are "consistent with the fact that they are a very young, mainly recently arrived immigrant population with more males than females."[22] With a median age of twenty-four in 2000, Latinos in North Carolina were much younger than the median age of thirty-five for the state's total population.[23] North Carolina, then, as one of the "new" destinations for Mexican immigrants in the post-1990s period, suddenly found itself in a situation with which it had little experience.

As headline in the *Washington Post* announced in 2000, the year Jesica and her family moved to North Carolina, "Hispanic Immigration Boom Rattles South: Rapid Influx to Some Areas Raises Tensions."[24] The article focused on North Carolina and the economic demand for entry-level workers, especially in poultry production, in an economy with just 2 percent unemployment at the time. Immigrants, particularly from Mexico, responded to the labor demand. Rather than facing the stereotypical black/white construction of ethnic relations, North Carolina suddenly had to learn to relate to Mexican, other

Latin American, and Asian immigrants. As one observer (a researcher at a Chapel Hill think tank) commented to the *Post*, "In the South, we're in the situation where what is basically a biracial community that was dealing with issues of prejudice has now become a multiracial community." A resident of Siler City, forty miles west of Raleigh, complained in the same article that his city was becoming "Little Mexico": "I don't want to say anything against anybody, but hey they just came in and took over." Another resident noted, "And these new people are not white Anglo-Saxons, which makes it harder, because after all, this is still the south." An article titled "Pockets of Protest Are Rising Against Immigration" appeared in the *New York Times* a year later, and it also focused on the tensions in North Carolina as a result of the rapid demographic changes related to immigration, especially from Mexico.[25]

Consequently, conditions were ripe for alarmist views of immigration to become associated with Jesica Santillan's presence in North Carolina and her organ transplants. However, the construction of Jesica ("the illegal immigrant") as a threat to medical resources for citizens and to the nation in general was built on more than thirty years of alarmist media representations of Mexicans and Mexican Americans. My research on national magazine covers and their accompanying articles found that the alarm has been conveyed through images and text that directly or metaphorically invoke crisis in the form of time bombs, invasion, reconquest, floods, war, and border breakdown.[26] For example, in December of 1974, the cover of the *American Legion Magazine* depicted the United States being overrun by "illegal aliens."[27] Most of those pictured were Mexicans storming the U.S.-Mexico border and inundating the nation's institutions, most notably welfare and those providing education and medical aid. Images like this became more frequent on the nation's magazines over the next three decades and contributed to the alarmist discourse on Mexican immigration.

On July 4, 1977, *U.S. News & World Report*'s cover also focused attention on Mexican immigration. The cover's text reads: "TIME BOMB IN MEXICO: Why There'll Be No End To the Invasion of 'Illegals.'" In my systematic examination of ten national magazines from 1965 to the end of 1999, this is the first instance in which the word "invasion" appeared on one of the magazine covers. This signalled a noteworthy escalation in the alarmist discourse on Mexican immigration. "Invasion" carries with it many connotations, none of them friendly or indicating mutual benefit. Friends do not invade; enemies invade.

The invasion metaphor evokes a sense of crisis related to an attack on the sovereign territory of the nation. Invasion is an act of war, and it puts the

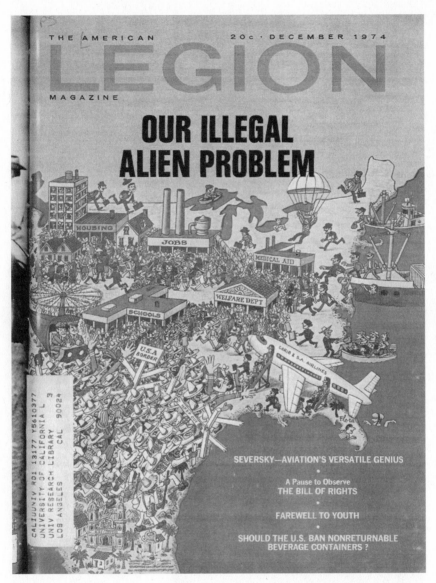

CALIUNIV R01 13177 Y5610377
UNIVERSITY OF CALIFORNIA L
UNIV RESEARCH LIBRARY 3
LOS ANGELES CAL 90024

The United States being overrun—an alarmist depiction of Mexican "invasion" on the cover of *American Legion Magazine*, December 1974. Illustration by James Flora. © The Estate of James Flora. Used by permission of the family of James Flora.

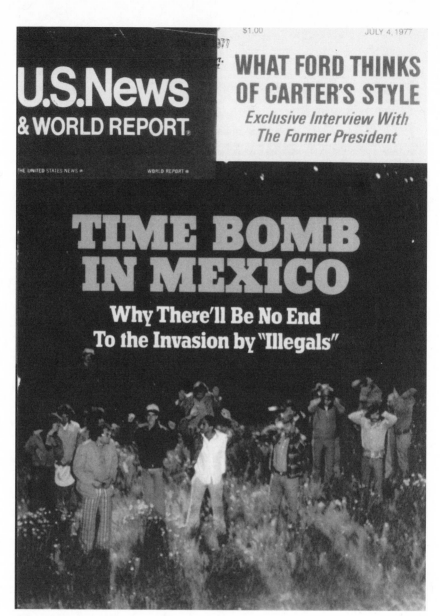

The cover of the July 4, 1977, issue of *U.S. News & World Report* portraying a nation at severe risk.

nation and its people at great risk. Exactly what the nation risks by this invasion is not articulated in the image's message. The war metaphor is enhanced by the prominence of the words "Time Bomb." The text conjures up an image of Mexico as the bomb that, when it explodes, will severely damage the United States. This damage, the message makes clear, will be the unstoppable flow of illegal immigrants to the United States.

Featuring immigrant women on the covers of national magazines, as did the *U.S. News & World Report* on March 7, 1983, and *Newsweek* on June 25, 1984, while warning of an "invasion" also sends a clear message about fertility and reproduction. Such images did not suggest an invading army, or even the stereotypical male migrant worker, but a more insidious invasion, one that includes the capacity of the invaders to reproduce themselves. Such images, and their accompanying articles, allude to issues of population growth and the use of prenatal care, children's health services, schools, and other social and medical services. Two decades later, Jesica's transplants would also be embedded in this broader discourse of invasion and depletion of medical resources.

A decade before Mexicans such as Jesica and her family began arriving in significant numbers in North Carolina, the media were raising the alarm about demographic changes occurring as Latin Americans and Asians became a majority of the nation's immigrants.[28] At the same time, the fertility of the native U.S. population, especially that of whites, began declining dramatically.[29] Around the late 1980s, the phrase "the browning of America" came into usage to describe such demographic changes. *Time* magazine described these changes in ways that dramatically underscore the binary of legitimate/ not legitimate members of society: "The 'browning of America' will alter everything in society, from politics and education to industry, values and culture. . . . The deeper significance of America becoming a majority non-white society is what it means to the national psyche, to individuals' sense of themselves and the nation—their idea of what it is to be American. . . . White Americans are accustomed to thinking of themselves as the very picture of their nation."[30]

In addition to the many such examples of the "Mexican immigrants as threat" narrative in national magazines, anti-immigrant images also became readily available on the Internet. The first of two examples that I have included here echoes the theme of Mexican immigration as an invasion; the second portrays undocumented immigrants as a burden on taxpayers because of their use of welfare and medical care.

The threat of Mexican immigrants, including undocumented immigrants

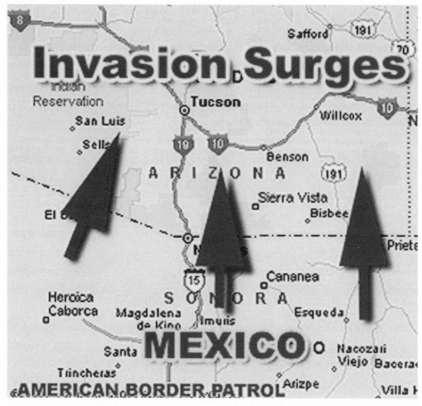

An Internet image (from the American Border Patrol Web site) portrays a surging invasion at the Arizona border.

such as Jesica Santillan, would again become the subject of an article by Samuel Huntington in 2004, this one in *Foreign Policy* appearing one year after Jesica's death. "In this new era," Huntington wrote, "the single most immediate and most serious challenge to America's traditional identity comes from the immense and continuing immigration from Latin America, especially from Mexico, and the fertility rates of those immigrants compared to black and white American natives."[31] Given the historical context, the description of Mexican immigrants as the "single most immediate challenge to America's traditional identity" is curious. At the time, the United States was still engaged in combat in Iraq, Al Qaeda maintained an international terrorist network, and Osama Bin Laden remained at large, as did many of his senior operatives. And yet Mexican immigrants, who primarily come to work in the United States under difficult social and political conditions, were labelled the greatest threat to the nation by many. The recent Minuteman

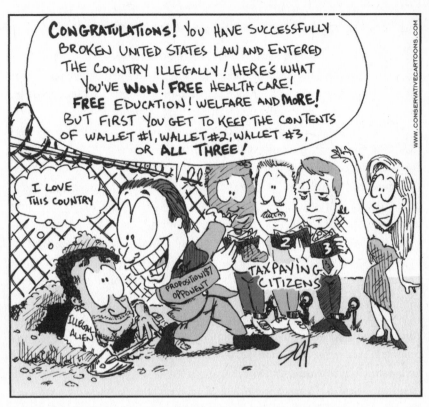

In the midst of heated debate over California's Proposition 187 in the mid-1990s, cartoonist Jim Huber caricatured "illegal aliens" as reaping free services and generous access to the wallets of "taxpaying citizens." Used by permission of the artist.

Project, enlisting citizens to conduct surveillance along the U.S.-Mexico border in Arizona, became a logical consequence of this construction of Mexican immigration as an "invasion."

The controversy over Jesica Santillan's organ transplants was swept up into this decades-long maelstrom of anti-Mexican immigration rhetoric. Mexican immigration had long been associated with narratives of threat, danger, invasion, and depletion of social services, including medical services. In February 2003, these grand narratives were readily available to apply to local events and people, such as Jesica Santillan and her organ transplants in North Carolina.

A Google search of the Santillan case on the Internet results in a rich array of public opinion. These views can be separated into two broad categories. First, one finds reactions of outrage over the medical incompetence that led to Jesica receiving organs of a mismatched blood type, which resulted in her death. Second, one finds reactions that revolve around and question the very idea that she received donated organs in the first place. It is this second category of reactions that concern me here.

Before the transplants, Jesica was portrayed in positive terms, as an "Angel" in dire medical straits requiring an organ transplant to avoid death at a young age, but this portrait soon changed.[32] The first hint that Jesica's organ transplant would become a touchstone in the political debate over immigration appeared shortly after her first transplant operation and just two days before she died. On February 20, 2003, Michelle Malkin published an article titled "America: Medical Welcome Mat to the World" on vdare.com, a Web site supported by the Center for American Unity.[33] In addition to writing such columns, Malkin was known as the author of the book *Invasion: How America Still Welcomes Terrorists, Criminals, and Other Foreign Menaces to Our Shores*,[34] and, according to Amazon.com, has appeared as a commentator on a wide range of programs, including on *Fox News*, on talk radio shows, on c-span's *Washington Journal*, and on the *McLaughlin Group*, ABC's *20/20*, and MSNBC. For Malkin, Jesica became an example of the undeserving "illegal" immigrants coming to America to take from deserving citizens. She questioned the appropriateness of Jesica receiving an organ transplant because of her immigration status and the cost to the health care system of providing follow-up care (she was still alive at the time). Although Jesica's mother's health insurance and a charity fund set up for Jesica paid for her operation (making Jesica's case highly atypical among uninsured undocumented immigrants), Malkin nevertheless questioned who would be responsible for expensive long-term care after the operation. The article emphasized the burden placed on hospitals, arguing that closures would result from their providing unreimbursed medical care for undocumented immigrants. The author raised the question of deportation, asking, "Will any federal immigration authority have the guts to enforce the law and send her and her family back home to Mexico."[35]

At the core of Malkin's case against Jesica receiving an organ transplant is the image of U.S. citizens as legitimate potential organ recipients who may not have received organs because Jesica did. (Of course, as the essay by Eric Meslin et al. has noted, in 2001, twice the number of undocumented Hispanics *donated* organs as *received* organs.) "According to national figures," Malkin wrote, using a more stark, nativist calculus, "16 patients die in the United States each day while waiting for a potentially life-saving transplant operation. How many American patients currently on the national organ waiting list were denied access to healthy hearts and lungs as a result of Santillan's two transplant surgeries? Who will tell their stories?"[36] Because of her national profile, Malkin's article would be cited in later articles concerned about the Jesica Santillan case.[37]

CITIZENS/FOREIGNERS, LEGITIMATE/ILLEGITIMATE

On March 6, 2003, Joe Kovacs published an article on WorldNetDaily.com that elaborated on the core issues in Malkin's article: Jesica's immigration status and U.S. citizens who must wait for organs. The article carried the titled "Coming to America: Transplants for Illegals Igniting U.S. Firestorm," with the subtitle "Case of Smuggled Mexican Teen-ager Prompting Public to Cry 'Citizens First,'" and focused on the story of Lauren Averitt, a young woman waiting anxiously for a lung transplant.[38] Lauren bore a certain resemblance to Jesica (at least in the photograph accompanying the article), and their stories converge at many points. Both were in desperate need of organ transplants. They shared the same blood type. And they had North Carolina in common; Lauren was born there, Jesica died there. The author, Kovacs, noted, "What's different about Lauren . . . is that no one smuggled her across the border to get her on a waiting list for new organs. She was born here in the United States in Wilmington, N.C., and now lives in South Carolina."[39]

Kovacs further emphasized that Jesica received her transplant before Lauren, which, in his view, subverted the natural order of things, citizens first, foreigners last: "The significance of such geographical disparity has sparked a firestorm of controversy across the continent, with many Americans venting outrage at how illegal aliens like Jesica are able to leap ahead of the many thousands of U.S. citizens patiently waiting and praying for their own personal miracle."[40] The article on Lauren (and Jesica) not-so-subtly drew upon the binaries of citizen/foreigner, legal/illegal, deserving/undeserving to make its points. Through such binary constructions, Lauren and Jesica came to embody opposing icons in the polarized debate over immigration.

A final example underscores the dichotomy between citizen and illegal alien. On May 31, 2003, Peter Brimelow weighed in on the Santillan controversy in an article appearing on the Web site vdare.com.[41] A restrictionist well known in the immigration debate because of his book *Alien Nation*,[42] Brime-

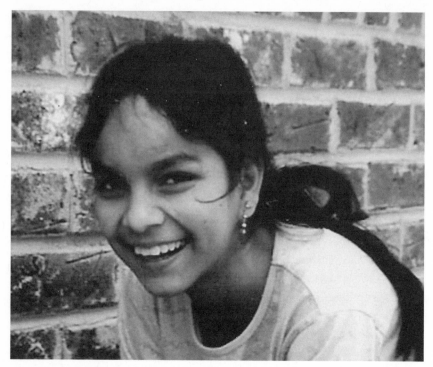

Jesica Santillan, whose "bungled" transplant in 2003 became a touchstone for broader debates about medical error, justice, and fairness in medicine and transplantation, and the American debate over immigration. Photograph used by permission of Mack Mahoney, founder, Jesica's Hope Chest Foundation.

low made his position clear in the title of this article: "That Santillan Saga: Lies, Damned Lies, Immigration Enthusiasts and Neosocialist Health Bureaucrats." He summed up the main point of the article this way: "The truth, of course, is that privileged access, paid for by Americans, was the subtext of the entire Santillan Saga. More than 75,000 Americans are on the federal transplant waiting list. Only 24,000 organs are available each year. Each year, while on the waiting list, more than 5,300 people die. So why give any organs at all to someone who is in the U.S. illegally?" Brimelow further insisted that the barriers to medical care experienced by Latinos are self-created: "Doesn't the 'Latino community' face these 'barriers' because they've chosen to immigrate to an English-speaking country—to a significant extent, in violation of that country's laws?"[43]

Another Web site put it even more bluntly. The top of the Web page reads: "Keep American organs in Americans!" under which there is an image of a

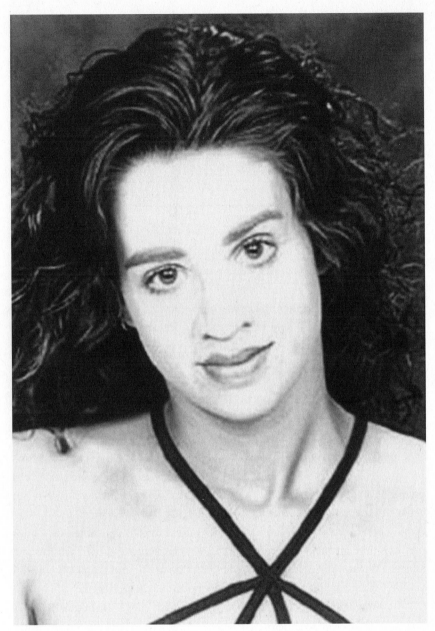

By contrast with the Santillan transplant story, Lauren Averitt's desperate need for a transplant was portrayed as the story of a deserving citizen. Photograph used by permission of WorldNetDaily.com.

Former Organic Donor Card

Sorry, but nobody made sure my organs would be used on FREE U.S. CITIZENS. So I'm taking them with me.

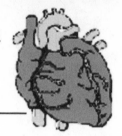

Name   Date

In response to the Santillan story, one Web site image angrily proposes a "Former Organ Donor Card" that insists that organs should only go to "Free U.S. Citizens."

beating heart, and under that is another caption that reads, "Where are *YOUR* organs going?" The text states: "To let an American die so some foreign national illegally in the country, or some convict behind bars can get the organ or organs needed to live, it is nothing more than an act of TREASON!" (emphasis in original).[44] The same Web site shows examples of donor cards specifically stating that the organs are for citizens only.

Some North Carolina residents also appeared to view Jesica and her transplants from the vantage point of citizen versus foreigner, "us" versus "them." One sixty-five-year old woman told the Raleigh *News and Observer* that she was reconsidering being an organ donor after hearing that Jesica and her family paid a smuggler to get them into the country. She would "prefer that her organs go only to U.S. citizens. 'I definitely do not want them to go to an illegal alien,' [she was quoted as saying]. 'I don't think they should be able to come in here and take our hospital and our medicine and turn around and sue us.'"[45] Another local resident quoted in the article made a similar observation, "Why were organs given to someone who is here illegally?"[46]

Of course, this discourse of citizen/foreigner/illegal immigrant masks the racial discourse discussed in Susan Lederer's essay in this book. Organ transplantation combines body parts from different people across crucial lines of difference. While not explicit in this discourse on immigration, this "transmogrification" may be an underlying subtext fueling racial/ethnic tensions in the Santillan case.

One of the perhaps unavoidable consequences of the publicity surrounding Jesica Santillan's organ transplants and death was that her life was reduced to that of icon, that is, she became "the Mexican immigrant" subject in the long-running debate over immigration in American public discourse. Jesica's story took on almost mythical proportions as it became a sounding board for views on current immigration patterns. Her story, despite the many complexities unearthed by the essays in this volume, dissolved into a number of structural oppositions, or essential binaries:

> belonging/not belonging
> us/them
> inside the nation/outside the nation
> English speaker/non-English speaker
> citizen/noncitizen
> native/foreigner
> legal immigrant/illegal immigrant
> deserving/undeserving
> transplant/no transplant
> life/death

Difference is constructed through such binary oppositions. Importantly, the terms in these binaries are not equal, but they exist in a power relationship such that one term is dominant and the other subordinate, one positive and one negative, one normal and one pathological.[47] These binaries help construct Jesica and other immigrants in her position as unacceptable members of society, as "space invaders," as Nirmal Puwar has put it.[48] Mary Douglas pointed out in her seminal work *Purity and Danger* that that which is out of place is often considered dangerous, as pollution, threatening the purity of those in place, that is, in their "proper" category.[49] Once constructed through such essentializing binaries, difference, in this particular case, is readily represented as a threat to Americans who die waiting for organs taken by people like Jesica (now metonymically representing a class of people, "illegal aliens") and as a threat to the health care system that their presence undermines. Jesica became a symbol of society's "Others," who are, as Michel Foucault notes, "for a given culture, at once interior and foreign, therefore to be excluded (so as to exorcise their interior danger)."[50]

Jesica Santillan's organ transplants occurred within the context of the often vitriolic debate over Mexican immigration. Her medical condition and need for organs to save her life became mired in discussions of her very presence in this country. She was portrayed as a threat to citizens who may have died because she received organs. Although Jesica's medical condition made her a humanitarian transnational citizen deserving of compassion and U.S. medical intervention, her nationality and immigration status made her an illegitimate donor recipient in the eyes of many. Jesica became a symbol of the threats to the nation posed by Mexican immigration, and her story raised all-too-familiar questions: Why is she here? How do citizens suffer because she is here? Who pays for her health care? Such questions underscore the difficulty of imagining Jesica as one of "us," a difficulty that was perhaps exacerbated by the fact that Jesica and her family were essentially voiceless in the entire affair (see the essay by Morgan et al. in this book). Jesica and her family were typically spoken for (in particular by Mack Mahoney, who became Jesica's benefactor) and about (in the press by reporters, pundits, medical practitioners, and a concerned public).

What is lost, or put aside, in this construction of Jesica Santillan as the prototypical "illegal alien," noncitizen, undeserving of citizen organs? Binaries are important for understanding identity constructions, but they do not reflect the complexity of lives "on the ground." The ambiguity and nuance of lived lives get lost in the construction of types in a social drama such as that surrounding Jesica. For one thing, Latinos are born in many different places; they differ in terms of national backgrounds, education levels, and gender, and in many other aspects of their lives. They are not reducible to simple citizen/noncitizen, insider/outsider binaries. Undocumented immigrants often find ways to become legal residents. Their children, if born in the United States, are automatically citizens. Jesica herself was not the prototypical "illegal immigrant seeking medical care" in that her mother had medical insurance and she had a fund set up to help meet her medical expenses. The fund was set up by a local citizen (Mack Mahoney) and contributed to by other local residents, blurring the sharp division between citizens and immigrants.

Left unexamined are the problems immigrants face when trying to obtain medical care, as Beatrix Hoffman's essay in this book details. For example, legal immigrants face obstacles to obtaining medical care and other social services as a result of the 1996 welfare reform laws, while undocumented immigrants are routinely denied most nonemergency medical services and programs.[51] Immigrants are less likely to be employed in occupations that provide private medical insurance. With access to nonemergency care difficult and without insurance, immigrants have little recourse but to pursue costly emergency-room service, which further exacerbates public animosities to their presence. Even with evidence suggesting that immigrants may provide more organs than they receive, and that Latinos in North Carolina are among the most likely groups to donate a family member's organs (about 78 percent of Latinos during the first six months of 2002, compared with 62 percent for other groups), there is still alarmist controversy over immigrants such as Jesica receiving organs.[52] Such public opinion, ignited by cases such as Jesica's, makes improving access to medical care for immigrants politically difficult.

Barely on the radar screen are discussions of the ethical issues related to medical care that Eric Meslin, Karen Salmon, and Jason Eberl speak about in their essay in this book. For instance, Jesica's case reflects how the rights and privileges of citizenship can be narrowly defined. But what about human rights and medical care?[53] Are there rights to lifesaving medical care that exist in a shared humanity, outside of citizenship defined in narrow legalistic terms?[54] Giorgio Agamben, in his book *Homo Sacer*, pointed to this conflict between citizen rights and human rights: "In the system of the nation-state, the so-called sacred and inalienable rights of man show themselves to lack every protection and reality at the moment in which they can no longer take the form of rights belonging to citizens of the state."[55] Unfortunately, alarmist discourse constructs Jesica, a Mexican immigrant with medical needs, in such a way that there is little space for broader considerations of human rights. Indeed, such considerations are anathema for many. Biocitizenship, as examined here, means that some members of society (immigrants such as Jesica) are less valued than others (citizens).[56]

NOTES

An earlier draft of this essay was presented at the conference "Beyond the Bungled Transplant—Jesica Santillan and High Tech Medicine in Cultural Perspective," organized by Keith Wailoo, Peter Guarnaccia, and Julie Livingston, at Rutgers University, New Brunswick, New Jersey, June 11–12, 2004. The final version benefited greatly from comments by the conference participants and later comments by Peter Guarnaccia. I am also indebted to Juliet McMullin, Mei Zhan, and Cathy Ota for their readings and suggestions.

1. Denise Grady, "Donor Mix-Up Leaves Girl, 17, Fighting for Life," *New York Times*, February 19, 2003.

2. Linda Villarosa, "Jesica Was One of 80,000 on Organ Waiting List," *New York Times*, February 19, 2003.

3. Randal C. Archibold, "Girl in Transplant Mix-Up Dies after Two Weeks," *New York Times*, February 23, 2003.

4. Walter Benjamin, *Illuminations* (New York: Harcourt, Brace and World, 1955); Roland Barthes, *Mythologies* (London: Cape, 1972); Stuart Hall, *Representation: Cultural Representations and Signifying Practices* (Thousand Oaks, Calif.: Sage Publications, 1997).

5. Kimberley Jane Wilson, "Transplant Details Raise Cruel Questions," published by the National Center for Public Policy Research, April 2003, <http://www.nationalcenter.org/P21NVWilsonOrgans403.html> (accessed May 4, 2004).

6. Brian Carnell, "Organ Donation: Should National Origin Matter?" February 24, 2003, <http://brian.carnell.com/articles/2003/02/000017.html> (accessed May 4, 2004).

7. Timothy J. Dunn, Ana Maria Aragones, and George Shivers, "Recent Mexican Migration in the Rural Delmarva Peninsula: Human Rights Verses Citizenship Rights in a Local Context," in *New Destinations: Mexican Immigration in the United States*, ed. Victor Zuniga and Ruben Hernandez-Leon (New York: Russell Sage Foundation, 2005), 155–83; Aiwha Ong, *Buddha Is Hiding: Refugees, Citizenship, the New America* (Berkeley: University of California Press, 2003); Raymond Rocco, "Transforming Citizenship: Membership, Strategies of Containment, and the Public Sphere in Latino Communities," *Latino Studies* 2 (1) (2004): 4–25; Gideon Sjoberg, Elizabeth A. Gill, and Norma Williams, "A Sociology of Human Rights," *Social Problems* 48 (2001): 11–47.

8. Adriana Petryna, *Life Exposed: Biological Citizens after Chernobyl* (Princeton: Princeton University Press, 2002).

9. Benedict Anderson, *Imagined Communities* (London: Verso, 1983), 15–16.

10. Leo R. Chavez, "Outside the Imagined Community: Undocumented Settlers and Experiences of Incorporation," *American Ethnologist* 18 (2) (1991): 257–78.

11. Carnell, "Organ Donation."

12. Ibid.

13. Siskind's Immigration Bulletin, "Duke Case Raises Questions About Transplants for Immigrants," March 9, 2003, www.visalaw.com/03mar1/9mar103.html (accessed May 4, 2004).

14. Judith Butler, *Bodies That Matter: On the Discursive Limits of "Sex"* (New York: Routledge, 1993), 2.

15. Leo R. Chavez, *Covering Immigration: Popular Images and the Politics of the Nation* (Berkeley: University of California Press, 2001)

16. Peter Brimelow, *Alien Nation: Common Sense about America's Immigration Disaster* (New York: Random House, 1995); Arthur M. Schlesinger Jr., *The Disuniting of America* (New York: Norton, 1992); Georgie Ann Geyer, *Americans No More* (New York: The Atlantic Monthly Press, 1996); Patrick J. Buchanan, *The Death of the West: How Dying Populations and Immigrant Invasions Imperil Our Country and Civilization* (New York: St. Martin's Press, 2002); Victor Davis Hanson, *Mexifornia: A State of Becoming* (San Francisco: Encounter Books, 2003).

17. Samuel P. Huntington, "The Special Case of Mexican Immigration: Why Mexico Is a Problem," *American Enterprise*, December 2000, 20–22.

18. David C. Griffith, "Rural Industry and Mexican Immigration and Settlement in North Carolina," in *New Destinations: Mexican Immigration in the United States*, ed. Victor Zuniga and Ruben Hernandez-Leon (New York: Russell Sage Foundation, 2005), 50–75.

19. Migration Information Source, "Fact Sheet on the Foreign Born: North Carolina," 2005, <http://www.migrationinformation.org/USFocus/state.cfm?ID=NC> (accessed March 12, 2005).

20. Ibid.

21. Ibid.

22. Paul A. Buescher, "A Review of Available Data on the Health of the Latino Population in North Carolina," *North Carolina Medical Journal* 64 (3) (2003): 97.

23. Ibid.

24. Sue Anne Pressley, "Hispanic Immigration Boom Rattles South: Rapid Influx to Some Areas Raises Tensions," *Washington Post*, March 6, 2000, A3.

25. Eric Schmitt, "Pockets of Protest Are Rising Against Immigration," *New York Times*, August 9, 2001.

26. Chavez, *Covering Immigration*.

27. On "illegal aliens" in U.S. legal history see Mae M. Ngai, *Impossible Subjects: Illegal Aliens and the Making of Modern America* (Princeton: Princeton University Press, 2004).

28. For a discussion of immigration control in earlier historical periods, see Eithne Luibheid, *Entry Denied: Controlling Sexuality at the Border* (Minneapolis: University of Minnesota Press, 2002).

29. Leo R. Chavez, "A Glass Half Empty: Latina Reproduction and Public Discourse," *Human Organization* 63 (2) (2004):173–88.

30. "Beyond the Melting Pot," *Time*, April 9, 1990.

31. Samuel P. Huntington, "The Hispanic Challenge," *Foreign Policy*, March/April 2004, 30–45.

32. See Beatrix Hoffman's essay in this book. See also Carolyn Rouse's and Lesley Sharp's essays for a discussion of how children become symbols for organ transplantation and other innovative medical treatments.

33. Michelle Malkin, "America: Medical Welcome Mat to the World," February 20, 2003, VDARE.com, The Center for American Unity, <http://www.vdare.com/malkin/welcome—mat.htm> (accessed May 5, 2004).

34. Michelle Malkin, *Invasion: How America Still Welcomes Terrorists, Criminals, and Other Foreign Menaces to Our Shores* (Washington, D.C.: Regnery Publishing, Inc., 2002).

35. Malkin, "America."

36. Ibid.

37. See Wilson, "Transplant Details Raise Cruel Questions"; and Peter Brimelow, "That Santillan Saga: Lies, Damned Lies, Immigration Enthusiasts and Neosocialist Health Bureaucrats," May 31, 2003, VDARE.com, <http://www.vdare.com/pb/santillan.htm> (accessed February 17, 2004).

38. Joe Kovacs, "Transplants for Illegals Igniting U.S. Firestorm: Case of Smuggled Mexican Teen-ager Prompting Public to Cry 'Citizens First,'" WorldNetDaily.com, March 6, 2003, <http://worldnetdaily.com/news/printer-friendly.asp?ARTICLE—ID=31379> (accessed May 4, 2004).

39. Ibid.

40. Ibid.

41. Brimelow, "That Santillan Saga." The quotations in this paragraph are from this article.

42. Brimelow, *Alien Nation*.

43. Brimelow, "That Santillan Saga."

44. "Where are YOUR organs going?" <http://www.geocities.com/americanorgans> (accessed May 4, 2004).

45. Christina Headrick and Vicki Cheng, "Some Link Citizenship, Transplants," *News and Observer* (Raleigh, N.C.), March 4, 2003, A1.

46. Ibid.

47. Hall, *Representation*, 258.

48. Nirmal Puwar, *Space Invaders: Race, Gender and Bodies Out of Place* (New York: Berg, 2004).

49. Mary Douglas, *Purity and Danger* (London: Routledge & Kegan Paul, 1966).

50. Michel Foucault, *The Order of Things* (New York: Vintage Books, 1970), xxiv.

51. Buescher, "Review of Available Data."

52. Headrick and Cheng, "Some Link Citizenship, Transplants."

53. Paul Farmer, *Pathologies of Power: Health, Human Rights, and the New War on the Poor* (Berkeley: University of California Press, 2003).

54. Dunn, Aragones, and Shivers, "Recent Mexican Migration"; Sjoberg, Gill, and Williams, "Sociology of Human Rights."

55. Giorgio Agamben, *Homo Sacer: Sovereign Power and Bare Life*, trans. Daniel Heller-Roazen (Stanford: Stanford University Press, 1998), 126.

56. Ong, *Buddha Is Hiding*.

4

SPEAKING FOR JESICA

BABES AND BABOONS

JESICA SANTILLAN AND EXPERIMENTAL

PEDIATRIC TRANSPLANT RESEARCH IN

AMERICA

LESLEY A. SHARP

Organ transplantation within the American context is regularly proclaimed as a miraculous medical procedure, and indeed for many patients
with life-threatening illness it can offer a remarkable extension of life. Bearing the potential to save, and thus enhance or extend individual lives, the
transplant miracle nevertheless depends on radical surgical interventions. In
anticipation of organ replacement, anesthetized patients must enter the operating theater, where their natal hearts and lungs, for instance, are removed,
their vital functions temporarily bridged by complex apparati until their surgeons can implant newly acquired parts. When transplantation is viewed in
this manner, it does in fact seem miraculous that annually, tens of thousands
of patients survive such procedures, their lives prolonged by days, months,
and even decades as a result of full organ replacement. These facts are even
more astounding when we consider that many of these patients are children.[1]

Our willingness to accept organ transplantation as an increasingly routine
procedure stems from a cultural imperative that biomedical expertise must
include the ability to repair breakdowns in fragile human bodies. Therefore,
medicine bears the promise of extending human lives, or, as it is commonly
phrased within the transplant arena itself, granting "second lives" or "re-
births" to organ recipients. When patients suffering from organ failure are
adults, surgical outcomes are assumed to bear additional promises associated
with longevity: these include greater mobility and, in turn, enhanced economic productivity.

An altogether different set of concerns emerge, however, when the patients in need are children. Within our society, we readily perceive a life cut
short as no life at all. Thus, children, as innocents, are frequently identified
as candidates for some of the most radical forms of medical intervention
known. This pairing of social expectations and medical responses springs

from shared understandings that we, as parents and extended kin, as community members, and as physicians, must do all that is possible to save children from the throes of death. Such is true even when children must endure great suffering in order to survive. Our actions are based on our desire that they experience adulthood and lead long and healthy lives. Middle-class values shape more specific social expectations and concerns, too: we hope that they complete advanced levels of schooling; find fulfillment in lucrative forms of work; encounter suitable partners and fall in love; survive long enough to bear witness to their own children's accomplishments; and outlive their elders, too.

Once defined as a maverick and thus dangerous clinical dream only fifty years ago, organ transplantation has rapidly transformed into a routinized medical practice. This transformation, however, would not have been possible were it not for ongoing experimental research involving both human and animal subjects. This progression, from renegade desire to medical success story, has depended overwhelmingly on an extraordinarily complex array of biotechnological interventions. The respirator, for instance, insures the viability of precious organs even when housed in the body of a brain-dead donor, the machine's pulsing action driving a steady flow of oxygenated blood and stimulating the heart's pulse. Anesthesia, in turn, stabilizes this "dead" body during surgery, dampening reactions that could threaten the "life" of vital organs. Furthermore, pharmaceutical cocktails composed of immunosuppressants, steroids, blood thinners, gastrointestinal medications, and vitamin supplements enable a transplanted graft to escape the assault of full-scale rejection once it has been placed in an organ recipient's body. Such procedures, now commonplace, nevertheless rest on a history of trial and error and, thus, failure and success. In more explicit terms, this means that a host of patients died while furthering the cause of transplantation.

The ability to sustain human life—whether that of a child or a seasoned elder—bears a heavy price: the success of all medical procedures, no matter how routine they may now seem, rests on earlier forms of experimentation. This experimental imperative pervades every area of medicine. Each time the novice practitioner attempts a procedure for the first time, the patient is, inevitably in some sense, an experimental subject. And with each innovation —be it a new medication, an emergent medical device, or even a slight innovation on an established surgical technique—individual patients again serve as medical guinea pigs. Often the most heroic acts are those known to involve the greatest risks: when attempting a new lifesaving procedure, the practitioner knows that it may well kill the very patient it is meant to help.

Organ transplantation offers an exquisitely clear example of what I label the "experimental imperative," and particularly so when framed by the boundaries of pediatric care. Organ transplantation in the United States is in fact driven by a tireless mandate to perfect continuously this ever-expanding and exacting craft. A range of specialties—including pharmaceutical research, organ procurement, and surgical implantation—constantly undergo revision, as new immunosuppressant drugs are tried out on patients, procurement specialists expand the age limits for organ donors, and surgeons attempt new procedures on younger, older, and sicker patients than was true only a few years before.

As an anthropologist and ethnographer who has focused for nearly fifteen years on the realm of "organ transfer,"[2] I find I am frequently drawn to the ethical conundrums that frame this extraordinary realm of medical expertise. Transplantation in the United States is driven by a strong professional ethos that insists on saving and extending human lives, sometimes, it seems, at all costs (and here "costs" may be financial, social, and emotional). Currently, an especially pronounced focus for concern is the ailing child. This is particularly challenging when the need for a heart or a set of lungs arises.

Within such contexts, among the most pressing issues at work involves the pairing of anxieties over organ scarcity with appropriate "fit." As I argue elsewhere, scarcity anxiety dominates the national discourse on organ transfer in the United States.[3] As reiterated in a plethora of research literature, hospital and other professional reports, and the mass media, the number of transplants performed in the United States has grown substantially over the course of only a few decades: the figure for 2004 exceeded 27,000, doubling that for 1989; and, as of June 2005, over 88,000 patients were registered on the national waiting list. In essence, only about one-third can expect to acquire an organ match, and many die waiting.[4] The problems associated with children are especially glaring because thoracic organs in particular must be small enough to fit within a child-size chest cavity. The body of a seven-year-old, for instance, can neither hold nor cope with the heart and lungs taken from an average-sized fifty-year-old adult. In essence, then, the desperation that plagues organ transfer in the United States is compounded in the pediatric context.

Set against these realities, the story of Jesica Santillan offers an especially compelling case through which to explore the significance of the child as a highly valued experimental "work object."[5] Throughout this essay, my frame of analysis is shaped by two related assumptions. First, as Jesica's story unwound, she was consistently perceived of (and thus portrayed) as a child.

Second, from the moment she was accepted as a patient at Duke Medical Center, until the time she died following her second transplant, her case might well be viewed as being consistently an experimental one. As a result, Jesica Santillan was transformed into an iconic cultural figure, one who emerges simultaneously as both a medical and a social experiment. Certainly this was a situation that Jesica and her family sought out, at great personal cost. In recent history, many desperately ill patients have hoped to access new and emergent medical technologies, navigating the blurred and rapidly shifting divide between research and practice in novel and agentive ways.[6] Clinicians, ethicists, and researchers, in turn, have had to rethink the ethical vulnerabilities and implications of their relationships with patients clamoring for experimental forms of care, as this blurring introduces new tensions into the relationship between researcher and subject.

I wish to clarify here that when I speak in this essay of "experimentation" I refer not simply to scheduled and approved clinical trials that have undergone interior and, frequently, careful exterior scrutiny by one or more human subjects research committees (such as an IRB or "institutional review board"), but also to less formal, and thus sometimes even on-the-spot, innovations. Such innovations are driven by the immediacy of medical emergencies that may require clinicians to attempt new techniques in order to stave off suffering or death of their patients. Experimentation—whether scheduled or spontaneous—is highly valued in medicine because experience and outcome inevitably generate new knowledge about what one should or should not do the next time around. I argue that both of Jesica's surgeries were experimental precisely because so few heart-lung transplants are attempted each year and because her team would have lacked much if any experience with this procedure. Her retransplant is by far the most "spontaneous" or renegade attempt, however, because by this point her medical team, headed by cardiac surgeon James Jaggers, was confronted with a patient whose chances of survival were deemed minimal by many critics working elsewhere within transplant medicine.

We might well view experimentation as a quotidian aspect of organ transfer in this country.[7] To paraphrase remarks I have heard echoed by numerous transplant surgeons at professional meetings and in casual conversation among peers, one is always experimenting by attempting new techniques within the transplant realm. The frontiers of surgical experimentation continually shift as once-novel procedures, like kidney transplants, become routinized. Relatively rare procedures performed by only a handful of surgeons only a handful of times—like the pediatric heart-lung transplant that Jesica received—underscore another understanding of experimentation. In such contexts, the potential for both miraculous outcomes and potentially fatal uncertainties pervades the therapeutic process for surgeon and patient alike.

As a means to make sense of these aspects of Jesica's story, in this essay I explore how children's bodies more generally have served as crucial experimental objects within so specialized a realm of technocratic medicine. As I will show, pediatric research at times offers an important bridge between animal research and adult treatments. With this in mind, I am most concerned with the following questions. What were the consequences of Jesica's paired statuses, first, as a minor and thus pediatric patient and, second, as an immigrant, noncitizen? In what ways, too, is she an iconic figure for transplant research? How relevant are the tales of other children who have gone before her? And how might we decipher the complex meanings assigned to children (and their bodies) during transplantation's experimental phases? Are children, for instance, more akin to animals or to adults in the ways in which they are handled clinically, represented visually, and discussed in the medical literature? And, finally, how might past experimental strategies assist us in rethinking the terrible tale of seventeen-year-old Jesica Santillan, who experienced (and ultimately died following) two sequential heart-lung transplants at Duke Medical Center in February 2003?

The ability to answer these questions necessitates exploring, first, public, and thus social, constructions of Jesica as a child, immigrant, and patient. After considering specific details of her story, I then turn to a more general discussion of experimental research in transplant medicine, and the particularly significant role occupied by children. As I do so, my goal is to offer a larger historical backdrop to Jesica's story so that I might then reanalyze Jesica as an iconic figure whose life (and death) were shaped by her transformation into a social and clinical experiment in America.

PLACING THE TRANSPLANTED CHILD IN CONTEXT

Jesica Santillan as Cultural Icon

A fact that has been reiterated by a number of authors within this volume (see Wailoo et al., Morgan et al., and Rouse) is that Jesica's two surgeries were performed just shy of her eighteenth birthday. Reasons given for why this was so range from the desperate nature of her clinical state, to the mandate of Jesica's charity that it only support minors, to the serendipity of when replacement organs became available. Jesica was consistently portrayed within a range of media, and by adults who spoke for her, as a young girl. Her patron,

Mack Mahoney, spoke of her exclusively in these terms. In an article in the *New York Times* in late February 2003, for instance, he is quoted as saying, "If we hadn't put the doctors square in the middle of the world stage . . . this baby would have died."[8] Others reporting on her story likewise drew on Jesica's youthfulness as a means to mark how frail and vulnerable she was. Following her death, a reporter for *Newsweek* described her in now all-too-familiar terms: "She was a small, frail child, barely over five feet and not much more than 80 pounds."[9] Those who worked for the local newspaper in Louisburg, North Carolina, employed similar language. In an online report focusing on Jesica's memorial service, Joe DeSantis, the managing editor of the *Franklin Times*, is reported as saying, "Well, they taught you and I in college that you're supposed to separate yourself from the story. . . . It's tough. . . . She's just the kind of kid you want to hug." Yet another newspaper employee, Joyce Pretty, described Jesica as "the bubbly girl who attended school with her [Pretty's] granddaughter."[10]

The fact that Jesica was considered (and also appeared) young served specific purposes on multiple fronts. Prior to her first transplant, her youthfulness and vulnerability captivated local audiences and led to an outpouring of emotional and financial support. Her innocence similarly justified arguments that someone of such humble origins deserved exorbitantly expensive and high-risk medical care. As a teenager, more specifically, she was easily perceived as suffering more than any child ever should, for she stood at the threshold of hopeful possibilities associated with impending adult status. Her apparent passivity also bolstered media portrayals of her childlike qualities. As studies by Carolyn Rouse and Helen Gremillion illustrate, chronically ill, compliant patients may continue to receive pediatric care well into their twenties, whereas defiant children may be expelled from clinics or "punted" to adult care because they are too difficult to manage.[11] Following the news of the botched blood match, Jesica's vulnerability was only further enhanced: the innocent child had now fallen victim to medical malfeasance, and, thus, at Duke at least, she certainly deserved another chance through the last-ditch effort of a second transplant. Even racist critics who denounced Jesica as a child of undeserving "illegal aliens" could draw on her status as a child. As the Santillans' daughter, she was living proof that procreation further enables "alien" proliferation within the United States.

In strictly clinical terms, Jesica's case was, at the very least, unusual. Significantly, heart-lung transplants are relatively rare in this country. Several factors account for this, and they include the surgical complexity of the procedure, the difficulty in acquiring an attached set of lungs and heart from a matching donor, and the small number of centers within the United States whose staff are qualified (and certified by UNOS) to attempt so difficult a surgery. The rarity associated with this category of transplant is reflected in the fact that the numbers performed annually have dropped by almost half since 1988.[12] Pediatric heart-lung transplants are even more exceptional. Jesica's team knew quite well how improbable Jesica's chances were for acquiring a heart-lung match from a pediatric donor and how exceptional a patient she would be in the history of pediatric care. Only twenty-nine heart-lung transplants were performed nationwide throughout 2003, and only six of these were pediatric; Jesica accounted for two of these because of her retransplant. This same year, the number of patients on the waiting list for this category hovered around 200.[13] As of June 2005, Jesica remains the only patient of any age to have received a second set of heart and lungs. As we can see, Jesica's first surgery was already a high-risk procedure, given the lack of experience at Duke (and at most transplant units throughout the nation, too) in performing the procedure. Whatever questions one might have concerning my assertion that the first surgery should be viewed as experimental, Jesica stood (or lay) quite firmly on experimental ground by the time she received her second transplant.

As the media sought to untangle so complex a tale, we find that Jesica's identity was consistently marked by this intertwining of her status as both a social and a medical experiment. Among the most pronounced themes that serve to unify these two domains is the redemptive quality of her story. Jesica quickly emerged as an iconic figure precisely because her life story typifies the (perhaps even stereotypical) tale of the Mexican who takes great risks to cross illegally a well-guarded border. As a minor, Jesica does so in the company of her parents, who then settle in the United States as undocumented migrants. Her story is unusual in that Jesica's ill health provides the impetus for the dangerous border crossing: she needs a type of transplant unavailable in Mexico, and thus her parents venture to the United States to save her.[14]

Medical attempts to save Jesica's fragile life reveal that the theme of redemption is at work on several fronts. For seemingly good-hearted, albeit paternalistic American citizens such as Mack Mahoney, Jesica's transplant would open a path to economic success coveted by Mexican immigrants who hope, through hard labor, to grant greater opportunities to their offspring. Members of Jesica's surgical team in turn were willing to perform this rare surgery precisely because they believed it might well save a dying (yet insured and financed) child. In this sense, their heroic efforts underscored that her citizenship was irrelevant: what mattered was that she was a sickly and vulnerable minor. In this sense, Jesica's story typifies the heroics associated with the expert clinical care of any child who is terminally ill. And, finally, her surgery offered still other forms of redemption for Duke Medical Center itself. Duke might, after all, with time, elevate its own status regionally and nationally as a center for high-risk pediatric surgery.

TRANSPLANT'S EXPERIMENTAL SUBJECTS

When viewed historically, it becomes clear that Jesica's tale is hardly unique; rather, her story is simply a recent example of a long trajectory of pediatric experimentation in the realm of transplant medicine and research. As I illustrate below, children are considered precious patients within the realm of organ transfer; ironically, this also renders them especially vulnerable to both scheduled and spontaneous forms of experimentation. In this sense, some exceptionally ill children's experiences overlap with those of animals. Within the experimental domain, they inevitably become, in Linda Hogle's words, "work objects,"[15] serving as bridges for newly acquired knowledge that might help establish future, successful outcomes in other children and adult transplant patients.

Imagining the Vulnerable Child

The contemporary realm of organ transfer in America is flooded with poster children, whose images grace a wide assortment of promotional materials. Relevant media include public outreach literature; videos, slideshows, television ads, and billboards; and professionals' PowerPoint presentations. These materials are generated by the staffs of tissue banks, organ procurement organizations (OPOS), and transplant units for use during those moments when they strive to celebrate or to commemorate the lives of either child transplant recipients or deceased organ donors. One impressive example includes the "CryoKid" campaign launched approximately a decade ago by CryoLife, a Georgia-based firm that specializes in human tissue preservation.[16] CryoKid posters and other supporting materials regularly feature photographs of smiling toddlers and older children, whose chest scars, for instance, may be clearly visible to the viewer, posed seated in a stroller or standing against the backdrop of an outdoor scene.[17] Yet another genre involves a now growing set of memorial projects erected in honor of transplantation's "heroes"—that is, donors whose body parts have either improved or saved the lives of a host of organ recipients. Yet again, children figure prominently at a range of sites. Relevant memorials include donor gardens (where, in some cases, trees are planted specifically in the names of particular deceased children), as well as the now burgeoning virtual cemeteries mounted on the Web.[18] Among the most famous of these virtual child memorials is associated with the Web site of the Nicholas Green Foundation.[19] In a host of ways, this site commemorates a seven-year-old boy who was shot by bandits in 1994 while on a family vacation in rural Italy. The decision by Nicholas's parents to designate their son as an organ donor made Italian, and then international, headlines.

Such examples illustrate a lesson I have learned through my extensive ethnographic research on organ transfer in the United States. That is, when parents are faced with the sudden, horrific, and numbing loss of a child, they frequently consent to organ donation in the hopes of saving the lives of other anonymous children who are in desperate need of replacement organs. In many instances, then, the child emerges as an iconic figure in two senses: as among the most needy of organ recipients and as the most precious of offerings of the "gift of life," a ubiquitous expression employed for organ donation in this country.

In quotidian terms, enormous social value is assigned to children within this culture, so much so that their loss is considered to be among the most tragic experiences that anyone could face. Whereas we most certainly mourn the loss of our elders, a child's death is considered especially horrible and a source of unending grief. As exemplified by the suffering of high-profile celebrities such as Eric Clapton and Danielle Steele, or historic figures such as Abraham and Mary Todd Lincoln, parents who outlive their children endure what many of us consider the worst form of suffering. Whereas we assume that our elders have been granted the opportunity to live life to its fullest, a child's death is a life unfulfilled. This collective sentiment is clearly conveyed, for instance, through cemetery imagery dating from over a century ago, when sculptures of mourning angels and severed columns were regularly erected at the graves of young children. Set against these heart-rending sentiments, lost children emerge as the victims of horrible circumstances. The lost child, then, is a subject who lacks agency. When mourned, he or she is memorialized as a beloved object of affection whom adults nevertheless failed to nurture and protect from life-threatening circumstances.

FROM CANINE AND BABOON TO BABIES' BODIES

Within clinical contexts, children likewise are viewed overwhelmingly as extraordinarily precious human beings whose lives must be protected at all costs. Physicians speak regularly of going to "heroic lengths" to save the lives of children who are severely physically damaged by a wide range of congenital complications or injuries. Physicians' efforts may target fetuses still in the womb[20] neonates,[21] as well as older pediatric patients. As minors, children of a range of ages fall under the protection of adults who may be called upon to make life-and-death decisions about their care. As Rouse's work in other clinical contexts illustrates, children by legal default often lack the agentive power to determine their own fates in medicalized contexts.[22]

Surgical efforts involving children are often understood as defining a special realm of medical expertise; this is because children's bodies are known to respond physiologically to many injuries in ways that differ from adults. Children's bones knit more rapidly, for instance, and young brains may be able to compensate more readily for lost capabilities, whereas adults with similar injuries often struggle with irreparable disabilities. Although certainly contested, a pronounced and long-standing assumption has been that neonatal susceptibility to pain is muted.[23] Thus, physicians may attempt complex procedures on newborns with little or no anesthesia, their actions driven by the understanding that, first, anesthesia in and of itself can be harmful and, second, that their fledgling nervous systems cope more easily than those of adults or older children when faced with an onslaught of invasive and, sometimes, experimental procedures.[24]

With these considerations in mind, a question of central concern is, under what circumstances is medical experimentation on children considered legitimate? An effort to explore this difficult issue necessitates defining the broader boundaries within which invasive experimental work on other subjects, including adult humans (who may or may not be able to grant consent), is conducted. Extraordinarily risky medical procedures are in fact routinely practiced (and, thus, first attempted) on a range of subjects other than medically imperiled yet presumably salvageable children. These subjects include other vertebrates (rodents, dogs, monkeys and apes, goats, and pigs figure prominently),[25] anencephalic infants,[26] dying and brain-dead patients,[27] human cadavers or their sectioned parts,[28] and, most recently, simulated, virtual bodies generated from computerized images of once living models.[29]

Cognizant yet ailing adults also regularly enlist in experimental protocols. Typically, following a battery of psychological tests, elaborate informed consent procedures, and in-house ethics reviews, such patients may offer their bodies to science, so to speak, knowing that a new or even previously untested procedure bears only some slight promise of extending their lives before they ultimately succumb to what is otherwise known as an incurable and fatal disorder. One need only consider recent research trials involving various artificial heart devices to grasp the ethical complexity—and medical hope—associated with this form of human experimentation.[30] Patients whose natal hearts have been replaced with the AbioCor mechanical device, for instance, have managed to survive anywhere from three to sixteen months, with their post-implant lives nevertheless plagued by strokes and, ultimately, multiple organ failure.[31] The willing investment of time, money, and faith by clinicians and their patients in such radically experimental procedures is possible because of the potential such experiments bear for generating new knowledge that could one day prolong or save other lives. Intensely painful and debilitating procedures may be hailed retrospectively as successful strides in transplantation research, strides that may eventually facilitate the shift from radical to routine approaches.

Sixty years ago, when transplantation presented myriad medical hurdles, research efforts necessitated testing various ideas and procedures on a range of nonhuman subjects, many of whom were dogs, chimps, and baboons. At some point, however, a small cavalier rank of surgeons crossed the species barrier, attempting what they hoped were promising techniques on the bodies of a select group of adults and children. One need only consider the highly publicized surgeries conducted by Christiaan Barnard in South Africa in 1967[32] to realize, too, that both transplant recipients and donors defined important work objects during early research phases. Attempts by Barnard (and others elsewhere) to save dying patients necessitated taking organs from the bodies of accident victims, some of whom were still connected to respirators. Within the South African context in particular (and in the United States as well; see Lederer, in this volume), race relations also figured in the transfer of organs from one body to another. In so racially polarized a setting as apartheid South Africa, the age, gender, and skin color of recipients and donors mattered. Thus, as Barnard's surgeries bear out, organ transfer can rapidly become a social experiment, too, a lesson that will prove especially helpful when I return to Jesica Santillan.

Medical Salvation in Pediatric Transplant Research
The earliest successful attempts at organ transplantation in the United States involved the transfer of kidneys between identical twins in 1954.[33] Heart and liver (and, later, lung) transplants, however, defined a far more complicated realm of medical desire if for no other reason than the fact that necessary organs had to be acquired from freshly dead patients-turned-donors. Early attempts at heart and liver grafting were disastrous. If recip-

ients survived the surgery, they soon died within days, weeks, or sometimes months as their bodies' immune systems inevitably rejected, on multiple fronts, organs of foreign origin.[34] Interestingly, child patients figure prominently in this phase of medical research.

This trend is described in detail by the imminent liver surgeon Thomas Starzl, whose professional career now spans half a century. Starzl's memoir, *The Puzzle People*, proves invaluable to understanding the inevitability of failure in early phases of planned experimentation. I offer below a few sample passages from Starzl's writings; in doing so, however, I intend no indictment of this physician or other members of his surgical team. Rather, the value of Starzl's account rests in the enlightening details he offers concerning the intended use—and, in retrospect, the seemingly inevitable deaths—of children as research subjects. Starzl's candor is rare, given the long-standing tradition within medicine to close ranks in cases involving hospital-based patient deaths.[35] More recent fears of litigation instigated by the surviving kin of deceased patients insures today that accounts with this level of detail no longer appear in the literature. Thus, it is important to stress Starzl's boldness and courage (rather than medical hubris) in his attempt to recount in print the stories of a range of patients. The excerpts I provide illustrate, then, the troubling sorts of events that precede achievements and breakthroughs. Given the nature of Jesica Santillan's own history, I focus on two specific sections from Starzl's book that detail the experimental use of two children of Spanish-speaking origins.[36]

Of special interest to me is the leap made from canine to juvenile research subjects, and Starzl's book in fact features photos of both children and a dog, all of whom the author describes as playing crucial roles in the early phases of transplantation. The first story relevant to my discussion begins in 1963, when, after conducting over 200 liver transplants on dogs, Starzl decided to attempt a pediatric liver transplant in a three-year-old boy name Bennie Solis.[37] Starzl's reflections on Bennie's life and death offer a particularly poignant example of pediatric experimentation, and he begins his account by describing Bennie thus: "Bennie Solis was a tiny spot in the universe, and a flawed one at that. The son of poor Spanish American parents, he was born with biliary atresia, a condition for which there was no medical or surgical treatment, nor any hope of divine intervention. His liver was incomplete."[38] Readers subsequently learn that Bennie was the victim of "battered child syndrome," a phrase coined by Starzl's colleague C. Henry Kempe. Kempe was a holocaust survivor, and thus Starzl underscores that "this was no ordinary pediatrician. He was a true defender of children" and one who strongly supported the decision to attempt a dangerous liver transplant on Bennie. Within Starzl's narrative, it appears that transplant surgery would somehow redeem Bennie. Although a victim of violence at home, his fate was now entrusted to the care of a medical team that valued his frail body for a purpose that could transcend his tragic home life. As Starzl explains, it was "Bennie's fate" to enable surgeons to bridge the gap between animal and human transplantation. Therefore, Bennie emerges as an iconic figure in the progress toward successful liver "homotransplantation."[39]

On March 1, 1963, Bennie's medical team attempted to transplant within him a liver acquired from still another child who had died during open-heart surgery. Starzl, writing thirty years later of the experience, explains, "In looking back, one can ask why Bennie, who himself was on life support with a ventilator, should not have donated a heart to the other child instead of receiving his liver. . . . Instead, the donor, who already was on a heart-lung machine, was cooled and maintained with an artificial circulation. The donor family gave permission for removal of the liver." Starzl then describes Bennie's tragic death in these moving terms:

> He bled to death as we worked desperately to stop the hemorrhage. The operation could not be completed. Bennie was only three years old and had not enjoyed a trouble-free day in his life. Now, his wound was closed and he was wrapped in a plain white sheet after being washed by a weeping nurse. They took him away from this place of sanitized hope to the cold and unhygienic morgue, where an autopsy did not add to our understanding of our failure. The surgeons stayed in the operating room for a long time after, sitting on the low stools around the periphery, looking at the ground and saying nothing. The orderlies came and began to mop the floor. It was necessary to prepare for the next case.[40]

Starzl has long been revered as one of the great pioneers in liver transplantation, and among his most celebrated characteristics is his ceaseless drive to refine his craft. Rather than abandoning the field after Bennie died, Starzl continued his work even when faced with seemingly insurmountable hurdles associated with the liver's complexity. By 1968, Starzl was able to report on the cases of seven additional patients, all of whom were children. Four died within two to six months postsurgery, spending the remainder of their lives in the intensive care unit. The other three, however, "were still alive and would remain so for long enough to demonstrate convincingly the potential value of this kind of treatment."[41]

One of these survivors was yet another child with a Spanish surname, Julie

Rodriquez, who was featured prominently alongside three other toddler girls in a two-page photo spread in *Life* magazine directly following the pages detailing the pathbreaking actions of Christiaan Barnard in South Africa.[42] At nineteen months, Julie received a new liver, and although she lived for 400 days, her body, like that of the other three remaining children, was riddled with cancerous tumors that arose in response to the medications that prevented graft rejection.[43] As with the story of Bennie Solis, Starzl breaks from a more clinical tone to describe in a heartfelt manner Julie's final days: "Yet this beautiful child seemed healthy most of the time. Doomed now, she became a familiar sight in the small parks near Colorado General Hospital where she went with her parents and doctors to play with the dogs who had undergone liver transplantation long before. The animals were brought out by Paul Taylor from the laboratory. The big people talked quietly and frankly to the other people. Julie talked to the dogs, who watched her as if they understood."[44] This passage is among the most touching in the book. There is, nevertheless, something deeply troubling about this image of a little girl who is too young to understand the seriousness of her medical predicament. So, too, is the sense of her isolation: too ill to play regularly with other children, Julie's primary playmates were dogs from her hospital who likewise served as experimental subjects for transplant research.[45]

Throughout these sections of his book, Starzl strives to make sense of his patients' deaths as set against the backdrop of experimental research. An inevitable focus of his musings concerns the question of culpability. As he explains, "the morality from the failed early trials and that which occurred later did not mean that liver transplantation was causing deaths. These patients were under a death sentence already because of the disease that had brought them to us."[46] Clearly, though, these children's final days were marked by an onslaught of highly invasive medical interventions. Typically, too, their deaths culminated in autopsies that nevertheless failed to reveal why early attempts at pediatric liver transplantation proved far less successful than canine ones. Furthermore, experimentation did not necessarily cease with post-transplant failure: some patients even became donors themselves following their own deaths. At the time, Starzl asserted publicly in medical circles that albeit *experimental*, his work was nevertheless primarily *therapeutic*, an argument that helped persuade others to support efforts that, in the end, proved highly successful.[47]

Starzl thus challenged those who insisted that "these little creatures had been denied the dignity of dying. Their parents [and Starzl, too,] believed that they had been given the glory of the striving."[48] In this respect, Starzl is no different from any other transplant surgeon. He is simply more candid and open in his reflections. Unfortunately, though, we remain unable to find in his book any indication as to why Starzl chose Bennie and Julie, for instance, over other children. When Starzl's account is considered alongside other high-profile cases involving child subjects, important clues begin to emerge that enable us to hypothesize about what additional hidden factors might have shaped the uncannily similar story of Jesica Santillan forty years later.

The Baby and the Baboon Heart

An odd characteristic of transplant medicine is that the procedure—whether experimental or routine—may well be proclaimed a success even if the patient dies after leaving the operating theater. This springs in large part from a widespread trend within clinical medicine to consider surgical and postoperative phases as temporally separate events. Whereas a transplanted heart can rapidly assume a regular beat when placed within a recipient's chest, or a transferred kidney may "pink up" once appropriately sutured in place, the subsequent causes of patient morbidity and mortality may be assigned to postoperative complications rather than to the surgery itself if the patient, at the very least, makes it to intensive care. The official causes assigned to patients' deaths often include infection or sepsis, stroke, embolism, or allergic responses to medications. Interestingly, too, for decades following well-publicized controversies involving patient deaths, hospitals may celebrate the achievements of associated surgeons whose actions were originally labeled as renegade and even unethical.

Such has proved true for Baby Fae, a seventeen-day-old female who, in 1984, received a baboon heart transplant at Loma Linda Hospital in California under the direction of surgeon Leonard L. Bailey.[49] The case generated a flurry of commentaries and acerbic critiques from clinicians and medical ethicists.[50] Of particular concern was the strong sense that Bailey's actions were premature and thus attempted against widespread medical opinion that researchers lacked the necessary knowledge to stave off immediate xenograft rejection. The fact that Bailey did not fall among the ranks of more prestigious investigators (such as Starzl and his peers), and, further, that Loma Linda's research was portrayed as being heavily financed by contributions from the Seventh-Day Adventist Church, and that Bailey, as a Seventh-Day Adventist, professed publicly to reject evolutionary theory, fueled the fire even further.[51] As one *New York Times* article noted, a public relations adviser at the hospital called the case "truly the biggest event for the Seventh-Day Adventist church and Loma Linda University."[52] At the time, the case focused on a renegade surgeon at an outlier research institution with an overarching religious agenda. And writing in 1988, ethicist and health lawyer George Annas characterized Bailey's operation as a "gross exploitation of the terminally ill."[53]

Over twenty years later, however, Loma Linda now celebrates Baby Fae as the third infant in pediatric history to receive a baboon heart transplant. As an in-house publication proclaims, "Baby Fae changed the course of history in Loma Linda. The institution was now recognized internationally. Loma Linda for a while became a household name. The magnitude and intensity of international interest had been genuinely overwhelming."[54] Indeed, Bailey's actions may have prolonged Baby Fae's life for twenty days; nevertheless, the quality of her life during that period is certainly questionable, given that she died of hyperacute graft rejection in response to a heart derived from a baboon. Such highly invasive procedures entail tremendous postoperative pain and discomfort, as does the experience of hyperacute graft rejection. Bailey's radical (and, as some would argue, botched) attempt generated a moratorium on xenotransplantation for another decade. His efforts nevertheless offered early clues that paved the way for more successful attempts at neonatal surgery in a range of contexts. In fact, only a year later, Bailey performed another human-to-human heart transplant on a child who was then the world's youngest patient, four-day-old Baby Moses, followed soon thereafter by yet another heart surgery on seven-day-old Baby Eve. Based on Bailey's experience with Baby Fae, Loma Linda sought to build a reputation as a center for neonatal transplant surgery at a time when no one else was attempting such procedures.[55] In other words, Baby Fae gave (or lost) her life while furthering scientific knowledge on several other medical fronts unrelated to xenografting.

Together, then, Baby Fae, Bennie Solis, and Julie Rodriquez (and, later, Jesica Santillan) emerge as iconic figures for a very special category of medical subject. Although their specific needs and stories are unique, they nevertheless fall within the legions of other experimental pediatric cases, some of which are hailed as wondrous successes, and still others as (often silent) failures. An important shared component of these specific children's stories is their celebrity, such that their personal levels of suffering and sacrifice were open to public viewing. Many other children have also succumbed to the surgeon's knife amid heroic efforts designed simultaneously to save them as individuals and to further medical knowledge in anticipation of the needs of other dying children. Because hospital public relations work is so expertly managed, we most often hear or read only about the success stories, and not the failures, unless kin take action and call a press conference. The question that remains, then, is whether there is something qualitatively different about experimental procedures attempted on children versus adults. When set against the stories recounted above, Jesica Santillan's emerges quite clearly as one of a failure gone public. Before I return to the specifics of Jesica's case, we must consider what values are embedded in instances where race and class converge with underage status in other experimental realms of medicine.

Children and Medical Research

A stumbling block within transplant medicine (and, one could also argue, research) is the "myth of democratization."[56] As I have found in the course of my research, practitioners of a range of stripes regularly assert that transplantation is "color blind," meaning that no one is excluded from transplant programs or waiting lists based on skin tone, ethnic background, or class standing. Social workers, in fact, occupy a special role on hospital-based transplant teams, devoting much of their time to assisting patients in overcoming significant financial burdens that might otherwise rule them out for so costly a medical procedure. In turn, the employees of the nation's myriad OPOS work long and hard to recruit minority donors while simultaneously promoting preventative health measures that could stave off organ failure within these same populations. Yet a persistent reality of transplantation, and in major urban centers in particular, is that donors rather than recipients are more likely to be people of color. Transplant centers thus crow over statistics that reflect a patient base representing a rainbow of ethnic or racial backgrounds. References to minority transplant candidates such as Bennie Solis, Julie Rodriquez, and Jesica Santillan are similarly evoked as potent symbols of the humanitarian qualities of this highly specialized—and extraordinarily expensive—realm of medicine. Transplant professionals are so deeply devoted to issues of equity that they may even exclude potential patients if they express racist sentiments. Children—including those of minority status—are doted on especially.

In contrast, and on other fronts, some authors have argued that the desire to protect the welfare of children has led to dangerous forms of neglect in various realms of medical experimentation. In 1968, Harry Shirkey coined the term "therapeutic orphan" as a means to foreground the lack of federal testing of pharmaceuticals for pediatric use.[57] As a result, doctors were forced to recalibrate dosages for children by extrapolating from directions intended for adults. Yet another chronic problem has been the limited availability of information on the side effects associated with pediatric doses for a wide assortment of drugs. Shirkey's arguments have driven a gradual, three-decade progression toward the development of government measures. These have culminated only recently in a bevy of mandates from Congress, the FDA, and other agencies that now require pediatric testing of new medications.[58] An immediate question to arise, however, concerns the ethics of recruiting children to participate in drug trials where child morbidity and even mortality are possible. Yet another significant concern is whether children of marginal social status might be targeted for drug testing, their susceptibility hinging, for example, on their dependence on semiliterate, legally unsophisticated, or economically desperate parents or other guardians who make such decisions for them. Informed consent by proxy is especially problematic if one's guardians are not fluent in English.

Several recent studies have investigated these particular concerns. Lainie Friedman Ross and Catherine Walsh, for instance, in surveying 529 studies published between July 1999 and June 2000 in three general pediatric journals, sought to uncover the level of pediatric reporting of minority involvement; 192 of the studies surveyed qualified for further examination.[59] The authors note that drug trials typically fall into one of two categories. They are framed either as pediatric "research" or as "therapeutic" trials (a language that clearly echoes Starzl's justification of Julie Rodriquez's involvement in liver transplantation). Some drugs, then, are tested on a sample population simply in order to determine their pediatric effectiveness and side effects where the subjects are otherwise assumed to be healthy children. In contrast, therapeutic trials are those that specifically target children who are already ill and who might well profit from the drug's effects.

Ross and Walsh's most striking finding is that minority, and especially black, children appear more likely to participate in research rather than therapeutic trials. Furthermore, their respective percentage of participation is grossly disproportionate to their representation within the U.S. census overall. The opposite is true for white children: that is, they are far more likely to be recruited for therapeutic trails, yet their low numbers even here do not reflect their strong representation within the more general U.S. population. In essence, then, minority children bear the burden of drug testing but individually are less likely to reap any benefits from the experience. The value of their participation is limited to helping other children who, when sick, may be administered the same drugs in the future.

In concluding their essay, these authors offer some hypotheses as to why the numbers are skewed. First, perhaps the overrepresentation of minority children in such studies hinges on the frequent location of academic medical centers in poorer urban settings. Yet another possibility is that the participants' guardians may lack access to decent health care services and insurance and thus they seek out medical assistance through drug trials. Finally, they posit that poor adults may be attracted to financial incentives. Nowhere in their essay is there any mention that drug trials might deliberately take advantage of such families through incentives or subtle forms of coercion, or else in knowing that they might be poorly informed of their legal rights, lacking the level of education or even linguistic fluency necessary to weed through a sometimes overwhelming number of documents during the informed consent process. Instead, an interesting subtext that runs throughout the essay is that poor or minority candidates appear more willing to "take advantage" of drug trials.

RETHINKING THE LIFE AND DEATH OF JESICA SANTILLAN

In this final section, I ask readers to return to my assertion that Jesica's case may be viewed from the outset as experimental on two fronts: that is, in both social and clinical terms. Furthermore, I assert that both the first and the second of Jesica's transplants qualify for experimental status. As argued earlier, combined heart-lung transplants are exceptional in this country and are rarely attempted on pediatric patients. Of primary concern to me, then, are the sorts of medico-ethical lessons we might learn from the Santillan case if we consider Jesica an experimental subject from whose suffering and tragic death one might still garner valuable clinical knowledge. As David Resnick wrote in a thoughtful essay that appeared in the *Hastings Center Report*, "Her story, as tragic as it is, can teach us important lessons about patient safety, medical fallibility, honesty, and trust."[60] I will build on this idea while also seeking more specifically to address other related yet hidden contradictions and consequences at work in the Santillan debacle.

The decision to frame my questions in reference to Jesica's experimental status allows us to step beyond the constant recirculation of debates over medical error and focus instead on the relevance of children as significant work objects in transplant research. Of special significance here is that Jesica was not only a child, but a child of a very particular sort: she was female, Latina, poor, and a noncitizen whose parents did not speak English. As a result, she bore enormous potential on two highly contradictory yet related fronts: as an icon of hope *and* in her susceptibility to medical experimentation. Her status as an object for research was initiated as soon as she entered the Duke medical system, because she so rapidly and readily embodied a flurry of clinical, social, and legal forms of symbolic capital.

Drawing on Resnick's detailed account of the story, I focus on several key aspects of the case. First, Jesica, not unlike other experimental subjects, was a child who suffered from life-threatening organ failure, a state that required radical surgical intervention if she were to survive. It is well known that by the time Jesica received her first transplant, she was gravely ill. In fact, the now iconic images of her featured in the press regularly portrayed a groggy or unconscious, bedridden child hooked up to a wide assortment of monitors and other forms of life support. Yet her status was tenuous not simply in physiological terms but in social terms as well. Her situation became even more precarious following her second transplant, soon after which it was apparent she had sustained a significant level of brain damage. Her story was further complicated when hospital staff struggled in vain to explain brain death to her parents through not one but three translators and a priest. Staff even went so far as to request Jesica's organs and tissue for other patients, even though she could not qualify as an organ donor.[61] In this sense her story is highly reminiscent of those of some of Starzl's earlier patients who became organ donors after their experimental transplants failed.

Particularly significant to Jesica's case is that she was the child of undocumented immigrants. This aspect of her story became the focus for virulent responses especially after her second transplant, where racist critics argued that Jesica was robbing deserving citizens of scarce organs.[62] Yet transplant centers nationwide now regularly report the increasing international quality of both organ donors and recipients. As I have learned in the course of my own ethnographic research, within the New York City metropolitan area, for instance, immigrants (who may reside here legally or illegally) frequently serve as organ donors when they sustain irreversible and life-threatening head injuries. More typically than not, such donors are drawn from the ranks of the urban poor.[63] Also, transplant centers nationwide accept recipients of foreign origin, and especially those who are able to pay out of pocket for their surgeries and other associated medical costs. For some time, one of the largest transplant centers in the New York City area maintained a unit that catered specifically to the needs of patients who were elite foreign nationals.

Against this background, Jesica Santillan was simultaneously typical and unusual. As her parents' child, she was marked as a member of the underclass. Yet she also inverted established patterns of health care access, entering the transplant realm not as a donor but as a needy yet insured recipient, and one who had a wealthy philanthropist as her patron and advocate. In turn, the double desire on the part of her medical team to save her life against all odds (be they clinical, economic, or social) may have driven the last desperate yet unorthodox request to procure her organs from her dead body for use elsewhere. In this final act, both physician and patient might have been redeemed, with Jesica "living on" in the bodies of still other recipients.[64]

After her transplant team botched her first surgery, Jesica had little (or even no) hope of survival. She was soon comatose, her body damaged by the devastating effects of mismatched blood types and other surgical complications. There was also acknowledgment in various quarters of the nation's medical community that a second attempt at a heart-lung transplant was futile. It was already certain the child would die, given the known effects of mismatched blood types. Thus, to some, the heroic effort to save Jesica's life through a second transplant appeared driven in large part by an attempt to counteract the devastating effects of negative publicity for Duke nationwide. It is reasonable to assume that, by this point, Jesica indeed had become little more than a medical guinea pig, where the only long-term clinical advantages of the second surgery lay in the knowledge reaped from the retransplantation of a set of lifesaving organs.

As we know from Starzl's account of Bennie Solis and Julie Rodriquez, it is humanitarian concerns for children that may well lead physicians spontaneously to try radical experimental procedures on those who are simultaneously the most frail and socially marginal of patients. The involvement of James Jaggers, Jesica's chief physician, certainly lends this sense of humanitarianism to the case. A preeminent cardiovascular surgeon, he is celebrated for his annual forays to Nicaragua where he performs pediatric surgeries for free through the charity organization Variety Children's Lifeline. Unpacking the relevance of humanitarianism further complicates the critique, because associated and extraordinary acts of generosity generally are *not* driven by a deliberate desire to harm a patient. Rather, the process is far more subtle. One desires to further one's knowledge in order to save myriad children's lives, yet appropriate, willing, and accessible subjects are also extraordinarily difficult to come by. It is not that minority children are deliberately preyed upon as candidates for radical transplant procedures but rather that they are more susceptible to the hidden costs of humanitarian aid.

Although clearly a mistake, even Jesica's first mismatched transplant should be viewed as experimental, precisely because it would certainly have shifted to this status once the mistake was recognized by her medical team. Tragically, even if Jaggers had recognized the mismatch at the moment of implantation, he still would have had no choice but to use the offered set of organs because, by the time they arrived at Duke, Jesica's natal heart and lungs had already been removed and she was on heart-lung bypass. Interestingly, however, surgeons based at Toronto's Hospital for Sick Children have in fact reported great success in transplanting mismatched hearts in infants (although they are no older than six months). Thus, the possibility that Jesica might somehow survive this medical mistake was there. Lori West, an American-trained cardiologist who runs the Toronto program, first attempted this radical procedure in 1995 when she felt far too many of her patients were dying for lack of an adequate supply of transplantable infant hearts. Based on her research findings involving infant mice, West suspected that human infants' immune systems might well be so underdeveloped as to be unable to recognize mismatched organs as foreign. By 2004, one of West's first patients had celebrated his seventh birthday. By this point, too, just under forty mismatched transplants had been conducted in Canada, the United Kingdom, and the United States.[65] Sadly, Jesica's immune system was far too advanced to ignore the presence of mismatched tissue. Given these dire circumstances, the only possibility for redemption for her surgical team and transplant center lay in risking Jesica to new surgical dangers, even though her chances of survival seemed negligible.

Jesica's story is thus a deeply complex one that defies the possibility of clear-cut explanations for why she died. Among the more complicated (and ironic) factors at work here is that, on the one hand—at least in terms of the manner in which the *first* transplant was portrayed in the media—the desire to attempt a heart-lung transplant on her frail body was a clear sign of medical heroics, an action carried out by a physician already known for his humanitarian bent. It is worth repeating that transplant surgery bears significant risks for any patient, who might well die either in the operating theater or from postsurgical complications. But the attempt to save Jesica's life was a worthy one because she was a child, and because of her socially marginal origins. In other words, by embodying the American dream, Jesica was indeed a *social* experiment: her transplanted organs would, in effect, give this frail transplanted soul an opportunity to thrive and grow on American soil. Our ability to save the life of so vulnerable a child as Jesica Santillan confirms as reality the American ethos of sheltering strangers and enabling them to succeed socially and economically in ways that stand in sharp contrast to oppressive circumstances that plague their nations of origin.

On the other hand, and this is where the irony rests, Jesica's marginality also opened her and her parents to medical abuse. Ultimately it is unclear how well informed Jesica's parents were, because a significant language barrier made it impossible for them to speak directly to their daughter's physicians and even, potentially, to her patron, Mack Mahoney. (It remains unclear how well Jaggers spoke Spanish.) The polarization of racial categories within the United States means that we are quick to identify abuses involving black children, but cases involving lighter-skinned, albeit still minority children, are potentially more likely to slip under the radar of ethicists and other medical watchdogs. Jesica's story is, nevertheless, eerily reminiscent of that of Bennie Solis, for instance. Bennie was, after all, not only a pediatric patient who suffered from a life-threatening form of organ failure, but he was also the son of Spanish-speaking parents. Both children, too, were unquestionably viewed as deserving heroic medical care precisely because their own situations were so dire: Bennie, because he was a victim of domestic violence, and Jesica because her parents were poor noncitizens who had taken great risks to enter the country specifically to seek medical care for their daughter. In a sense, it did not really matter if either of these children or others like them died. Either way, those involved in their care would know that they had offered these children the best possible medical care available to them through world-class hospital facilities. In the public eye, the Santillan case backfired because of a gross medical error.[66] However, we see that, when set against a host of pediatric experiments, Jesica's story defines in quintessential ways the power of pediatric bravado. If nothing else, in the long run we are certain to learn much about the effects of mismatched blood types in an older child and the aftermath of so risky an attempt at pediatric heart-lung retransplantation.

"THE DIGNITY OF DYING AND THE GLORY OF STRIVING"

In closing this essay I return to Starzl's protest that Julie Rodriquez most certainly did not die in vain. As the stories of Julia, Bennie Solis, Baby Fae, and Jesica Santillan attest, pediatric transplant surgery—be it experimental or routine—is driven by the courageous desire to end suffering by granting new life to often terminally ill children. This sentiment is echoed in Starzl's own reflections on Julie Rodriquez, whom he asserts "became a metaphor for courage and human progress."[67] Nevertheless, the very actions that bear such promise also generate other forms of anguish. Transplant surgery is without question a major assault on the body, and it carries mortal risks and lesser though still serious medical complications. If, in Renée Fox and Judith Swazey's words, transplantation, especially in its more radical or experimental forms, demands of surgeons "the courage to fail,"[68] then such risks are even more pronounced when children are concerned, precisely because of the high social value we assign to them.

When Jaggers and his team realized that they had "bungled" Jesica's initial surgery, their subsequent actions were driven by an intense desire to set things right. When her death was imminent, among their most pronounced desires would have included hopes of a "good death" for this child.[69] Sadly, though, if, as Beverley McNamara and her colleagues argue, "the Good Death is not a single event, but a series of social events,"[70] the circumstances leading to Jesica's demise defined yet another layer of medical failure. Already vulnerable on multiple fronts—as an ailing child, an undocumented migrant, and the daughter of non-English-speaking parents who could ill afford the costs of her care—Jesica became a sorry victim to a complex web of medical, technocratic, and social processes that lay well beyond her control. Like other pediatric cases before her, Jesica failed to thrive while tethered to an array of complex machines. As the target of intense public scrutiny, she nevertheless has reemerged as an iconic figure—and perhaps even a martyr—within the complicated realm of pediatric transplant research.

NOTES

Support from the following institutions enabled me to conduct research relevant to this essay: The Soros Foundation's Project on Death in America; the Wenner-Gren Foundation for Anthropological Research (Grant no. 7017); the Faculty Grants Committee at Barnard College, several of whose generous awards were underwritten by the Mellon Foundation; The Hastings Center for Bioethics, where I was a North American Visiting Scholar in July 2004; and The Russell Sage Foundation, where I was a Visiting Scholar during the 2003–4 academic year. Kari Hodges, Sonya Rubin, and Scott Michener provided invaluable research and other forms of assistance throughout various phases of manuscript preparation. I also wish to extend my warmest thanks to members of the seminar that generated this collected volume: Keith Wailoo, Peter Guarnaccia, Julie Livingstone, Carolyn Rouse, Leo Chavez, and Nancy King gave especially detailed and insightful comments.

1. In 2003, the year of Jesica Santillan's surgeries, 25,464 people received organ transplants; children ranging in age from under one year to seventeen years accounted for 1,795 of these patients. The 11–17 age range was the largest group at 784 transplants. Twenty-nine heart-lung transplants were performed, of which four fell within the age group of under one year to seventeen. As noted later in this essay, Jesica accounted for two of these four pediatric transplants because she received a second transplant soon after her first. For a detailed breakdown of these data see <www.optn.org/latestData/rptData.asp> (accessed June 18, 2005).

2. In employing the expression "organ transfer" I underscore the inseparable

relationship that binds the three-step process of donation, procurement (that is, harvesting), and transplantation. Within this essay I speak exclusively of the use of the whole or major organs (in the early years this meant the liver, heart, and kidneys; today, surgeons make regular use as well of lungs, the pancreas, and intestine). I thus exclude from this discussion tissues (a category that includes bone, skin, cornea, ligaments, tendons, heart valves, and veins) because the system of procurement is radically different, and tissues do not play a significant part in those aspects of early experimentation central to my discussion here.

3. Lesley A. Sharp, *Strange Harvest: Organ Transplants, Denatured Bodies, and the Transformed Self* (Berkeley: University of California Press, 2006).

4. Again, for up-to-date, online statistical data compiled by the United Network for Organ Sharing (UNOS), which oversees the distribution of organs in this country, see <www.optn.org>.

5. Linda F. Hogle, *Recovering the Nation's Body: Cultural Memory, Medicine, and the Politics of Redemption* (New Brunswick: Rutgers University Press, 1999).

6. See, for example, Steven Epstein, *Impure Science: AIDS, Activism, and the Politics of Knowledge* (Berkeley: University of California Press, 1996).

7. I wish to thank Nancy King for urging me to think carefully and critically about my use of the term "experimentation." Her thoughtful comments helped me to refine the definition I offer here.

8. Jeffrey Gettleman and Lawrence K. Altman, "Girl in Donor Mix-Up Undergoes Second Transplant," *New York Times*, February 21, 2003, A1.

9. Jerry Adler, "A Tragic Error," *Newsweek*, March 2, 2003, 20.

10. This story, titled "Transplant Patient Left Lasting Impression on Louisburg Community / Two Memorial Services Held for Jesica Santillan on Sunday," was posted at <www.wral.com/news/1996817/detail.html> on February 21, 2003, and updated on February 24, from Louisburg, North Carolina.

11. Helen Gremillion, *Feeding Anorexia: Gender and Power at a Treatment Center* (Durham: Duke University Press, 2003); Carolyn Rouse, "The Politics of Uncertain Suffering, Race, and Medicine: Racial Health Disparities and Sickle Cell Disease" (manuscript).

12. As reported by UNOS, a total number of 867 heart-lung transplants were performed between January 1, 1988, and December 31, 2004, of which 152 were pediatric. Interestingly, the annual number has dropped steadily since 1988: that year is marked by 74 surgeries; by 2000 it was 48; and in 2003 and 2004 it was 29 and 39, respectively. See <www.optn.org/latestData/rptData.asp> (accessed June 18, 2005).

13. The source of the data reported here is <www.optn.org/latestData/rptData.asp> (accessed April 22, 2005, and June 18, 2005).

14. As Megan Matoka Crowley reports, only kidney transplants are routine in Mexico; see her *Producing Transplanted Bodies: Life, Death, and Value in Mexican Organ Transplantation* (Durham: Duke University Press, in press).

15. Hogle, *Recovering the Nation's Body*.

16. For details on the CryoKid campaign, see the Web site <www.cryolife.com/corporate/cryokids>.

17. It is common practice for transplant centers throughout the country to feature in promotional material patients in daytime clothing and in outdoor settings as a means to underscore either their progression toward health or the idea that they have fully conquered their illness and now lead full social lives.

18. Lesley A. Sharp, "Commodified Kin: Death, Mourning, and Competing Claims on the Bodies of Organ Donors in the United States," *American Anthropologist* 103 (2001): 1–21; Lesley A. Sharp, "Denying Culture in the Transplant Arena: Technocratic Medicine's Myth of Democratization," *Cambridge Quarterly of Healthcare Ethics* 11 (2002): 142–50. For information on the newly erected National Donor Memorial at the UNOS headquarters in Richmond, Virginia, see <www.donormemorial.org>.

19. For information on this foundation and associated memorial projects, see <www.nicholasgreen.org>.

20. Monica J. Casper, *The Making of the Unborn Patient: A Social Anatomy of Fetal Surgery* (New Brunswick: Rutgers University Press, 1998).

21. Suzanne J. Kessler, *Lessons from the Intersexed* (New Brunswick: Rutgers University Press, 1998).

22. See Rouse's essay in this volume and Rouse, "Politics of Uncertain Suffering."

23. David B. Chamberlain, "Babies Don't Feel Pain: A Century of Denial in Medicine," *Journal of Prenatal and Perinatal Psychology and Health* 14 (1999): 145–68.

24. Since the 1980s and 1990s, however, the norms surrounding anesthetizing infants and pain has changed, yet parallel issues persist around questions of sentience, as, for example, in anencephalic infants.

25. L. L. Bailey et al., "Orthotopic Cardiac Xenografting in the Newborn Goat," *Journal of Thoracic Cardiovascular Surgery* 89 (1985): 242–47; Sharp, "Denying Culture"; Thomas E. Starzl et al., "Baboon-to-Human Liver Transplantation," *The Lancet* 341 (8837) (1993): 65–71; Thomas E. Starzl, S. Iwatsuki, and B. W. Shaw et al., "Orthotopic Liver Transplantation in 1984," *Transplantation Proceedings* 17 (1985): 250–58.

26. George J. Annas, "From Canada with Love: Anencephalic Newborns as Organ Donors?" *Hastings Center Report* 17 (1987): 36–38; John C. Fletcher, John A. Robertson, and Michael R. Harrison, "Primates and Anencephalics as Sources for Pediatric Organ Transplants," *Fetal Therapy* 1 (1986): 150–64; Michael R. Harrison and Gilbert Meilaender, "Case Studies: The Anencephalic Newborn as Organ Donor (two commentaries)," *Hastings Center Report* 16 (1986): 21–23; Rene Lafreniere and Mary H. McGrath, "End-of-Life Issues: Anencephalic Infants as Organ Donors," *Journal of the American College of Surgeons* 187 (1998): 443–47; Sharon E. Sytsma, "Anencephalics as Organ Sources," *Theoretical Medicine* 17 (1996): 19–32; James Walters, Stephen Ashwal, and Theodore Masek, "Anencephaly: Where Do We Now Stand?" *Seminars in Neurology* 17 (1997): 249–55.

27. Rebecca D. Pentz and Anne L. Flamm, "Letters: The Newly and Nearly Dead," *Hastings Center Report* 33 (2003): 4; Rebecca D. Pentz et al., "Revisiting Ethical Guide-

lines for Research with Terminal Wean and Brain-Dead Participants," *Hastings Center Report* 33 (2003): 20–26; Robert D. Truog, "Dying Patients as Research Subjects," *Hastings Center Report* 33 (2003): 3; T. M. Wilkinson, "Last Rights: The Ethics of Research on the Dead," *Journal of Applied Philosophy* 19 (2002): 31–41.

28. Mary Roach, *Stiff: The Curious Life of Human Cadavers* (New York: W. W. Norton and Co., 2003).

29. Thomas J. Csordas, "Computerized Cadavers: Shades of Being and Representation in Virtual Reality," in *Biotechnology and Culture: Bodies, Anxieties, Ethics*, ed. Paul E. Brodwin (Bloomington: Indiana University Press, 2000), 173–92; Catherine Waldby, "Virtual Anatomy: From the Body in the Text to the Body on the Screen," *Journal of Medical Humanities* 21 (2000): 5–107.

30. Lesley A. Sharp, *Bodies, Commodities, and Biotechnologies* (New York: Columbia University Press, 2006).

31. "First Heart Implant Dies," *Courier-Journal* (Louisville, Ky.), December 1, 2001; Sharp, *Bodies, Commodities, and Biotechnologies*. For details on patients' stories provided by the manufacturer and transplant centers working with the AbioCor, see <www.CHFpatients.com>.

32. "The Gift of a Heart," *Life*, December 15, 1967, 24–27.

33. Renée C. Fox and Judith P. Swazey, *The Courage to Fail: A Social View of Organ Transplants and Dialysis*, 2nd rev. ed. (Chicago: University of Chicago Press, 1978); Renée C. Fox and Judith P. Swazey, *Spare Parts: Organ Replacement in Human Society* (Oxford: Oxford University Press, 1992).

34. See Emily Martin, "Toward an Anthropology of Immunology: The Body as Nation State," *Medical Anthropology Quarterly* 4 (1990): 410–26.

Organ graft rejection occurs in phases, ranging from acute or immediate bodily responses (which arise within hours and days) to more chronic forms, which can span months or years. Thus, to speak of a transplant's success is a tricky enterprise, especially given that organ recipients take immunosuppressants precisely because they are in a constant state of rejection. When a patient dies several months following a radical transplant, other body systems may bear the blame. It is important to realize that chronic rejection may bring on a host of other potentially fatal consequences. The mismatching of blood type, which Jesica Santillan experienced, would stimulate immediate, life-threatening, hyperacute rejection responses. (I wish to thank Tom Diflo for clarifying this during our second conference.)

The language of bodily invasion by tissue of "foreign" origin also demands special note within the context of a discussion of Jesica Santillan. As Emily Martin ("Toward an Anthropology of Immunology") notes, immunology is rife with language that resonates with current models of the nation-state from a specifically U.S. perspective.

35. Mark Kramer, "Medical Mortality Review: A Cordial Affair," in *Invasive Procedures: A Year in the World of Two Surgeons* (New York: Harper and Row, 1983).

36. Not all—or even the majority—of Starzl's pediatric patients were of Spanish origin. Racial differences—and social tolerance—nevertheless define a theme that

figures prominently in Starzl's personal life. A significant portion of *The Puzzle People: Memoirs of a Transplant Surgeon* (Pittsburgh: University of Pittsburgh Press, 1992), for instance, focuses on his courtship and second marriage to Joy Conger, an African American woman; Starzl himself is white.

37. Starzl, *Puzzle People*, 96–100.

38. Ibid., 97.

39. Ibid. 97–99.

40. Ibid., 99–100.

41. Ibid., 165.

42. "Four Little Girls Stave off Death with Liver Transplants," *Life*, December 15, 1967, 28–29.

43. Starzl, *Puzzle People*, 166–67.

44. Ibid., 167.

45. A subject of great interest to me is the transplant memorial; it is possible that the first public project created for this purpose was in fact erected in Julie's memory. As Starzl describes, a Swedish artist named Dietrich Grunewald, who was living in New Mexico, created a portrait titled *In Memoriam Julie Rodriquez, January 2, 1955, to August 26, 1968*. The image depicts a child "bathed in sunlight, picking long-stemmed flowers." It hung for approximately five years in the transplant ward of Colorado General Hospital, where Starzl worked; when it was harmed during a move, Starzl relocated it to his bedroom at home (see Starzl, *Puzzle People*, 166).

46. Ibid., 165.

47. Ibid., 163–64.

48. Ibid., 165.

49. Lawrence K. Altman, "Baby Fae, Who Received a Heart from a Baboon, Dies after 20 Days," *New York Times*, November 16, 1984; Lawrence K. Altman, "Baby with Baboon Heart Better; Surgeons Defend the Experiment," *New York Times*, October 30, 1984; Lawrence K. Altman, "Confusion Surrounds Baby Fae," *New York Times*, November 6, 1984; Lawrence K. Altman, "First Human to Get Baboon Liver Is Said to Be Alert and Doing Well," *New York Times*, June 30, 1992; L. L. Bailey et al., "Baboon-to-Human Cardiac Xenotransplantation in a Neonate," *Journal of the American Medical Association* 1985, no. 254 (1985): 3321–29.

Interestingly, Loma Linda figures prominently, too, in the history of early attempts to acquire organs from anencephalic infants (see Lafreniere and McGrath, "End-of-Life Issues"). Loma Linda later suspended this program in response to disputes over the ethics of acquiring body parts from still-living donors.

50. George J. Annas, "Baby Fae: The 'Anything Goes' School of Human Experimentation," *Hastings Center Preport* 15 (1985): 15–17; A. Capron et al., "The Subject is Baby Fae (Commentaries)," *Hastings Center Report* 15 (1985): 8–17; Olga Jonasson and Mark A. Hardy, "The Case of Baby Fae," *Journal of the American Medical Association* 254 (December 20, 1985): 3358–59; Thomasine Kushner and Raymond Belliotti, "Baby Fae: A Beastly Business," *Journal of Medical Ethics* 11 (1985): 178–83; Richard A.

McCormick, "Was There Any Real Hope for Baby Fae?" in *Human Organ Transplantation: Societal, Medical-Legal, Regulatory, and Reimbursement Issues*, ed. Dale H. Cowan et al. (Ann Arbor: Health Administration Press, 1987), 361–62; Kenneth P. Stoller, "Baby Fae: The Unlearned Lesson," *Perspectives on Medical Research* 2 (1990), online journal <www.curedisease.com>, published by Americans/Europeans/Japanese for Medical Advancement.

51. Australian Broadcasting Corporation (ABC), "Artificial Hearts," in *The Health Report, Radio National Transcripts* (Australia, 1996); S. J. Gould, "The Heart of Erminology. What Has an Abstruse Debate over Evolutionary Logic Got to Do with Baby Fae?" *Natural History* 97 (24) (1981); Kushner and Belliotti, "Baby Fae"; McCormick, "Was There Any Real Hope for Baby Fae?"; Stoller, "Baby Fae."

52. Lawrence Altman, "The Doctor's World: Confusion Surrounds Baby Fae," *New York Times*, November 6, 1984, C1.

53. Cited in Darcy Henton, "Baboon Heart Transplants Defended," *Toronto Star*, October 16, 1988, A12.

54. University & Medical Center Loma Linda, "LLUMC Legacy: Daring to Care. Chapter 3: Perspective on Neonatal Heart Transplantation [revised 3.18.01]," <www.llu.edu/info/legacy/Legacy4.html> (accessed April 22, 2005).

55. Ibid.

56. Sharp, "Denying Culture."

57. Harry Shirkey, "Therapeutic Orphans (Editorial Comment)," *Journal of Pediatrics* 72 (1968): 119.

58. Gregory Hazard, "Please Sir, I Want Some More: Congress' Carrot-and-Stick Approach to Pediatric Testing Leaves Therapeutic Orphans Needing More Protection," *Journal of Contemporary Health Law and Policy* 20 (2004): 467–508; Loretta M. Kopelman and Timothy F. Murphy, "Ethical Concerns about Federal Approval of Risky Pediatric Studies," *Pediatrics* 113 (2004): 15–23; Lainie Friedman Ross and Catherine Walsh, "Minority Children in Pediatric Research," *American Journal of Law and Medicine* 29 (2003): 319–36.

59. Ross and Walsh, "Minority Children in Pediatric Research."

60. David Resnick, "The Jesica Santillan Tragedy: Lessons Learned," *Hastings Center Report* 33 (2003): 19.

61. This is true today for all organ recipients because they have been administered immunosuppressants that render the organs susceptible to cancers and other infections that might be passed on to other patients.

62. See, for instance, the commentaries and blogs mounted by such Web sites as <www.vdare.com> and <www.talkaboutgovernment.com>.

63. Sharp, "Commodified Kin"; compare Resnick, "Jesica Santillan Tragedy," 15–20; Nancy Scheper-Hughes, "The Global Traffic in Human Organs," *Current Anthropology* 41 (April 2000): 191–211, 218–24 (reply); Nancy Scheper-Hughes, "Parts Unknown: Undercover Ethnography on the Organs-Trafficking Underworld," *Ethnography* 5 (2004): 29–72.

64. As I describe at length elsewhere, in "giving the gift of life" through organ donation, the surviving kin of deceased organ donors frequently understand the donor (especially where a child is concerned) as living on in the bodies of anonymous strangers, a sentiment that is actively promoted by procurement teams as an incentive for donation among family members suddenly faced with a terrible tragedy (Sharp, "Commodified Kin").

65. Tom Anderson, "Change of Heart," in *Sixty Minutes II* (2004).

66. Institute of Medicine, *To Err is Human: Building a Safer Health System* (Washington, D.C.: National Academy Press, 1999).

67. Starzl, *Puzzle People*, 166.

68. Fox and Swazey, *Courage to Fail.*

69. Nancy Johnson et al., "Towards a 'Good' Death: End-of-Life Narratives Constructed in an Intensive Care Unit," *Culture, Medicine and Psychiatry* 24 (2000): 275–95; McNamara, Charles Waddell, and Margaret Colvin, "The Institutionalization of the Good Death," *Social Science and Medicine* 39 (1994): 1501–8.

70. McNamara, Waddell, and Colvin, "Institutionalization of the Good Death," 1501.

JESICA SPEAKS?

ADOLESCENT CONSENT FOR

TRANSPLANTATION AND ETHICAL

UNCERTAINTY

CAROLYN ROUSE

In February 2003, freelance writer Nancy Rommelmann fixated on daily news accounts of Jesica Santillan's deteriorating health. Rommelmann had a thirteen-year-old daughter who looked strikingly like seventeen-year-old Jesica, and the resemblance had been enough to fuel a paralyzing obsession. After Jesica died, Rommelmann was able to contact the Santillan's benefactor, Mack Mahoney, and Mahoney decided that Rommelmann should be the one to write Jesica's story. Rommelmann flew to North Carolina, was warmly greeted by Nita and Mack Mahoney, and for the next week embarked on a journey that ended with her abruptly fleeing from Mahoney's paternalism. To Rommelmann's horror, Mahoney wanted the Santillans to sign away their rights to Jesica's story. Explaining why her husband believed he should be the one to own the account of the ordeal, Nita Mahoney bemoaned that she and Mack were the ones who found and loved Jesica, and they were the ones who contributed extensive resources and time to her care. For the Mahoneys it seemed as though story ownership was an appropriate form of reciprocity for their investment in hope.[1]

The legal struggle over who should own the rights to Jesica's posthumous story mirrors a much more troubling issue: Who controlled Jesica's story while she was alive? Mahoney, it seems, had such tremendous influence over the Santillans that one wonders what agency Jesica actually had to determine her course of treatment or even how she wanted to live her life. From the botched transplant archives one gets the sense that Jesica was swept up in the hopeful narratives generated by a community, a medical system, her parents, and benefactors, but missing is any clear indication of what Jesica thought of her disease or her terminal status or whether she understood the risks involved in a heart-lung transplant.

I wondered whether in this case there was what Myra Bluebond-Langner in *The Private Worlds of Dying Children* describes as "mutual pretense."[2] Bluebond-Langner discovered that terminally ill children as young as three years old understand that they are dying yet they often hide this knowledge from their parents and medical practitioners.[3] For many of the children, playing along with socially acceptable pretenses of hope made them feel secure that they would not be left alone. Given Bluebond-Langner's observations, it seems appropriate to ask, what was Jesica's understanding of her terminal disease? Did she believe a transplant would improve her life? Unfortunately, in an exhaustive examination of media surrounding Jesica Santillan I found only a few quotes attributed to Jesica by Mack Mahoney. Mahoney reported, for example, that after Jesica's first transplant she whispered into his ear, "Yo no puedo respirar. Estoy muriendo." ("I can't breathe. I'm dying.").[4] If she thought she was dying, did she want heroic or palliative care? Did she wish she had never received the first transplant? Did she wish she had spent more time with peers rather than her family and her benefactors? Given the increasing number of experimental interventions for devastating illnesses, is mutual pretense a sufficient enough cultural explanation for denying sick adolescents the legal right to decide whether they wish to participate in risky treatments? Or should sick adolescents be considered equal partners in deciding how they want to live and die? The current recommendation from the Institute of Medicine's Committee on Clinical Research Involving Children is to encourage researchers to develop an adolescent assent process that mimics in substance and form the adult consent process.[5] The committee recognizes that the current goal of involving children in decisions is "less a reality than an aspiration," yet the committee does not go so far as to recommend granting mature adolescents legal rights in order to *ensure* patient consent.[6] For me, Jesica Santillan's story typifies a bind experienced by many chronically ill teenage minors. Like Jesica, they are legally too young to make medical decisions that will affect their future quality of life.

The decision to limit adolescent agency in the case of medical consent is based upon the premise that adolescents are not yet ready to assume adult responsibilities. Adolescence is generally understood as a developmental period during which children practice adult independence, openly challenge authority, and become increasingly self-aware (individuation) while remaining dependent on adults to meet their basic needs.[7] Cross-cultural studies of adolescence, however, demonstrate that whether a society recognizes a distinct stage between childhood and adulthood is largely dependent on cultural beliefs and economic structures.[8] In some parts of the world, children move directly into adult roles at the onset of puberty. In cultures where a well-educated workforce is required, adolescence can extend well into a young adult's early thirties. Research indicates that adolescence is not a universal stage of development but rather a classification emerging from a variety of cultural and social forces.[9]

What seems to be a contradiction in medicine, however, is that while institutions use the age of majority to determine the age of consent, more and more pediatric physicians are encouraging parents of chronically ill teenagers as young as thirteen to cede responsibility for disease management to their sick children. These physicians believe that if children do not assume responsibility for managing their disease in their early teens, they will have a difficult time transitioning to adult institutions where care is organized around presumptions about patient self-reliance.[10] Chronically ill adolescents, in other words, are treated according to two contradictory paradigms regarding their psychological development; the legal one that deems them incompetent until eighteen years of age and the clinical one that deems them competent before eighteen, given the right parenting and psychosocial support. As the population of chronically ill adolescents grows, it is necessary to ask, given what clinicians believe about teenage competence, what social and cultural forces are at play that continue to limit the ability of chronically ill adolescent minors like Jesica to make medical decisions? And does this limitation make sense, given that risky interventions have the power to determine entirely different futures?

I felt I might be able to better understand Jesica's thoughts about her transplant and her life through research I had been conducting on adolescents with sickle cell disease. My research addressed adolescent transitioning, which is the transitioning of chronically ill children from pediatric to adult care. I was interested in everything from what sorts of assumptions undergird the division between child and adult health care services to how adolescents deal with their illness. The Santillan story encouraged me to investigate how the sickle cell community, which includes patients, medical professionals, patient advocates, and families, conceptually organize the intersection between adolescence, chronicity, and risky experimental treatments, namely bone marrow transplantation. In order to do this, I developed an ethical thought experiment, which I discuss later in this essay. My queries introduced a range of possibilities regarding what cultural ideologies may have determined Jesica's personal narrative.

Without a heart-lung transplant, Jesica was predicted to die suddenly from restrictive cardiomyopathy. Preparing for a possible future for Jesica meant restricting her activities in the present. For fear that school might hasten her demise, Jesica spent most of her days with Nita Mahoney, Mack's wife, who did not speak Spanish, while her mother, Magdalena, and "father," Melecio, worked and her eight-year-old sister, Dulce, and six-year-old brother, Ulises, went to school. During those long hours Jesica would call Mack, whom she called "my Mack" and who speaks Spanish, up to twenty times a day. He seemed to be her one personal connection to the world beyond her immediate family. She would also draw in a diary. Rommelmann describes the entries in the diary: "There was no writing in it, only drawings, of a rose being pierced by a knife, Latin girls with boobs bursting out of skimpy tops and boys in muscle cars, temporary tattoos that read 'Naughty As I Want To Be' and 'Sweet Thing,' and pictures of Shakira and Enrique Iglesias torn from magazines."[11] Jesica had a rich adolescent life that many people either did not see or refused to see. Her lack of breasts and other signifiers of maturity made it easy to ignore the fact that she was only months away from the legal age of majority when she died.

Jesica's innocence was a necessary element of Mack Mahoney's hagiography. In order for Mack to be a saint, Jesica needed to be an angel, and Jesica's mother and father needed to be worthy of redemption. In fact, Mack purchased clothes for Jesica that made her look more like a child than an adolescent. Mack noted to Rommelmann, "I would not buy her some of the stuff she wanted, hip-huggers and midriff tops. I told her, that stuff makes you look like a little slut."[12] Even after Jesica's death, Mack Mahoney continued to try to control the Santillans' public image, even demanding that Magdalena Santillan marry Melecio Huerta, the man Jesica identified as her father. Rommelmann reports, "When I asked if Magdalena wanted to get married, Mack gave me a look that said I was naïve, 'It don't matter what she *wants*,' he said. 'These people essentially have a sixth-grade education; where they come from there aren't even roads. They'll do what I tell them to do.'"[13]

Perhaps Mack Mahoney's desire to control the Santillans' public image was related to his need to attract financial supporters. Mahoney, the consummate salesman, mobilized numerous sponsors to donate time and building supplies to produce the first Jesica House. Mahoney's foundation then sold the house, and the profits went toward financing Jesica's treatment. On the Internet there is a picture of a smiling Jesica putting her handprints in wet cement during the house's construction. But what was required for Jesica to be the object of a community's pity? According to the mission statement of Mahoney's foundation, Jesica's Hope Chest, Inc., A Foundation for Critically Ill Children, Jesica needed to be a child. The first sentence of the mission statement specifies that "Jesica's Hope Chest, Inc. . . . is dedicated to helping critically ill children up to the age of (18) eighteen years old (but not past the child's eighteenth birthday)."[14]

The reason the foundation refuses to support adolescents beyond the age of eighteen is related to what Lesley Sharp in her essay in this volume identifies as the disproportionate social value placed on children. The social benefits bestowed upon children, free education and in many states free health care, express this disproportionate value. These benefits are considered gifts rather than inalienable rights, which means benefits can and do get withheld under particular circumstances. Similar to her undocumented status, Jesica's age meant that her social rights and privileges were ambiguous, leaving her vulnerable to the sentiments of those with the power and authority to decide whether she was worthy of receiving a transplant.[15]

As we see in the case of the juvenile justice system, some adolescents are treated as children, or less harshly, while others are treated as adults. Human Rights Watch reports that black youth under the age of eighteen are twelve to twenty-five times more likely to be incarcerated in an adult facility than white youth. Hispanic youth are seven to seventeen times more likely to be serving in an adult facility than white youth.[16] As Leo Chavez argues in his essay in this book, perceptions about which adolescents are worthy of a social good, like a donor organ, are based upon understandings of legitimacy and citizenship. These disparities mean that child status during adolescence is treated as a privilege rather than an inalienable right.[17] Within medicine, age and social status are entangled in what medical sociologist Mary-Jo Good calls the "biotechnical embrace," or the hope generated around the development of new therapies for particular diseases.[18] The value we place on certain children inspires us not only to provide unequal social benefits but also to disproportionately invest in novel therapies to alleviate children's suffering.[19]

In order to remain iconic of a community's hope, Jesica, who appears angelic in photos distributed to news organizations, needed to be infantilized. There was no room in this rescue narrative for Jesica to be agentive, to possibly reject the idea of a heart-lung transplant, or to reject a life held in abeyance for the sake of an uncertain future. In return for Jesica's compliance, individuals donated money to Mahoney's foundation not simply for her treatment but for the developing hagiography, and the physicians at Duke University Hospital agreed to give Jesica access to one of the rarest and riskiest transplant procedures.

There are a number of reasons why Jesica may have lacked control of her personal narrative. First, she trusted her parents, who loved her and who sacrificed so much in order for her to receive care at Duke University Hospital. As children, we often do not differentiate ourselves from our parents, and Jesica may never have developed a perspective about her future that differed from that of Magdalena Santillan. Her lack of education and her sheltered existence also may have contributed to her inability to differentiate herself from her parents and benefactors.

Second, often an adolescent's agency is usurped in order for hospitals to enact an institutional narrative. Richard Cook notes in his essay in this book that the successful performance of risky cutting-edge treatments, like a heart-lung transplant, garner respect and business for a hospital. Once the scientific community and the public have chosen to embrace a novel treatment like a heart-lung transplant, then treatment risks, including possible long-term complications, are made to seem rational. As Nancy King points out in her essay in this volume, the benefits of transplantation are often overestimated by the medical community, and this overestimation seems to benefit medical institutions more than individuals.

Third, adolescents do not just complicate institutional narratives, they complicate physician narratives as well. At a sickle cell bone marrow transplantation meeting at the National Institutes of Health in 2003, a physician involved with one of the first transplants in 1998 reported that the adolescent test subject was noncompliant with postoperative treatments and therefore continued to suffer complications. Her solution was to try to transplant children before they reach adolescence so that the parents would assume responsibility for treatment compliance. While family-centered care remains an organizing principle in health care, it continues to be socially acceptable for pediatric physicians to assume a paternalistic role with their patients. For example, if a pediatric patient fails to adhere to treatment, a physician can involve a judge, who has the power to strip the parents of their parental rights. If an adolescent fails to comply with treatment, it is difficult to determine whether it is the fault of the parent or the patient. Not knowing where to locate blame, physicians often lack a strategy for enforcing compliance. Physician anxiety about patient noncompliance is not, as David Rothman argues, simply a demonstrated lack of respect for patients and their autonomy or lack of acknowledgement that medical uncertainty exists, but is, in many ways, motivated by concern that under their care a patient may needlessly die or become disabled.[20] The physician narrative and the institutional narrative share many features. However, the physician narrative is generally more patient-centered, or more concerned with long-term patient outcomes, than the institutional narrative.

With risky experimentation, institutions calculate risk differently than

physicians. Institutions consider the financial and symbolic costs and benefits, whereas physicians generally try to calculate the patient's personal costs
and benefits when determining whether to encourage a patient like Jesica to
participate in a lifesaving transplant. After a physician has decided that the
benefits of treatment outweigh the risks, then the next step is to encourage
the patient to consent. One method to encourage consent is to tell anecdotal
stories of individuals who survived transplants fairly unscathed. I observed
an oncologist describe to a mother of a four-year-old with a brain tumor his
institution's success rate with bone marrow transplantation. His explanation
began with, "We've transplanted sixteen patients," then he quickly recited the
low survival-rate statistics almost as an aside. Finally, he closed by saying, "A
boy we transplanted in the fall is back in school getting A's and B's." The fact
that one patient survived and was leading what the doctor presented as a
normal life was enough for this mother to agree to a transplant. The four-
year-old was ultimately refused a transplant because her kidney function was
poor, and eventually she died, but the fact that without a transplant her
chance of survival was zero made it difficult for the mother not to accept the
physician's hopeful narrative as a rational choice. As I discovered with my
thought experiment, while loved ones often find it difficult to dismiss over-
estimations, patients more willingly reject treatments with low survival rates
or that drastically reduce quality of life. In her article "Acknowledging the
Hypocrisy," Christine Hanisco describes a number of recent cases in which
adolescents tried to refuse medical treatment:

> In Massachusetts, a sixteen-year-old boy ran away from home to avoid
> chemotherapy treatment despite his parents' consent. In California, a
> fifteen-year-old girl fled her home after being physically forced to succumb
> to chemotherapy, despite both her parents' and her lack of consent. An-
> other fifteen-year-old who, with parental consent, chose to discontinue his
> medication and decline a third liver transplant, was forcibly removed by
> police from his home and hospitalized. Another fifteen-year-old, suffering
> from end-stage cystic fibrosis, was placed on a ventilator despite his re-
> peated wishes against life-prolonging measures, such as intubation and
> mechanical ventilation.[21]

In all these cases, minors rejected the narratives of hope generated by the
medical community. For all these individuals medical intervention caused
them more suffering than the disease and therefore it made sense to stop
treatment. For example, the fifteen-year-old girl, a Hmong refugee, did not
want chemotherapy because it threatened her ability to bear children, which,

for traditional Hmong, is an essential part of a woman's identity. She also described the pain caused by chemotherapy as "torture."[22] If Jesica had been given the legal right to choose, which would have required that her physicians explain directly to her that she had less than a 40 percent chance of surviving the transplant and an even smaller chance of living without secondary complications, would Jesica have similarly rejected the transplant and embraced an alternative understanding of a life well lived?

In an attempt to better understand what agency chronically ill adolescents have, given competing cultural narratives about hope and patient autonomy, I conducted a thought experiment at a sickle cell association meeting in 2004. Sickle cell disease is a congenital disease that primarily affects blacks in the United States. A one base pair substitution on the part of the DNA that codes for hemoglobin causes the otherwise round hemoglobin to sickle. This fragile sticky hemoglobin often blocks capillaries, causing a decrease in blood circulation and oxygenation to various organs. Long-term damage to lungs, kidneys, and/or brain results in high rates of morbidity and mortality. The average age of death in the last thirty years has risen from around twenty to around forty-five. Regardless of the increase in life expectancy, there is reason to want to cure rather than simply treat sickle cell disease. Patients continue to suffer from severe painful crises that require hospitalization, and for some, silent strokes cause decreased mental and physical function over time.

In the early 1980s, a sickle cell patient with leukemia who received a bone marrow transplant was cured of both her leukemia and sickle cell disease. Since that time, some hematologist/oncologists have been encouraged by the outcomes of the over 200 transplants for sickle cell disease worldwide. The procedure requires that the patient first be given high doses of toxic chemotherapy drugs in order to destroy the patient's bone marrow. After the marrow is destroyed, and while the patient hovers near death, the patient receives the donor marrow, which slowly draws him or her back from the precipice. A regimen of immunosuppressants must be started in order for the patient not to reject the foreign marrow, but with bone marrow transplants, patients can slowly be weaned from these drugs. Possible complications include death or graft-versus-host disease (GVHD), which occurs when the donor marrow attacks the host body. About 50 percent of bone marrow transplant patients develop GVHD, which manifests in a number of ways, causing everything from chronic to acute, minor to severe, illness and sometimes death.

In order to understand how cultural beliefs about adolescence and the biotechnical embrace shape adolescent agency in the clinic, I interviewed thirty-five medical professionals, researchers, community advocates, and patients over three days. Specifically, I interviewed five patients, eleven doctors, six nurses, four psychosocial staff, seven researchers, and two community-based activists. Each participant signed a consent form, interviews were taped and transcribed, and each participant was offered a gift of See's Candies following the interview. The National Sickle Cell Association allowed me to use a booth generally reserved for pharmaceutical companies.

For the experiment I described three hypothetical dilemmas and asked my informants to respond:

> Dilemma One: Jasmine is 15 years old. Her physician has told her that she is an excellent candidate for a bone marrow transplant. *She wants the transplant, but her parents refuse to give their consent.* For her the risk seems small. Two friends received transplants and are now doing well. Her parents believe the risk is too high. *Should Jasmine be allowed to get a transplant without her parents' permission and why?*

> Dilemma Two: Simon is 15 years old. His physician has told him that he is an excellent candidate for a bone marrow transplant. *Simon's parents want Simon to have the transplant, but Simon does not want to have the transplant. Should Simon be required to undergo the transplant and why?*

> Dilemma Three: Jasmine is now 28. She was not allowed to have the bone marrow transplant, and she was not offered another opportunity to have a transplant. *At 28 Jasmine is severely ill and spends 6 months of every year in the hospital. Given her present condition, should Jasmine have been allowed to have the transplant at 15 and why?*

The dilemmas seem deceptively pedestrian without any medical context. The chances of surviving a bone marrow transplant disease-free decreases from approximately 90 percent for patients under ten years of age to 80 percent for patients over ten. Physicians prefer to perform transplants on children under ten because overall survival is almost 100 percent and disease-free survival is around 90 percent. For older patients, ten to sixteen years old, overall survival is around 88 percent and disease-free survival is around 80 percent. In a study of parental decision-making, only 49 percent would accept the current mortality risks for bone marrow transplantation in theory.[23] In practice, physicians report that parents are even more reluctant to agree to a transplant than the literature indicates. Even using the current predictors for future disease severity—early swelling of the hands, high levels of white blood cells, and anemia during the second year of life—parents will often reject a transplant unless their child has had serious disease-related events, including stroke and recurring acute chest syndrome (sickling in the lungs), one of the leading causes of death.[24] Therefore, discussions of bone marrow transplantation take on credible urgency when patients are between the ages of ten and sixteen, at which time a patient's disease severity becomes clear. Most myeloablative transplants, which involve destroying all of the patient's bone marrow, have protocols that exclude patients over the age of sixteen. Nonmyeloablative transplants, where only some of the patient's bone marrow is destroyed, creating a mixed hematopoietic chimerism, or a marrow that produces sickled and normal cells, are currently being tested on patients in their thirties. The procedure for nonmyeloablative transplants remains highly experimental.

Jesica's treatment narrative was shaped by four powerful cultural beliefs about the body and medicine. First, that it is rational to want to preserve the body at any cost. Second, that all medical interventions reduce suffering. Third, that adults are better able to determine what medical interventions will enhance a mature minor's quality of life. Fourth, that physicians are the authorities when it comes to determining when a parent or patient is making a rational medical choice. Responses to my ethical thought experiment were framed in large part by these same cultural beliefs. Medical professionals, research scientists, and patient advocates ($n=30$) seemed to accept these values as rational. Sickle cell patients ($n=5$), on the other hand, expressed a different understanding of rational action in medical decision-making. The patient responses differed enough that I broke the samples into two groups, and my response rate calculations are based upon this division. Before describing this disparity and its significance, I will present the results.

Assuming that Jasmine was mature and able to understand the transplant procedure and risks, 30 percent of the medical professionals, researchers, and community advocates said that Jasmine should be allowed to have the transplant without her parents' consent. When I included the sickle cell patients, who comprised about 15 percent of the entire sample, that figure increased to 40 percent. Patients overwhelmingly believed that the underage Jasmine should have the power to consent to her medical care. Fifty percent of nurses, compared to 9 percent of physicians, said they would try to bypass parental authority. This occupational disparity demonstrates that one's professional relationship to patients and the health care system influences beliefs about adolescent rights. When responding to the dilemmas, nurses, for example, generally assumed the role of patient advocate. In contrast, physicians attempted to balance the interests of the parent and patient against the interests of the institution. This pragmatic approach was not simply an attempt to instantiate institutional power and medical authority. Rather, many of the physicians did not think that transplants were panaceas and therefore worthy of a court battle. One respondent, a white, male physician, commented: "Many transplanters are cowboys. I had a patient with [a chronic condition] that went to do a transplant in a nearby state. [The doctor] said, 'Sure I can do a transplant for his disease. What is that by the way?' Honestly. . . . This is conveyed to me by the mother. I mean they're transplanting end-stage brain tumors for God's sake. I think that's unethical."

Two male respondents, a physician and a research scientist, argued that scientists and judges should be given the authority to decide whether Jasmine should receive a transplant. Both respondents believed that medical and legal authority should be considered as relevant, if not more relevant, than parental autonomy. Justifying his response the physician, who was from Nigeria, said, "I come from a background that says, 'It takes a village to raise a child.'" The scientist, who was a genetics researcher from Ghana, argued that in clinical dilemmas such as these adults and children should be required to demonstrate their medical knowledge in order to earn the right to consent. Sixty-three percent of all nonpatients (19 out of 30 cases) clearly stated that parental approval trumps Jasmine's desires for a transplant. The number one reason cited was that transplantation requires a strong support network and if the parents are unsupportive, Jasmine's recovery would be compromised. Most transplant patients require a year of pre- and postoperative care and therefore, my informants reasoned, if Jasmine's parents harbor any resentment, they may not fully participate in helping her recover.

An overwhelming 73 percent of all nonpatients (22 out of 30) felt that Simon should not be forced to undergo the procedure. Most argued that, given the pain and postoperative treatment regimens, it would be unlikely that an unwilling patient would benefit from the transplant. The 17 percent who said that Simon should be required to undergo a transplant believed that Simon's resistance was probably based on his lack of knowledge, immaturity, and/or fear, which they considered illegitimate bases for rejecting a medically indicated transplant. Three respondents, or 10 percent, argued that an outside authority should decide for the family. These respondents included the two men from West Africa, as well as a female physician from India who believed strongly that parents should have authority over their children until the age of eighteen. Her belief in the sanctity of parental autonomy applies only in cases where the benefits of transplantation are unclear: "I feel that this decision is very medical rather than ethical. So I'm biased. I feel that this depends on the medical situation of the patient." She believed that parents and physicians should have equal authority, and in the case of a dispute, the decision should be made by an outside authority.

Respondents were almost equally divided over whether prognosis (or hindsight, depending on perspective) should determine whether Jasmine should be given the power to consent to a transplant at fifteen. Fifty-three percent believed that if Jasmine's terminal status at twenty-eight had been predictable, then she should have had the right at age fifteen to consent to a risky transplant. That number includes the 30 percent who initially agreed that Jasmine should be given the right to consent and the 23 percent who changed their answer given the information about her medical status at twenty-eight. Others believed that even with tools of prognostication the choices are not so clear. For example, some argued that there are so many variables that affect future morbidity and mortality that the predictive measures will never be 100 percent accurate, and in addition, new therapies are on the horizon and so waiting for the next cutting-edge treatment makes sense. Finally, a number of respondents felt that extenuating circumstances make every adolescent consent case unique, and therefore many felt that their answers might change based upon variables such as the severity of Jasmine's and Simon's sickle cell disease, the current state of the art with respect to treatments, and the quality of Jasmine's and Simon's support network.

The medical professionals, researchers, and community advocates viewed underage consent as either a question of rational choice, patient autonomy, or individual versus institutional checks and balances. Very rarely did this group consider parental autonomy the final judgment. Only three argued that parental autonomy is necessary given an adolescent's essential lack of maturity. The other twenty-seven believed Jasmine and Simon were competent enough to make an informed decision but considered parental rights a necessary part of a structural checks and balances system.

Overall, the issue for the majority of respondents was not patient maturity. Suggested in all the answers were different understandings of what it means to save a life. For some, saving a life means keeping a body alive. I would put into that category respondents who framed the issue as a "medical" rather than an "ethical" decision. By the use of the term "medical" they meant decisions that should be determined by evidence-based medicine. These individuals drew a firm distinction between rational and irrational choice. The second category of respondents includes those who believed that lifesaving means giving adolescent patients the agency to determine their own futures, to paint their own lifescape, even if that means taking extreme risks. Finally, the third category includes those who believed that saving a life is not just about saving a physical body but about saving a social body as well. These respondents acknowledged the arbitrariness of the law, but understood its value in freeing physicians and institutions from responsibility for risk-taking. A male physician originally from India said, "Well, you know, parents are given complete control over the destiny of their children, and that is the ethical framework in which all of civilization, not only western civilization is based, so. . . ." He added, "Any line that you draw in the sand is a line drawn in the sand. The wind can blow it away you know" (laughs). This physician recognized the arbitrariness of the age of majority but respected that it exists as a solution to impasses. Under no circumstances would he go to court over either of these ethical dilemmas, primarily because of the medical uncertainty surrounding transplantation but also because the legal lines protect all parties. His appreciation of medical uncertainty seemed to fuel his desire for clearly demarcated structural and legal boundaries. This became apparent in his final comments regarding why he believes Jasmine's prognosis should not be a factor.

> Dr. Kassim: Hindsight is twenty-twenty is the only reason I can tell you why.
> Carolyn: But they are trying to find new ways of developing prognostic tools. . . .
> Dr. Kassim: Sure, but that is still really in development you know. Okay, so . . . I gave a talk on unrelated donor transplant to the ethics institute at the University of Minnesota. Jeff Kahn and all those people and Art Caplan had been there before.

Unrelated donor transplants are much riskier than related donor matches, and so this doctor's talk addressed the question, If sickle cell disease can be treated through chronic transfusion therapy and hydroxyurea (and other less significant therapies), is transplantation a legitimate option?

> Dr. Kassim: I talked to them for an hour and I said, "Answer my question, is it ethical to do unrelated donor transplant for sickle cell disease?" They said, "Ah, nice talk." You know. . . .
> Carolyn: They avoided the question! (laughs). . . .
> Dr. Kassim: They said, "Can we write a paper?" I said, "What do you mean?" You're ethicists. You're suppose to tell me what to do!" They said, "No. Ethicists can allow you to phrase the question. We can't give

you the answer." So, that would be why I have this little bias, and I'm sorry that I haven't answered any of your questions the way you wanted me to! (laughs).

Physicians in this study like this pediatric hematologist make up the bulk of those who desire clear structural and legal boundaries. It is an overwhelming responsibility to put a patient's life at risk. Physicians readily prescribe medications because doing so shifts responsibility for potential disease or disability from the physician to the patient, the drug manufacturer, or pathophysiological chance. With experience, physicians modify treatment protocols to match what they observe in the clinic, but particularly with respect to new treatments supported by a respected scientific study, it is difficult to, for example, not prescribe a cholesterol-lowering drug or a new pain reliever. It is not simply a reductionistic approach to the body; physicians are truly unnerved by the thought that something they did or did not do could end in a patient's death or disability. When I introduced the issue of medical uncertainty during another interview with a white male physician from the West Coast, this was his response:

Dr. Allen: You know, hydroxyurea has made a huge difference in their overall survival.
Carolyn: It's really changed who dies and who doesn't.
Dr. Allen: Well, according to Steinberg's paper last summer, there is a 40 percent decrease in death.
Carolyn: And you see that in your clinic?
Dr. Allen: Oh, yeah, I see kids that were admitted all the time and they're not coming in at all anymore.

The fact that sickle cell patients are often treated by physicians who know very little about sickle cell disease also changes how aggressively some physicians pursue different treatments and therapies, including bone marrow transplantation. Earlier in the conversation this same hematologist mentioned, "If the choices were to have a transplant or go off to Indiana where there isn't a sickle cell patient in the state, then. . . ."

For the patients, patients and parents were the only legitimate decision-makers. Once a patient or guardian understood the risks and benefits, then, from the perspective of the patients, the institutional concerns were simply obstacles. All the patients had disabused themselves of the belief that there is one rational treatment choice and had accepted instead that treatment decisions were based on a series of trade-offs. Medical decisions were never right or wrong but rather better or worse based upon patient perspective. In order to support their reasoning, all cited numerous examples of doctor error in diagnosis and treatment. In most cases they had already lost confidence in the medical system, recognizing that both systems and individuals fail.[25] In response, they had developed medical decision-making strategies that they felt liberated them from dominant discourses about the miracles of medicine. These strategies were rooted not in a rejection of biomedicine but rather in an acknowledgment of the tremendous uncertainties in medicine. Because of these uncertainties, they felt that patients, even adolescents, should be given the respect and authority to decide on their course of treatment even if it went against standard protocols.

One of the patient respondents, Doris (a Jamaican woman and director of a sickle cell support network), who rejects most of the sickle cell treatments encouraged by her physicians, said, "If a person really wants to do it (have a transplant), let them at least try. My thing is like, hydroxyurea, I personally make a choice I don't want it. I'm going to try something else."

> Carolyn: So, you were offered it?
> Doris: Yeah, I didn't want it. Because to me, that would be like adding more stuff to my system than my system probably can't deal with. That's the way I look at it. I said, "Let me try another route and then I will see how that works."

Another sickle cell patient, Jan, stated that she, too, refuses standard therapies. She sought refuge in religion from chronic blood transfusions after deciding that they were wrong: "After I had my second child and they wanted to give me blood. I was so sick of taking blood transfusions. My sister who lived in the Los Angeles area at the time said, 'Why are you crying?' And I said, 'Because I've got this bag of blood hanging here and I'm so sick of taking blood I don't know what to do.' She said, "Talk to a Jehovah's Witness. They do not take blood.' The next year, I got into a Bible study and everything."

Jan, a thin, light-skinned women in her fifties, exuded vitality. Her energy and longevity masked her precarious health. In addition to her frequent pain episodes, she has had double vision in one eye and near blindness in another, and she has had thirteen operations, including two hip replacements. Despite her disabilities, Jan was pursuing a degree in counseling. Her goal was to educate physicians about the patient's perspective. She said, "Don't treat the person as though they are not involved, okay. That is their life, alright. So don't sit back and make decisions on a child who is able to think, alright. They are able to think and function and say, 'I've read something about this. I know some things about this. If I don't have all the information and everything then help me there so that I *do* make the right decision.' That's what I'm saying." The ways in which patient responses differed from responses given by other members of the sickle cell community can best be summed up by Tamika. Tamika, similar to most of the sickle cell patients, had a difficult time maintaining one perspective about whether patients or parents should be awarded autonomy. Responding to Simon's dilemma, Tamika said:

> There might be a reason why this child does not want to have the transplant. He might be scared, he might be nervous. That's a kind of hard question actually because the parents' want him to have it and he doesn't want to have it. I think that if that child has sickle cell, and that's the way that child feels, than the child shouldn't have to have it. Because I'm like this . . . I have the disease myself and everybody says, "Oh, you know, there might be a cure for sickle cell," and stuff like that. I was born with this disease, I'm gonna leave here with that disease, and the reason why I feel like that is because this is something that God gave me. Also, when they say that they find cures and stuff like that, I always hear that there is a side effect. I have enough problems I don't need any more. Honestly.

Eventually the conversation went like this:

> Tamika: If Simon died, it was Simon's time to go [Carolyn and Tamika laugh]. It was Simon's time to go.
> Carolyn: Just accept it.
> Tamika: Right. Because I've been in the hospital, and I've been overdosed and stuff like that. And they would have to pump my stomach and bring me back. I could have died, but it wasn't my time to go. So, if Simon died, it was Simon's time to go I believe.

Tamika's fatalism was mirrored by all but one of the patients.

CONCLUDING THOUGHTS

Could Jesica have had the same fatalistic attitude toward life? If so, given the opportunity to make her own medical decisions, what types of choices would she have made? Was the pain of a transplant and almost inevitable complications something she chose for herself or something others chose for her? By participating in a hopeful narrative generated by her parents, a scientific community, and her benefactors Jesica insured that she would not suffer alone, but at what cost to the quality of her short life? Some might argue that the sheltered Jesica was too immature to consent, but perhaps her immaturity resulted from our failure in general to involve chronically ill adolescents in decisions that shape their future. Perhaps we limit the agency of sick adolescents out of fear that they will imagine a destiny that does not embrace biotechnology. Perhaps chronically ill teenagers who have most likely experienced the best and worst of health care recognize the limits of medicine with unnerving clarity.

With respect to the ethical dilemma, the respondents in my study determined what constitutes rational or ethical choice based upon their understanding of what it means to save a life. For some, to save a life means to preserve the physical body regardless of the quality of that life. These respondents felt that decisions about transplantation must rely upon evidence-based risk assessments. Authority, in other words, should be granted to the one whose medical decisions are rooted in scientific reason. Others felt that transplantation decisions must rely upon the patient's own risk assessments, which factor in interpersonal experience.[26] These respondents believed that Jasmine and Simon should have the right to consent regardless of the supposed risks or benefits. For others, the fact that bone marrow transplants continue to be highly risky and experimental means that no decision is rational and therefore all decisions should be in the best interest of the institution. Denying adolescents the right to consent, they felt, is somewhat arbitrary, nevertheless having a legal age of consent is helpful for demarcating lines of authority.

As more and more risky therapies become available for chronically ill adolescents, the question of a mature minor's role in deciding his or her future should give us pause. Many medical interventions for serious diseases are not cures but a series of trade-offs for different types of suffering, and chronically ill children, like Jesica, often suffer in ways that medical science neither recognizes nor can alleviate. While culturally hope is a driving force behind innovative medicine, hope can also limit the ways we imagine a patient's future. Perhaps Jesica wanted the transplant because the risks of complications were preferable to living with the knowledge that she was terminal. Or perhaps she did not want the transplant and would have preferred finding ways to adapt to living with restrictive cardiomyopathy. While the first scenario was validated by the medical community, the Santillans, Mack Mahoney, and numerous benefactors, the second scenario received no cultural validation. The dominant discourse of hope limited Jesica's ability to determine her own future, yet the investment in these hopeful narratives ultimately shortened her life.

The ethical thought experiment demonstrated that even though hope is sold in the medical marketplace, members of the sickle cell community are profoundly aware of the uncertainty surrounding chronic illness and different types of interventions. The respondents who sided with the parents, in the case of Jasmine, based their decision in large part on the legal age of consent, which they recognized is a line drawn in the sand. On the other hand, many of the same respondents expressed concerns about adolescent patient compliance, not simply to treatment, but to scientific reason. One physician said, for example, that he would side with the parents if they expressed concern about treatment risks. But, he stated emphatically, if Jasmine's parents rejected a transplant for religious reasons, he would take them to court immediately. So, even though many professionals would find it acceptable to grant adolescents the right to consent, they do not feel comfortable granting rights to adolescents who reject the narratives of medicine and rationality. Hope, positivism, and the cultural value of children are powerful social forces that clearly contributed to Jesica's diminished ability to shape her treatment narrative and life story.

NOTES

I wish to thank Susan Lieff, Ph.D., and the Sickle Cell Disease Association of America for their support and generosity.

1. Nancy Rommelmann, "Grief's Gravity," *Los Angeles Weekly*, February 20–26, 2004.

2. Myra Bluebond-Langner, *The Private Worlds of Dying Children* (Princeton: Princeton University Press, 1978), 210–30.

3. Psychologists have determined that most seven-year-olds understand that death is irreversible and universal and that the dead are unable to function. From this, I think we can extrapolate that young children recognize at least some of the risk implications of a treatment that may result in death. See Mark W. Spence and Sandor B. Brent, "Irreversibility, Nonfunctionality, and Universality: Children's Understanding of Three Components of a Death Concept," in *Children and Death: Perspectives from Birth Through Adolescence*, ed. John E. Schowalter, Penelope Buschman, Paul R. Patterson, Austin H. Kutscher, Margot Tallmer, Robert G. Stevenson (New York: Praeger, 1987), 19–29.

4. Allison Fass, "Duking It Out," Forbes.com, June 9, 2003, <http://www.forbes.com/forbes/2003/0609/074.html>. This encounter was cited in a number of articles on the Internet.

5. Marilyn J. Field and Richard E. Behrman, eds., *Ethical Conduct of Clinical Research Involving Children* (Washington, D.C.: National Academies Press, 2004), S-6 (prepublication copy, uncorrected proofs).

6. Ibid.

7. G. Robinson, "Families, Generations, and Self: Conflict, Loyalty, and Recognition in an Australian Aboriginal Society," *Ethos* 25 (3) (1997): 303–32.

8. L. M. Burton, "Ethnography and the Meaning of Adolescence in High-Risk Neighborhoods," *Ethos* 25 (2) (1997): 208–17; R. G. Condon, "The Rise of Adolescence: Social Change and Life Stage Dilemmas in Central Canadian Arctic," *Human Organization* 49 (3) (1987): 266–79; L. Neyzi, "Object or Subject?: The Paradox of 'Youth' in Turkey," *International Journal of Middle East Studies* 33 (2001): 411–32.

9. Margaret Mead, *Coming of Age in Samoa: A Psychological Study of Primitive Youth for Western Civilization* (New York: Morrow, 1928); Mary Bucholtz, "Youth Culture and Practice," *Annual Review of Anthropology* 31 (2002): 525–52.

10. Sociologist Joseph Telfair has written extensively on the role a clinic can play in helping adolescent patients achieve independence in the case of sickle cell disease. He believes strongly that adolescents who become self-sufficient early are more likely to have better treatment outcomes as adults.

11. Rommelmann, "Grief's Gravity."

12. Ibid.

13. Ibid.

14. Jesica's Hope Chest, Inc., Web site, <http://www.4jhc.org/jhcmission.html>.

15. While I do not disagree with Rosamond Rhodes (see her essay in this volume) that physicians are the best judges of how scarce organs should be allocated based upon medical criteria, I do question how accurate they are in assessing other criteria including future patient adherence or other soft measures used to determine if a patient is worthy of a transplant. In order to be considered worthy, vulnerable populations are often forced to perform in the clinic in ways that undo problematic stereotypes. For poor undocumented people like the Santillans, they were also forced to perform for the public in order to receive the financial resources necessary for Jesica's transplant.

16. Statistics for black and Hispanic youth were compiled by Human Rights Watch based upon the 2000 census data: "U.S. Incarceration Rates Reveal Striking Racial Disparities," Human Rights Watch, February 27, 2002, <http://hrw.org/backgro under/ usa/race/pdf/race-bck.pdf>.

17. The Convention on the Rights of Children, which was adopted by the United Nations General Assembly on November 20, 1989, outlines what the drafters believe are children's inalienable rights. Rights include the right of children under the age of eighteen to be treated differently from adults by the justice system and to have the right to healthcare and education. Missing from this charter is a clear recognition that, cross-culturally, teenagers assume very different roles. In some cultures it is not uncommon for girls under eighteen years of age to be married. In other cultures, children work to help provide for the family.

18. Mary-Jo Delvecchio Good, "The Biotechnical Embrace," *Culture, Medicine, and Psychiatry* 25 (4) (December 2001): 395–410.

19. The political economy of hope is well articulated in Ernst Bloch, *The Principle of Hope* (Cambridge, Mass.: MIT Press, 1986); and Hirokawa Miyazaki, *The Method of Hope: Anthropology, Philosophy, and Fijian Knowledge* (Stanford, Calif.: Stanford University Press, 2004).

20. David J. Rothman, *Strangers at the Bedside: A Brief History of How Law and Ethics Transformed Medical Decision-Making* (New York: Basic Books, 1991).

21. Christine M. Hanisco, "Acknowledging the Hypocrisy: Granting Minors the Right to Choose Their Medical Treatment," *New York Law School Journal of Human Rights* 899 (Summer 2000) (16 N.Y.L. Sch. J. Hum. Rts. 899).

22. Ibid. ("torture").

23. Christiane Vermylen, "Hematopoietic Stem Cell Transplantation in Sickle Cell Disease," *Blood Review* 17 (3) (September 2003): 163–66.

24. Ibid.

25. Regardless of damage control for medical system failures (see essays by Gross and Bosk in this volume), the disparities in healthcare and health outcomes by race have left an indelible mark in the consciousness of most sickle cell patients, many of whom have witnessed these disparities firsthand.

26. Kleinman and Kleinman argue for an approach to studying human suffering that considers the indeterminacy and uncertainty of individual experiences of suffering. See Arthur Kleinman and Joan Kleinman, "Suffering and Its Professional Transformation: Toward an Ethnography of Interpersonal Experience," *Culture, Medicine, and Psychiatry* 15 (3) (September 1991): 275–301.

FAME AND FORTUNE

THE "SIMPLE" ETHICS OF

ORGAN TRANSPLANTATION

NANCY M. P. KING

Jesica always wanted to be famous. It's just a shame she had to be famous this way.—Mack Mahoney, Santillan family benefactor, Raleigh News and Observer, 2004

As the essays in this volume show, the story of Jesica Santillan's bungled transplant raises many questions about medical technology, bioethics, and American society. These questions appear in Jesica's story as both new and yet familiar.

What interests me most is their familiarity. These questions return again and again, in stories about medical advances and family tragedy, because they haven't really been answered. And the questions are familiar for another reason, too: they go hand in hand with the stories of individuals like Jesica, whom we come to know through the peculiar variety of fame exemplified in her story and examined in this volume. These stories are characterized not only by fame but also by fortune—that is, both money (organ transplantation both generates and requires a great deal of it) and luck (being on the right list in the right place at the right time with the right blood type and the right story to show that you deserve your organ and will treat it well). The familiar and recurring questions, when asked about transplantation, show us that fame and fortune, a historically simple formula for success, is deceptively simple—in reality, devilishly complicated in terms of technology, society, and ethics.

Three narratives help illuminate this complexity. First, the story of how organ transplantation has evolved from experiment to expected treatment, even while it is still a profoundly imperfect technology, represents some key aspects of how we regard scientific progress. Second, the stories that are told about patients and doctors involved in life-and-death technologies like organ transplantation seem to teach us something about what we collectively value —both by what such stories include and by what they omit. And finally, the way our storytelling unfolds, when we are presented not only with Jesica's story but also with those of her many sisters—not only Libby Zion, Baby Fae, and Julie Rodriquez (see the Lerner and Sharp essays in this volume) but also Karen Ann Quinlan, Nancy Cruzan, Jamie Fisk, Ladan and Laleh Bijani, and, most recently, Terri Schiavo—raises questions about the relationships between individual and societal viewpoints and responsibilities. How do—or should—individual stories really matter?

Twenty-five years ago, Jamie Fisk's father took to newspapers the story of his adorable toddler daughter's incurable liver disease and Blue Cross/Blue Shield of Massachusetts' refusal to pay for her transplant.[1] Amazingly, this appeal to consider liver transplantation as the standard of care for biliary atresia came fewer than twenty years after Bennie Solis, the first toddler to be given a new liver for the same disease, died during the surgery (see Sharp essay in this volume). Today, Jesica Santillan and her mother appear on television public service announcements in North Carolina promoting organ donation through a foundation called Jesica's Hope Chest.[2] Jesica's death in February 2003 is not mentioned.

Organ transplantation has had a short and spectacular history as a technology. Thanks to attractive poster children from Jamie to Jesica, it has gone from expensive, uncertain, innovative, and not covered by insurance to so standard and familiar that people are no longer said to die from organ failure. Instead, they are said to die for lack of transplantable organs (see Rhodes essay in this volume). Yet organ transplantation is still expensive; it still has many of innovation's characteristics, even as it is considered routine; and it is, most definitely, an uncertain, burdensome, and medically complex "halfway technology."[3]

Both because Jesica would have died if she had not received a transplant and because she died after her mismatched transplant, it is easy to forget that life after transplantation is challenging in many respects (see Cook essay in this volume).[4] "In six years, I've had a stroke, a possible rejection episode, two bouts with double pneumonia, a nasty (and potentially life-threatening) cryptococcal fungal infection, and taken over $100,000 in anti-rejection drugs," said Geov Parrish, recipient of a kidney-pancreas transplant, in 2001. Even more challenging is the other key aspect of this halfway technology—it's temporary: "[M]y six-year-old non-native organs have a finite life span," Parrish added. As transplantation technology, immunosuppression, and aftercare improve—which, through innovation, they surely will—difficult medical, societal, and ethical questions about repeat transplantation can only increase. As Parrish poignantly asks about himself, "I'm left with one of those too-simple questions: How much is the extension of a life worth?"[5]

Even though it is a resource-intensive halfway technology, organ transplantation does offer patients a reasonable likelihood of an outcome that is often significantly better than available alternatives. In light of continual technological advances, it may be exceedingly difficult to remember that there is no certainty attached to any outcome. This difficulty is not unique to transplantation but is shared by many medical technologies. Two good examples represent the most common and the rarest of technologies, respectively: Cardiopulmonary resuscitation, or CPR, and the artificial heart.

CPR is routinely depicted on television as highly effective rescue technology.[6] It works—way too often on TV, of course, in comparison to real life—or it fails and death follows. What is left out of the picture is the patient whose heartbeat is restored but whose brain has been irreversibly damaged, or who cannot be weaned from the respirator after resuscitation. End-of-life decision-making in health care has for many years been plagued by the reality of what lies in between definitive failure and definitive success, even though CPR has become routine. At least some patients and families with experience as the beneficiaries of medical technology now refuse resuscitation because they fear what will happen if it doesn't work. And even those without experience rely on stories about its failure to inform their decisions. In the 1980s, people said, "Don't let me become another Karen Ann Quinlan." In the 1990s, they instead referred to Nancy Cruzan. Today, of course, the person many of us don't want to live like is Terri Schiavo.[7] It is noteworthy—but perhaps not surprising—that the invocation of these women's names condenses intricate narratives of family tragedy into simplified images of helpless and dependent young women whom technology has both saved and failed.

At the other end of the spectrum, the AbioCor totally implantable artificial heart has been tested in humans for whom no other technologies were left to try, and whose deaths were expected very soon. Patients who were "cardiac cripples" clamored to become research subjects, viewing the artificial heart experiment as their last hope. One of those subjects experienced complication after complication. After his death, his widow sued the manufacturer of the device and the academic medical center where the research was conducted. She said that she and her husband had expected that if the experiment did not work, he would simply die. They did not anticipate the possibility of a twilight existence with such a poor quality of life. She claimed that her husband was not informed of this kind of bad outcome, which he viewed as a fate worse than death.[8]

Medical innovation is always attended by optimism—if it weren't, it wouldn't happen. Almost by definition, innovations lack a reasonable expectation of success. Yet the innovator's intention is to benefit the patient. Newsworthy innovations generally involve very sick, even desperately sick, patients who are regarded (and may regard themselves) as having little or nothing to lose. The novelty of the proposal and the confidence of the innovator combine to produce overoptimism about success—usually in the absence of much supporting evidence.[9] And then, apparently promising innovations, piloted out of necessity and lack of information, can easily become standardized by virtue of enthusiasm and by default. Scholars like John McKinlay and Thomas Chalmers acknowledged this in their classic writings well over twenty years ago.[10]

One of the key issues in the transition of a medical technology from new to standard is what actually should be counted as success. In transplantation, most of the time the alternatives are pretty poor choices. That makes transplantation better than nothing, better than lousy, and better than being dead. But a lack of satisfactory alternatives, by itself, doesn't necessarily make transplantation a good technology. Instead, it ensures that transplantation, like other innovative medical technologies, will always involve the maximum tolerable amount of uncertainty (see Cook essay). It also promotes what I call "desperation creep": an inevitable, heartfelt, disturbing, and ever-expanding argument that the only thing that is good for patients is the speedy development of new technology. Taking time to move forward carefully is, by this argument, equated with enslavement to the "insensitive" demands of science, and with causing patients unnecessary suffering by denying them the chance to gamble on the new.

Surprisingly (to me at least), this portrait of innovations is generally not regarded as problematic; instead it is sexy. The lone ranger transplant surgeon is often a cowboy hire, known—and courted—for the ability and willingness to push the envelope and capture both attention and financial support. (Note the use of "lone ranger" and "cowboy" to describe not only physicians, in the Rouse essay in this volume, but also Mack Mahoney, in the Morgan et al. essay in this volume.) This portrait is especially seductive in surgery, a practice area that has historically been largely exempted from standardized research pathways. Our fascination with surgical innovation makes it frequently both prestigious and lucrative for major medical centers. Innovative practitioners are sought after and valued as teachers, mentors, and faculty stars. They participate in the same media mechanisms their patients use to make themselves visible, desirable, worthy of public attention. To give just one example, Dr. Ben Carson, a prominent Johns Hopkins neurosurgeon who specializes in separating conjoined twins, appeared in the movie comedy *Stuck on You* as the surgeon separating the conjoined brothers.

Perhaps not surprisingly, however, as they grow older and more experienced, cowboy surgeons display an interesting tendency to look back on their innovations with some dismay. Toward the end of their careers as spectacular surgical innovators, primarily in organ transplantation, both Thomas Starzl and Frannie Moore became increasingly reluctant cutters.[11] Moore, in particular, questioned the ethics of early efforts at surgical innovation, most of which resulted in patients' deaths. While acknowledging that successful medical innovations depend on just such failures, and that many or most such deaths were—like Jesica's—deaths that would have been inevitable without intervention, Moore worried, and rightly so, that innovations' growing pains had nonetheless inflicted suffering on those patients (see Lederer and Sharp essays in this volume).[12] He would have understood why the widow of the artificial heart recipient sued.

Even the younger cowboys sometimes question the nature and pace of medical progress—though here, too, it is only failure that pricks the conscience. The movie-struck Ben Carson was a consulting member of the surgical team that undertook the unprecedented separation of adult craniopagus conjoined twins in Singapore in July 2003. After the Bijani sisters died in surgery, he publicly criticized the way the team had planned and undertaken the procedure.

The enormous public attention focused on the Bijani sisters provides yet another example of the optimism and simplification that seem to accompany medical innovations. Ladan and Laleh Bijani, adult twins conjoined at the head, were one of only a few sets of adult conjoined twins who aggressively sought separation. Born in Iran and committed to different careers, they had consulted with surgeons all over the world and had always been told that their anatomy made the attempt too dangerous. Finally, new imaging technology convinced Dr. Keith Goh, a neurosurgeon experienced in separating conjoined infants, that the attempt was worth making. The publicity-seeking propensities of Raffles Hospital, the for-profit hospital in Singapore where he practices, may have also had an impact.[13]

The Bijani sisters' story soon became world news. The hospital asked for donations on their behalf; the Iranian government helped pay for the procedure; and the international surgical team donated their services. When the twins bled to death in surgery from an unanticipated kink in their shared arteriovenous anatomy, an enormous public debate erupted about the twins' determination that death was preferable to remaining conjoined. Their vivid and dramatic story was too easily reducible to dichotomies: autonomy versus beneficence; patients' choices versus doctors' responsibilities; elective versus indicated procedures; caution versus hope; freedom versus death. Yet most dichotomies are far too simple.

The story of the Bijani twins, like Jesica's story, exemplifies the complexity of uncertainty and optimism in medicine. The intent to benefit patients, the need to believe in the possibility of success, even the rewards (both spiritual and material) of altruism can deeply imbue providers with unwarranted optimism, affecting how they themselves think about the potential harms and benefits, how they present them to patients, and thus how the decision appears to and is discussed by everyone. This was as true in Jesica's case as it was for the Bijani twins.

Because it focuses so naturally on individual patients, donors, and surgeons, organ transplantation can readily promote a fallacious moral simplicity, attending to the trees while ignoring the forest. It is quite possible that one of the most important accomplishments of such "simplifying stories" is to deflect public attention from the inherent uncertainty of medicine (even though experienced patients themselves can appreciate it, as Rouse demonstrates in this volume); from close examination of the necessary social and bureaucratic complexities of health care delivery (see Cook and Gross essays in this volume); and from the problem of evaluating medical judgment (see Lerner essay).

While we watch the trees, the forest that surrounds us, unseen, represents not only the actual complexity of medical technologies but also the historical trajectory of innovation and the moral status of resource-intensive technologies in a landscape of unmet needs: How much is the extension of a life worth? The problem of how to address both the rights and interests of individual moral actors and the priorities and needs of populations and communities in health care (see Scheper-Hughes essay in this volume) is complicated by our collective interest in captivating, newsworthy cases above all else. Jesica Santillan, Jamie Fiske, and the Bijani sisters were "identified lives," gaining attention while others in equal need of it could not. Indeed, the history and ethics of the allocation of scarce resources like transplantable organs has always depended on the simplifications made possible by focusing on identified lives (see Wailoo and Livingston essay in this volume).[14]

In the 1960s, before transplantation was common, bioethics got off to a bad early start in the form of "God committees," which doled out access to a scarce resource: kidney dialysis. An infusion of federal funding for dialysis soon solved the problem of how to choose who was "worthy" of that life-extending, but physically and psychologically demanding, halfway technology. But by that time, the components of the choice—and the way petitioners for access sought to convince the gatekeepers of their "worthiness"—had become all too familiar in the transplant arena (see Rhodes, Gross, and Lederer essays in this volume).[15]

These days, the requirements that would-be organ recipients must meet include money, assertiveness, medical suitability, having a connection to primary care, compliance, social support, and the promise of a sufficiently stable future to maximize the life of the organ. Not surprisingly, these requirements translate into a psychosocial screening process that tries hard to avoid the moral pitfall of social worth determinations but still manages to seem, in practice at least, like a job interview in which the interviewers worry about whether the applicant will "fit in."

And if "a Henry David Thoreau with bad kidneys" hasn't got much of a chance to make a good impression on the judges, and the prostitute or the playboy even less, well then, the young and the photogenic, innocent victims of life's unfairness, always seem to do fine.[16] *Their* desperation can make *us*— potential donors, benefactors, surgeons, institutions, the public at large—feel generous and noble, both when we give and when we approve of what is given. Giving something to support the identified lives of transplant recipients is, apparently, far more satisfying than paying taxes, or writing a check to a charity, or improving sanitation and the public water supply, or making prenatal care and vaccinations available to all in need.

Thus, the public is becoming accustomed to the heroic stories of living donor transplantation: the North Carolina teacher who gave a kidney to her student; the New York physician who gave a kidney to her patient; the couples who give kidneys, or liver lobes, or lung lobes, to each other's spouses; the North Carolina man who donated bone marrow to both of his brothers; the wife whose donation of a kidney to her husband has saved their marriage; the friends who are organ donor and recipient; the donor and recipient who become friends. In the 1980s, when talking with an organ procurement official in Massachusetts, I was given a promotional pen stamped with the slogan, "Organ donors recycle themselves." Today, organ procurement organizations regularly urge people to become organ and tissue donors by means of national campaigns featuring "many really moving stories from around the country."[17]

Jesica's story is such a one, despite—or perhaps because of—her death. As the Raleigh *News and Observer* put it in February 2004: "Save for one horrible mistake a year ago Saturday, Jesica Santillan might have lived as a triumph of community support and medical science—an immigrant child doomed to die from a congenital heart defect, rescued by a heart-lung transplant."[18] That quote alone is a perfect example of how transplantation promotes a focus on the identified life, overstates the potential benefits and understates the potential harms of a halfway technology, and creates a neatly oversimplified dichotomy of death and rescue that fails to acknowledge the complexity of the moral framework of health care choices.

Difficult decisions always involve more than the dyad of doctor and patient. Many people, institutions, and entities had stakes in Jesica's story, for a variety of reasons. Her celebrity gained her a benefactor;[19] her benefactor used her celebrity to ensure that Duke University Hospital acknowledged its error in her case and reformed its procedures relating to transplantation (see Morgan et al. and Diflo essays in this volume). The "firestorm of publicity" surrounding Jesica's death may have temporarily helped sidetrack efforts to limit awards in medical malpractice lawsuits, and even to call attention to the need to prevent medical errors in hospitals.[20]

And at least in part because of Jesica's story—but also because of the increasing numbers of telenovelas on North Carolina television and tiendas and taquerias all across the state—medicine and medical education in North Carolina has increasingly taken account of Latino culture, customs, and language over the last five to ten years. Nonetheless, familiar and unanswered questions continue to appear in this new cross-cultural context. To give just one example, after Jesica was declared dead by neurological criteria, her family requested a second opinion about the diagnosis. It appeared from newspaper accounts that the explanation given to the family about how the determination of brain death is made, what exactly brain death is, and what it means, was poor. Determining death by neurological criteria generally requires the separate assessments of two physicians, according to specific physiological measurements, after a specified interval to ensure that the findings are not being affected by any medication. Thus, a detailed and sympathetic explanation of "brain death" might have showed the family that a second opinion had, in a way, been obtained; instead, the hospital simply refused the request.

This story is familiar because, ever since "brain death" was established as a diagnosis in the 1960s—for reasons intimately connected both with medicine's increasing technological "success" and with the need for transplantable cadaver organs[21]—health care providers and patients alike have had trouble envisioning it as "real" death. Indeed, it has been well demonstrated that health care providers' own confusion leads to poor explanations, careless language ("She's brain-dead but we're keeping her alive on the machines till the family can get here."), and misunderstanding by families and the general public.[22] Death itself is a familiar question that has not been answered.

Given this evidence of complexity in Jesica's story—and even some acknowledgment of that complexity as a means of beginning to effect change—perhaps it could be argued that, contrary to my thesis, looking hard enough at individual trees can lead us back into sight of the forest. I wish it were so. Though it can be a powerful spotlight, the artificially simplified "stakeholder" perspective on morally freighted cases and issues seems to serve principally to maintain a problematic overoptimism: things could have gone right, lives would have been saved, all can really be perfect.

Yes, compelling cases with "mediagenic" patients like Jesica do indeed command public attention. But that attention is often largely in the form of advocacy and punditry. Compelling cases are just as lousy as lawsuits as a means of designing anything that is lasting or of substance—safe automobiles, ethical codes for physicians,[23] or, in this case, morally sound public policy that addresses health care costs and needs. Instead, compelling cases usually place the public and policymakers squarely on the pendulum that seems constantly to swing between promoting and curbing medical technology.[24] The pendulum view sees technology as either perfect or perfectible: fix the trees and the forest will go away.

Bioethics scholars—myself included—are always hoping that working in the trees is going to get us a better view of the forest. But bioethics scholars are like everyone else: we generally find it easier and more congenial to contemplate a tree. Remember that bioethics has been struggling for some time now to address complicated, unwieldy, and long-unanswered organizational and policy questions about health and social justice. And we haven't (or at least I haven't) yet figured out how to "unsimplify" a discussion that has already gone public—how to move beyond advocacy and punditry to generate public interest and policy progress in system-level considerations, like access and cost in health care.

This is hard stuff, but as a society we defer the discussion at our peril. Indeed, not only are these questions not going away, they are increasingly globalized. Medical tourism, and attendant concerns about medical citizenship as described throughout this volume, now complicate health care allocation decisions worldwide, forcing us into international discourse about global health as surely as do air travel–fueled fears of pandemics. In the United States, we continue to notice patients who travel here for health care and are viewed as consuming scarce resources, like the undocumented immigrants receiving or awaiting donated organs, or as jumping the queue, like the transplant recipient whose Saudi-funded operation recently caused controversy in California.[25] But the Bijani sisters were medical tourists, too. These days, patients from all over the world move all over the world seeking scarce and costly treatments that are still cheaper or more available than what they can get at home. Others, like the Bijani twins, travel in search of medical innovation. Still others travel to enroll in clinical research.[26] Seeking global discourse on matters such as these may—like transplantation itself—appear a luxury in the face of enormous worldwide disparities in basic health care and health.[27] But Jesica's story, if it teaches us anything, shows us that nothing about health care can truly be isolated from the forest of familiar questions we have not yet navigated successfully. Every society on earth addresses these familiar questions about death and life; we need to start learning from one another's stories.

Finding a different focus on what matters in health care and in life—developing the capacity to get beyond our dependence on identified lives to fire our moral imagination and activate our sense of moral obligation—should ultimately lead to changes in individual and public decision-making about the development, promulgation, and use of resource-intensive halfway technologies like transplantation. Uncertainty and tragedy are inescapable, in health care and in life. Instead of pretending to escape uncertainty and tragedy, we have to face them. Unless we acknowledge that our task is not perfection, we may keep trying too hard to solve the wrong health care problems.

Can we ever get to that discussion by talking about Jesica? We've seen that identified lives like Jesica's are usually shaped and flattened into the simple coin of public discourse. But identified lives can also be seen as rich, detailed stories, with narrators who have points of view, minor characters with stories of their own, and intricately woven threads leading outward and upward to other stories and to unanswered questions. All humans trade stories, and trade in stories. So perhaps we could, with a little extra effort, fashion Jesica's story into a narrative that leads us, by new paths, to some new answers.

You, the reader, have by this time perused the essays in this volume, all of which tell different versions of Jesica's story. What should we do with her story now? You tell me.

NOTES

1. Clark C. Havighurst and Nancy M. P. King, "Liver Transplantation in Massachusetts: Public Policymaking as Morality Play," *Indiana Law Review* 19 (1986): 955–87.

2. Melissa Draper, "Jesica's Mom Has New TV Role," Raleigh *News and Observer*, January 2, 2004, N6.

3. Lewis Thomas, *Late Night Thoughts on Listening to Mahler's Ninth Symphony* (New York: Viking Press, 1983).

4. Rosemary Quigley, "A Weeklong Electronic Journal of a Double-Lung Transplant Recipient," *Slate* magazine online, <http://slate.msn.com/id/2096727/entry/2096 844/>.

5. Geov Parrish, "Defending My Life," *Seattle Weekly*, May 31, 2001, 17–23, reprinted in *The Social Medicine Reader*, 2nd ed., vol. 2, *Health Policy, Markets, and Medicine*, ed. J. Oberlander et al. (Durham: Duke University Press, 2005), 119–27.

6. S. J. Diem, J. D. Lantos, and J. A. Tulsky, "Cardiopulmonary Resuscitation on Television—Miracles and Misinformation," *New England Journal of Medicine* 334 (1996): 1578–82.

7. Maria Newman, "Schiavo Dies Nearly Two Weeks after Removal of Feeding Tube," *New York Times*, March 31, 2005.

8. Stacey Burling, "Life, but at What Cost?" *Philadelphia Inquirer*, September 29, 2002; Stacey Burling, "Mechanical-Heart Patient Comes to Regret His Life-Saving Choice," *Philadelphia Inquirer*, July 14, 2002; Stacey Burling, "Widow Sues Artificial-Heart Maker" *Philadelphia Inquirer*, October 17, 2002.

9. Atul Gawande, "Desperate Measures," *New Yorker*, May 5, 2003, 70–81; Nancy M. P. King, "Experimental Treatment: Oxymoron or Aspiration?" *Hastings Center Report* 25 (4) (1995): 6–15.

10. Nancy M. P. King and Gail E. Henderson, "Treatments of Last Resort: Informed Consent and the Diffusion of New Technology," *Mercer Law Review* 42 (1991): 1007; Nancy M. P. King, "The Line between Clinical Innovation and Human Experimentation," *Seton Hall Law Review* 32 (2002): 573–82.

11. Gawande, "Desperate Measures."

12. Francis D. Moore, "The Desperate Case: CARE (Costs, Applicability, Research, Ethics)," *Journal of the American Medical Association* 261 (1989): 1483–84.

13. Nancy M. P. King, "The Stories We Tell Ourselves," *Hastings Center Report* 33 (5) (2003): 49.

14. Guido Calabresi and Phillip Bobbitt, *Tragic Choices* (New York: W. W. Norton, 1987); D. A. Redelmeier and A. Teversky, "Discrepancy between Medical Decisions for Individual Patients and for Groups," *New England Journal of Medicine* 322 (1990): 1162–64.

15. George Annas, "The Prostitute, the Playboy, and the Poet: Rationing Schemes for Organ Transplantation," reprinted in Oberlander et al., eds., *Health Policy, Markets, and Medicine*, 150–57.

16. Annas, "Prostitute," 2005, quoting Sanders and Dukeminier ("a Henry David Thoreau with bad kidneys"); the reference to prostitutes and playboys is from ibid.

17. Draper, "Jesica's Mom Has New TV Role."

18. Sarah Avery and Michael Easterbrook, "A Year of Grief, Changes," *Raleigh News and Observer*, February 8, 2004, A1.

19. Nancy Rommelmann, "In Jesica's Name," *Independent Weekly*, May 19, 2004

(reprinted from "Grief's Gravity," *Los Angeles Weekly*, February 20–26, 2004, http://www.laweekly.com/features/1973/griefs-gravity/.

20. Tom Clavin, "How Can You Protect Yourself?" *Parade* magazine, May 23, 2004, 4–7.

21. A. M. Capron and L. R. Kass, "A Statutory Definition of the Standards for Determining Human Death: An Appraisal and a Proposal," *University of Pennsylvania Law Review* 121 (1972): 870.

22. S. J. Youngner, R. M. Arnold, and R. Shapiro, eds., *The Definition of Death: Contemporary Controversies* (Baltimore: Johns Hopkins University Press, 1999); G. Greenberg, "As Good As Dead," *New Yorker*, August 13, 2001, 36–41.

23. *Barber v. Superior Court*, 195 Cal. Rptr. 484 (CA Ct. App. 1983).

24. A. Mastroianni and J. Kahn, "Swinging on the Pendulum," *Hastings Center Report* 31 (3) (2001): 21.

25. On undocumented immigrants receiving or awaiting donated organs, see Mark Bixler, "Illegal, Uninsured, but Alive," *Atlanta Journal-Constitution*, April 25, 2004; on the Saudi-funded operation and the controversy in California, see Charles Ornstein, "Hospital Halts Organ Program," *Los Angeles Times*, September 27, 2005.

26. Jerome Groopman, "The Reeve Effect," *New Yorker*, November 2003. Available at <http://www.jeromegroopman.com/reeve.html>.

27. Paul Farmer, *Infections and Inequalities: The Modern Plagues* (Berkeley: University of California Press, 1999).

ACKNOWLEDGMENTS

In mid-2004, Peter Guarnaccia, Julie Livingston, and I brought together this extraordinary group of authors (from transplant surgery and medicine, anthropology, medical sociology, history, medical ethics, philosophy, health law, and health policy) for a series of conversations about the infamous "bungled transplant" and its implications for health care and society. From the start, we saw the notorious operation on Jesica Santillan at Duke University Medical Center in February 2003 as a powerful microcosm—a case study of the complex interactions among medical practice, biomedical science, and American culture, politics, and society. After a follow-up authors' meeting in May 2005, this book emerged.

The rich conversations among authors would not have happened without generous support from the James S. McDonnell Foundation's Centennial Fellowship in the History of Science—a long-term grant to Keith Wailoo to encourage the exploration of precisely the kinds of interconnections among science, medicine, politics, and society that the Santillan story embodied. The book, accordingly, offers new understandings of the far-reaching impact of modern immunology on medicine and on culture and politics. Its essays take us from the biology of immunosuppression (which has fueled the dramatic growth of organ transplantation as a field), through the administrative, technical, social, and ethical complexities associated with organ matching today. They introduce readers to the stunning array of cultural complexities involved with moving organs from donors to recipients across different social gradients, and to the moral, legal, and philosophical questions of eligibility and justice embedded in that process. They take us into contentious political questions surrounding the transplantation process—questions of citizenship, immigrants' access to health care, the regulation of medical practice, and the toll of error in high-tech medicine. And because the girl at issue in the "bungled transplant" case was a Mexican citizen living illegally in the United States, the story links the seemingly narrow, technical story of blood-type mismatch to a modern global story of mobility and the commerce in organs. In tracing these multiple dimensions, the book reflects one important goal of the McDonnell Fellowship—to promote innovative cross-disciplinary scholarship and to advance the understanding of the biomedical sciences and their sweeping implications in the modern world. In addition, a Robert Wood Johnson

Investigator Award has supported the work of several contributors in this volume, as well as my own research on themes of race, ethnicity, and disparities in health care.

The McDonnell Fellowship has supported many research assistants who have been critically important in helping create the book. They are Joseph Gabriel, Michele Rotunda, Jane Park, William Gordon, Justin Lorts, and Dominique Padurano. In particular, Stefani Pfeiffer and Rachel McLaughlin applied great energy and skill to the task of organizing our authors' meetings. Several colleagues helped to enliven these meetings when the book was in its infancy. They include Ted Marmor, Jean DeKervasdoue, Steven Feierman, Alastair Bellany, Mark Schlesinger, Brian Elbel, Samira Kawash, Ben Sifuentes-Jauregui, Onell Calderas, Jeff McMahan, and Ed Cohen. Finally, Julie, Peter, and I owe a profound thanks to the essay contributors for their patience, hard work, insight, and brilliance in developing this exceptional work of collaborative reflection.

Keith Wailoo, November 2005

CHARLES L. BOSK is professor of sociology and graduate group chair of sociology at the University of Pennsylvania. He is author of *Forgive and Remember: Managing Medical Failure* (1979); *All God's Mistakes: Genetic Counseling in a Pediatric Hospital* (1992), and the forthcoming *What Would You Do? The Collision of Ethics and Ethnography* (2006). He has a Robert Wood Johnson Foundation Investigator Award in Health Policy Research to pursue a project titled, "Restarting a Stalled Revolution: Patient Safety, Systems Error, and Professional Responsibility."

LEO R. CHAVEZ is professor of anthropology and director of the Chicano/Latino Studies Program at University of California–Irvine. He is the author of *Shadowed Lives: Undocumented Immigrants in American Society*, 2nd ed. (1997), and *Covering Immigration: Popular Images and the Politics of the Nation* (2001). His recent articles include "A Glass Half Empty: Latina Reproduction and Public Discourse," *Human Organization* (2004).

LISA VOLK CHEWNING is a Ph.D. student at Rutgers University. Her focus is in organizational communication with a minor emphasis in sociology. She also serves as project manager on a federally funded grant studying the most effective way to develop health campaigns about organ donation.

RICHARD I. COOK is associate professor in the Department of Anesthesia and Critical Care and director of the Cognitive Technologies Laboratory at the University of Chicago. A practicing anesthesiologist, he is internationally recognized as an expert on complex systems failure, the impact of technology on expert performance, and accident investigation and analysis. He was a member of the board of the National Patient Safety Foundation from its inception until 2006 and is frequently a consultant on patient safety. His most cited publications are "Operating at the Sharp End: The Complexity of Human Error," with David Woods, and "Gaps in the Continuity of Care and Progress on Patient Safety," with David Woods and Marta Render.

THOMAS DIFLO, a transplant surgeon, is associate professor of surgery and director of renal transplantation at the New York University Medical Center. His ongoing research projects involve the mechanisms of chronic rejection and the expression of matrix metalloproteinase enzymes, and the effects of immunosuppression on wound healing. He is author of several papers on transplant ethics and has been involved in documenting the international organ trade, with a particular interest in the use of prisoners' organs for transplantation in China.

JASON T. EBERL is assistant professor of philosophy and codirector of the master's program in the Department of Philosophy, Indiana University–Purdue University, Indianapolis; and an affiliate faculty member of the Indiana University Center for Bioethics.

JED ADAM GROSS, a joint J.D.-Ph.D. student at Yale University, is former managing editor of the *Yale Journal of Health Policy, Law, & Ethics*. He is author of "Getting Disability Insurance to Work: Social Security Benefits as a Means Toward Independent Living," *Quinnipiac Health Law Journal* (2003) and "Trying the Case Against Bioethics," *American Journal of Bioethics* (2006). His research interests include the cultural and political economy of organ allocation policy, scientific and medical evidence in the courtroom, and how the common law responds to technological change.

PETER GUARNACCIA is a medical anthropologist and professor at Rutgers University, jointly appointed in the Department of Human Ecology and at the Institute for Health, Health Care Policy, and Aging Research. He is author (with Lewis-Fernandez and Rivera Marano) of "Toward a Puerto Rican Popular Nosology: Nervios and Ataques de Nervios," in *Culture, Medicine, and Psychiatry* (2003), and (with Martinez Pincay, Ramirez, and Canino) of "Are Ataques de Nervios in Puerto Rican Children Associated with Psychiatric Disorder?" in the *Journal of the American Academy of Child and Adolescent Psychiatry* (2005). He is coeditor-in-chief of *Culture, Medicine and Psychiatry* (2002).

JACKLYN B. HABIB is a project manager for AARP. She received her masters in communication at Rutgers University and previously served as a project manager on a federally funded grant examining the most effective way to develop organ donation health campaigns in university and organizational settings.

TYLER R. HARRISON is assistant professor in the Department of Communication at Purdue University. A specialist in organizational structure and conflict, Dr. Harrison is principal researcher on a federally funded project developing and evaluating organ donation campaigns in the workplace. He has also consulted for the hospitality industry, as well as medical groups, on using communication skills to manage conflict and improve relationships in the workplace. He is author (with Susan E. Morgan and Thomas Reichert) of *From Numbers to Words: Reporting Statistical Results for the Social Sciences*.

BEATRIX HOFFMAN is associate professor of history at Northern Illinois University. She is author of *The Wages of Sickness: The Politics of Health Insurance in Progressive America* (2001) and of "Health Care Reform and Social Movements in the United States" in the *American Journal of Public Health* (2003). With support from a Robert Wood Johnson Foundation Investigator Award in Health Policy Research and the

National Endowment for the Humanities, she is currently at work on a history of the right to health care in the United States.

NANCY M. P. KING is a health lawyer and professor in the Department of Social Medicine in the School of Medicine at the University of North Carolina, Chapel Hill. She is author of *Making Sense of Advance Directives*, rev. ed. (1996), and coeditor of *Beyond Regulations: Ethics in Human Subjects Research* (1999) and *The Social Medicine Reader*, 2nd ed. (2005). She is also author of "Accident and Desire: Inadvertent Germline Effects in Clinical Research," *Hastings Center Report* (2003), and "The Line Between Clinical Innovation and Human Experimentation," *Seton Hall Law Review* (2003).

SUSAN E. LEDERER is associate professor of the history of medicine, also appointed in history at Yale University. She is also the author of *Subjected to Science: Human Experimentation in America before the Second World War* (1995) and *Frankenstein: Penetrating the Secrets of Nature* (2002). Her book *Flesh and Blood: Organ Transplantation and Blood Transfusion in Twentieth-Century America* is forthcoming.

BARRON H. LERNER, a physician and historian, is the Angelica Berrie-Arnold P. Gold Foundation Professor of Medicine at the Columbia University Mailman School of Public Health. He is the author of *Contagion and Confinement: Controlling Tuberculosis along the Skid Road* (1998), *The Breast Cancer Wars: Hope, Fear and the Pursuit of a Cure in Twentieth-Century America* (2001), and *When Illness Goes Public: Celebrity Patients and How We Look at Medicine* (2006)—the last supported by a Robert Wood Johnson Foundation Investigator Award in Health Policy Research. Dr. Lerner also contributes regular essays on medicine and history to the *New York Times*.

JULIE LIVINGSTON is associate professor of history at Rutgers University. A historian with a degree in public health, her work explores the human body as a moral condition in southern Africa. She is author of *Debility and the Moral Imagination in Botswana* (2005), and numerous articles on aging, disability, and HIV/AIDS in Botswana.

ERIC M. MESLIN is director of the Indiana University Center for Bioethics, assistant dean for Bioethics and professor of medicine and of medical and molecular genetics at the Indiana University School of Medicine; and professor of philosophy in the School of Liberal Arts at Indiana University–Purdue University, Indianapolis. He is coeditor (with J. F. Childress and H. T. Shapiro) of *Belmont Revisited: Ethical Principles for Research with Human Subjects* (2005).

SUSAN E. MORGAN is associate professor in the Department of Communication at Purdue University. Her research has focused primarily on the development and evaluation of health communication campaigns, and most recently, public under-

standings of organ donation issues. Her interests in organ donation and in inter-
cultural communication intersect in her widely recognized empirical work on the
willingness of African Americans to register as organ donors. She is author (with
Tyler Harrison and Thomas Reichert) of *From Numbers to Words: Reporting Statistical Results for the Social Sciences* (2002), as well as numerous articles on organ
donation that have appeared in both medical and social science journals.

ROSAMOND RHODES is professor of medical education and director of bioethics education at Mount Sinai School of Medicine and professor of philosophy at The Graduate Center, CUNY. She has coedited *Physician Assisted Suicide: Expanding the Debate*
(1998), *Medicine and Social Justice: Essays on the Distribution of Health Care* (2002),
and *The Blackwell Guide to Medical Ethics* (2006).

CAROLYN ROUSE, associate professor of anthropology at Princeton University, is the
author of *Engaged Surrender: African American Women and Islam* (2004). She is also
the author of "Paradigms and Politics: Shaping Health Care Access for Sickle Cell
Patients through the Discursive Regimes of Biomedicine, *Culture, Medicine, and
Psychiatry* (2004), and "If She's a Vegetable, We'll Be Her Garden: Embodiment,
Transcendence, and Citations of Competing Metaphors in the Case of a Dying
Child," *American Ethnologist* (2004).

KAREN R. SALMON is a first-year law student at the New England School of Law.

NANCY SCHEPER-HUGHES is professor of anthropology at University of California,
Berkeley, where she also directs Organ Watch. As a critical and so-called militant
anthropologist, Scheper-Hughes is concerned with the violence of everyday life.
She is author of *Death Without Weeping: The Violence of Everyday Life in Brazil*
(1993) and *Saints, Scholars and Schizophrenics: Mental Illness in Rural Ireland*
(2001). Her essay in this volume draws on material from her forthcoming book,
Parts Unknown: The Global Traffic in Organs, based on a ten-year, multisited ethnographic study of the global traffic in humans (living and dead) for their organs
and tissues.

LESLEY A. SHARP is professor of anthropology at Barnard, as well as associate pro-
fessor of anthropology and sociomedical sciences at the Mailman School of Public
Health of Columbia University. She is the author of "Organ Transplantation as a
Transformative Experience: Anthropological Insights into the Restructuring of the
Self," *Medical Anthropology Quarterly* (1995); "Commodified Kin: Death, Mourning, and Competing Claims on the Bodies of Organ Donors in the United States,"
American Anthropologist (2001); "Bodies, Boundaries, and Territorial Disputes: Investigating the Murky Realm of Scientific Authority," *Medical Anthropology* (2002);
and two book-length studies concerning indigenous healing and political consciousness in Madagascar. Her recent books are *Strange Harvest: Organ Trans-*

plants, Denatured Bodies, and the Transformed Self (2006) and *Bodies, Commodities, and Biotechnologies* (2006).

KEITH WAILOO is a professor at Rutgers University and is jointly appointed in the Department of History and in the Institute for Health, Health Care Policy, and Aging Research. He is author of *Drawing Blood: Technology and Disease Identity in Twentieth Century Medicine* (1997), *Dying in the City of the Blues: Sickle Cell Anemia and the Politics of Race and Health* (2001), and (with Stephen Pemberton) of *The Troubled Dream of Genetic Medicine: Innovation and Ethnicity in Tay-Sachs, Cystic Fibrosis, and Sickle Cell Disease* (2006). In 2004, he coedited (with Mark Sclesinger and Tim Jost) a special issue of the *Journal of Health Politics, Policy, and Law*, titled "Transforming American Medicine," and is currently completing a history of race and cancer, and a study of the cultural politics of pain medicine. This work has been supported by a Robert Wood Johnson Foundation Investigator Award in Health Policy Research and by the James S. McDonnell Foundation Centennial Fellowship in the History of Science.

INDEX

California, 120, 132, 185, 189, 195, 207, 239, 243, 244, 248, 285, 313, 335, 358

Callendar, Clive, 152, 196

Canada, 13, 215, 262, 320

Cancer, 7

Carolina Donor Services (CDS), 8, 64–65, 66, 70, 107, 108, 109

Carson, Ben, 352–53

Casey, Robert, 131

Celebrated cases in medicine, 46–47, 67, 82–96, 97, 98, 99, 101, 102, 111, 142–57, 349–58. *See also* Averit, Lauren; Baby Fae; Bijani conjoined twins; Casey, Robert; Clark, Barney; Cruzan, Nancy; Dunn, Belynda; Fisk, Jamie; Kramer, Larry; Mantle, Mickey; Quinlan, Karen Ann; Rodriguez, Julie; Schiavo, Terri; Solis, Bennie; Tucker, Bruce; Zion, Libby

Center for American Unity, 286

Chalmers, Thomas, 352

Change of Mind (film), 150

Charity, 10–11. *See also* Philanthropy

Chavez, Leo, 10, 25, 39, 136, 246, 248, 250, 257, 333

Chemotherapy, 335–36

Chicago, 149, 240, 243, 245

Child-Pugh score, 166, 167

Children's Miracle Network, 246

Childress, James, 269

China, 13, 223, 230; use of prisoners' organs, 76–77

Chua, Amy, 183

Citizenship. *See* Immigration; Medical citizenship; Santillan, Jesica: and citizenship

Civil Rights Act, 142

Clarian Health Partners, 268

Clark, Barney, 12, 139 (n. 26)

Clifton, Hardie, 196

Clifton, Sherry, 196

Clinton, Bill, 16 (n. 17), 132, 162, 163, 243

Cobb, Montague, 151

Cokkinos, Dennis, 151

Colorado, 312

Comarow, Avery, 131, 133

Conjoined twins, 352–53. *See also* Bijani conjoined twins

Connelly, Michael, 100

Cook, Richard I., 7, 34, 35, 75, 90, 105, 107, 108, 124, 131, 181, 182, 198, 199, 334, 352, 354

Cooley, Denton, 144, 149, 151

Corchado, Alfredo, 250

Cruzan, Nancy, 350, 351

Cuba, 215

Darvall, Denise, 147

Das, Veena, 221

Da Silva, Alberty, 214

Davis, Dena, 260

Davis, Duane, 110

Dayrit, Manuel, 227

Death, 31, 313; "brain death," 8, 39, 143, 149–50, 185, 208, 228, 300, 308, 356–57; of child, 33, 307, 320, 326 (n. 45); legal death, 6, 146. *See also* Santillan, Jesica: death of

De Castro, Leonardo, 208, 228

DeSantis, Joe, 304

Devlin, Lord Patrick, 270

Dialysis, 121, 160, 216, 218, 228, 354. *See also* End-Stage Renal Disease Program; Organ transplantation: kidney

Diflo, Thomas, 7, 124, 125, 133, 137, 356

Douglas, Mary, 291

Dreffer, Ronald L., 196

Duke University Medical Center, 1–8, 13, 19, 21, 26, 29–36, 39, 46, 63–67, 70, 74–75, 82, 86, 101–2, 107–11, 120, 134–35, 158–60, 187, 237, 244–48, 267–77, 276 306, 319, 333; institutional response to error, 77–79, 94, 111–14, 356

Dunn, Belynda, 126–29, 136

Durham, N.C., 1, 2, 12–13, 37, 171, 205, 210

Dwyer, James, 258–59, 260

Eberl, Jason, 293

Efficacy, 159, 164, 165, 168, 169, 172–77

Egypt, 195

End-of-life decision-making, 9, 12, 30, 31, 351

Justice, 7–8, 9, 36, 94, 130, 158–79, 205, 224, 257–62, 357; clinical justice, 159, 163–65, 170–77

Justice, Department of, 191

Juvenile diabetes, 124

Kant, Immanuel, 264
Kantrowitz, Adrian, 144
Kasperak, Mike, 144
Kempe, C. Henry, 310
Kentucky, 168
Kermode, Frank, 40
King, Nancy, 11, 24, 29, 91, 137, 247
Klett, Joseph, 143, 144
Kobzeff, Luba, 120–21, 132, 136–37
Kovacs, Joe, 287
Kramer, Larry, 127–28, 130
Kravinsky, Zell, 207–8
Kuwait, 196

Lawsuits. See Malpractice; Tort reform
Lebanon, 196
Lederer, Susan, 9, 188, 290, 309, 353
Lehman, Betsy, 88
Lerner, Barron, 7, 122, 350, 354
Leukemia, 336–37
Levi-Strauss, Claude, 99, 232
Livingston, Julie, 8, 30, 35, 167, 182, 268, 354
Lock, Margaret, 131
Locke, John, 257
Los Angeles, 218, 240
Louisburg College, 3, 259
Louisiana, 132, 142, 168
Lower, Richard, 144–46, 152. See also Tucker, Bruce; Tucker v. Lower

Madeira, Rodney, 184
Mahoney, Mack, 3, 7, 11, 14, 21, 26–29, 34, 38, 39, 93–94, 101, 141 (n. 45), 171, 174–75, 210, 237, 246–47, 256, 292, 304–5, 309, 319, 321, 329–32, 345, 350, 352, 356
Mahoney, Nita, 329, 332
Malkin, Michele, 286–87
Malpractice, 1, 14, 31, 82, 84, 85, 86, 87, 88, 90, 102, 119, 310; insurance, 5; reform, 4–5

Mann, Geoffrey T., 149
Mantle, Mickey, 75, 131
Martin, Edward, 196
Massachusetts, 189–90, 335, 350, 356
Matthews, Esther, 151
Mauss, Marcel, 232
McCormick, Renee, 26
McCullough, Larry, 269
McKinlay, John, 352
McNamara, Beverley, 322
Media coverage, 19–45, 67, 85, 86, 88, 89, 93, 97, 101, 102, 122, 125, 126, 127, 143, 144, 146, 147, 149, 151, 170, 174, 181, 188, 189, 198, 199, 247, 248, 292, 300, 321; anchoring and, 21; objectification and, 21; and "mediagenic" individuals, 24, 357. See also Jesica Santillan: media coverage and representations of

Media:
—popular: ABC, 286; American Enterprise, 279; American Legion Magazine, 280; Cable News Network (CNN), 25, 26, 28, 30, 34; Charlotte Observer, 35; C-SPAN, 286; Dallas Morning News, 250; Ebony, 148–49; Fox News, 286; Franklin Times, 3, 304; International Herald Tribune, 213; Life, 160, 312; McLaughlin Group, 286; MSNBC, 32, 35, 36, 286; Nation, 149; NBC, 110; News and Observer (Raleigh, N.C.), 245, 349, 356; Newsweek, 3 (n. 9), 31, 35, 93, 120, 122, 125, 187, 283, 304; New York Daily News, 88; New York Times, 3, 28, 31, 37, 85, 148, 171, 187, 188, 189, 280, 304; Pittsburgh Press, 189, 194, 196, 197; Richmond Times-Dispatch, 146; San Antonio News-Express, 2; Time, 184, 283; USA Today, 193, 199; U.S. News and World Report, 3, 131, 280, 283; Wall Street Journal, 213; Washington Post, 32, 33, 37, 143, 189, 195, 198, 279–80
—professional: Duke Med News, 109; Foreign Policy, 284; Journal of the National Medical Association, 151; Lancet, 208, 209, 227; Michigan Law Review, 186

Medicaid. See Health care system: and Medicaid

Wake Tech. Libraries
9101 Fayetteville Road
Raleigh, North Carolina 27603-5696

WAKE TECHNICAL COMMUNITY COLLEGE

3 3063 00130394 9

WITHDRAWN

DATE DUE

OCT 15 2008		

OCT   '07